Clinical Reasoning in Veterinary Practice

Clinical Reasoning in Veterinary Practice

Problem Solved!

Second Edition

Edited by

Jill E. Maddison

Department of Clinical Science and Services, The Royal Veterinary College
London, UK

Holger A. Volk

Department of Small Animal Medicine and Surgery, University of Veterinary Medicine Hannover
Hannover, Germany

David B. Church

Department of Clinical Science and Services, The Royal Veterinary College
London, UK

WILEY Blackwell

Registered Offices
John Wiley & Sons, Inc., 111 River Street, Hoboken, NJ 07030, USA
John Wiley & Sons Ltd, The Atrium, Southern Gate, Chichester, West Sussex, PO19 8SQ, UK

Editorial Office
9600 Garsington Road, Oxford, OX4 2DQ, UK

For details of our global editorial offices, customer services, and more information about Wiley products visit us at www.wiley.com.

Wiley also publishes its books in a variety of electronic formats and by print-on-demand. Some content that appears in standard print versions of this book may not be available in other formats.

Library of Congress Cataloging-in-Publication Data Applied for

[ISBN PB: 9781119698203]

Cover Design: Wiley
Cover Images: © Tinnakorn jorruang/Shutterstock, gurinaleksandr/Getty Images

Set in 11/14pt LiberationSans by Straive, Pondicherry, India
Printed and bound by CPI Group (UK) Ltd, Croydon, CR0 4YY

C9781119698203_120224

Contents

About the Editors, vii

List of Contributors, ix

Preface, xi

Acknowledgements, xiii

1 Learning to learn and its relevance to logical clinical problem-solving, 1
   Ivan Newman

2 Introduction to logical clinical problem-solving, 7
   Jill E. Maddison and Holger A. Volk

3 Vomiting, regurgitation and reflux, 35
   Jill E. Maddison

4 Diarrhoea, 55
   Jill E. Maddison and Lucy McMahon

5 Weight loss, 73
   Jill E. Maddison

6 Abdominal enlargement, 89
   Jill E. Maddison

7 Weakness, 103
   Holger A. Volk, David B. Church and Jill E. Maddison

8 Fits and strange episodes, 125
   Holger A. Volk

9 Sneezing, coughing and dyspnoea, 153
   David B. Church

10 Anaemia, 181
Jill E. Maddison and Lucy McMahon

11 Jaundice, 199
Jill E. Maddison and Lucy McMahon

12 Bleeding, 215
Jill E. Maddison

13 Polyuria/polydipsia and urinary incontinence, 237
Jill E. Maddison and David B. Church

14 Gait abnormalities, 261
Holger A. Volk, Elvin R. Kulendra and Richard L. Meeson

15 Pruritus, scaling and otitis, 285
Andrea Volk

16 Problem-based approach to problems of the eye, 305
Charlotte Dawson

17 Problem-based approach to small mammals – rabbits, rodents and ferrets, 323
Joanna Hedley

18 Problem-based clinical reasoning examples for equine practice, 353
Michael Hewetson

19 Principles of professional reasoning and decision-making, 391
Elizabeth Armitage-Chan

Index, 407

About the Editors

Jill E. Maddison
BVSc DipVetClinStud PhD FACVSc SFHEA MRCVS

Jill is a small animal veterinarian with expertise in internal medicine and clinical pharmacology. She is currently Professor of General Practice at the Royal Veterinary College (RVC) and Director of Professional Development overseeing the college's continuing education programmes. She is actively involved in undergraduate teaching and continuing professional development (CPD) at the RVC in the areas of clinical reasoning in small animal medicine and clinical pharmacology. She has lectured extensively on these topics to veterinarians around the world and published on a wide variety of topics related to internal medicine, pharmacology and veterinary education.

Holger A. Volk
PhD DipECVN

Holger studied veterinary medicine at the University of Veterinary Medicine Hannover, Germany and at the Ecole Nationale Vétérinaire de Lyon, France. He is a board-certified clinical neurologist, passing the ECVN exams in 2008. He is actively involved in clinical research and has published extensively in the area of clinical neurology. Holger is currently Head of Department of Small Animal Diseases, University of Veterinary Medicine Hannover. He has been a recipient of the prestigious Bourgelat Award from BSAVA and the International Canine Health Award from the Kennel Club. His main research interests are Chiari-like malformation and syringomyelia in Cavalier King Charles Spaniel and canine and feline epilepsy.

David B. Church
BVSc PhD MACVSc FHEA MRCVS

David is currently Professor of Small Animal Studies at the Royal Veterinary College. He has spent more than 30 years in small animal specialist practices and is the author of more than 200 peer-reviewed publications and numerous textbook chapters on companion animal endocrinology and small animal medicine. He has been a long-standing advocate of the benefits of veterinarians developing a logical approach to clinical reasoning to complement their pattern recognition skills. As a co-founder of VetCompass, he is also passionate about developing mechanisms to define and understand the disorders encountered in general practice and how to optimise their management.

List of Contributors

Elizabeth Armitage-Chan

Department of Clinical Science and Services, The Royal Veterinary College, London, UK

David B. Church

Department of Clinical Science and Services, The Royal Veterinary College, London, UK

Charlotte Dawson

Department of Clinical Science and Services, The Royal Veterinary College, London, UK

Joanna Hedley

Department of Clinical Science and Services, The Royal Veterinary College, London, UK

Michael Hewetson

Department of Clinical Science and Services, The Royal Veterinary College, London, UK

Elvin R. Kulendra

North Downs Specialists Referrals, Bletchingley, UK

Jill E. Maddison

Department of Clinical Science and Services, The Royal Veterinary College, London, UK

Lucy McMahon

Anderson Moores Veterinary Specialists, Winchester, UK

Richard L. Meeson

Department of Clinical Science and Services, The Royal Veterinary College, London, UK

Ivan Newman

Specialist Study Skills Tutor, Dyslexia Assessment & Consultancy Ltd, London, UK

Andrea Volk

Lecturer in Veterinary Dermatology, University of Veterinary Medicine Hannover, Hannover, Germany

Holger A. Volk

Department of Small Animal Medicine and Surgery, University of Veterinary Medicine Hannover, Hannover, Germany

Preface

The second edition of our book has been a wonderful opportunity to update relevant content, expand the areas of clinical practice discussed and, perhaps most importantly, improve the layout and formatting using Universal Design for Learning principles. This edition has benefited from extensive reader feedback about the first edition which we are very grateful for. We hope that this second edition will help enhance clinical and professional reasoning skills of veterinary students and veterinarians around the world. Keep on problem-solving!

Acknowledgements

We are indebted to the support and feedback we have received from veterinary students and colleagues at the RVC and the Centre for Veterinary Education at the University of Sydney. Special thanks to Alex Currie, Sue Bennett and Karen Humm who all provided insightful input or feedback. We are particularly grateful to Dr Ivan Newman, whose work with students with learning differences has been seminal in the development of the format of the book to enhance its accessibility for all.

CHAPTER 1

Learning to learn and its relevance to logical clinical problem-solving

Ivan Newman

Specialist Study Skills Tutor, Dyslexia Assessment & Consultancy Ltd, London, UK

The why

- Animals present to veterinarians with clinical signs, not diagnoses. Therefore, the aim of this book is to enhance your clinical reasoning skills by providing you with a consistent and transferable problem-solving framework that can be applied to common clinical signs in veterinary practice.
- Most of the chapters relate to small animal practice, but there are also chapters demonstrating how to use the problem-solving framework in exotic animals and horses as well as a chapter discussing a framework for professional reasoning.
- Before we start, though, we should review why having a consistent problem-solving framework can be so powerful for veterinary students starting on their clinical journey as well as veterinarians who have knowledge and experience but may struggle when medical cases become more complex or unusual.

Learn more effectively

This chapter will help you learn more effectively, both to build your veterinary knowledge and more generally. Of course, as learning carries on beyond graduation, many of the ideas described here will be useful for years to come and so are relevant to those of you who

Clinical Reasoning in Veterinary Practice: Problem Solved!, Second Edition.
Edited by Jill E. Maddison, Holger A. Volk and David B. Church.
© 2022 John Wiley & Sons Ltd. Published 2022 by John Wiley & Sons Ltd.

may be studying for post-graduate qualifications. The chapter examines:

- How we learn – using our senses in combination to boost memorisation
- How to use this book
- Study skills strategies for veterinary knowledge.

Let's get going

How do we learn? Our five senses play a major part in how and what we learn, as much of what we learn is based on memory; using them together results in much better memory outcomes than only using one or even two senses.

Consider this sequence of learning something new: reading alone; reading with hearing; reading with hearing plus kinaesthetic (doing or acting out); reading with hearing plus kinaesthetic (doing or acting out) and repetition. As we proceed through this sequence, we understand and remember more and for longer (Flanagan 1996) – what could be called the 'staircase' of memorisation.

We remember:
- 20% of what we read
- 30% of what we hear
- 40% of what we see
- 50% of what we say
- 60% of what we do
- And as much as 90% of what we read, hear, say, see and do.

That last bullet point is worth emphasising; we can achieve exceptional results by combining multiple senses (see Figure 1.1).

Of particular relevance to this book, placing information within 'frameworks' further boosts memorisation. In the context of veterinary studies, imagine you are in a lecture, in person or online, and the presenter just verbally describes a procedure step-by-step. How much do you remember? Perhaps not too much. Now imagine that the presenter talks you through the procedure step-by-step using a diagram, ideally using colour. Are you likely to remember more? Probably. Now imagine that you later talk yourself through the procedure, using your finger to trace the diagram's steps. Is your memory better? Again, probably. Now additionally you perform the procedure either in mime or a practical session. How is your recall now? Quite likely better still. Finally, if you add in teaching the procedure to someone else, you will achieve the highest level of memorisation.

Figure 1.2 illustrates this idea of increasing ability to memorise. Note that the graphic itself provides a sequence/framework that can be learned, and it uses colour and directional symbols to support the above description and underlying concept.

Figures 1.1 and 1.2 embody alternative representations of broadly the same idea. This repetition is intentional; repetition is important in building memory, especially if that repetition occurs multiple times shortly after original exposure to the material (Ebbinghaus 1885; Flanagan 1996). This is one of the key elements of the problem-solving framework we will discuss – repetition and consistency of clinical reasoning steps regardless of the clinical problem.

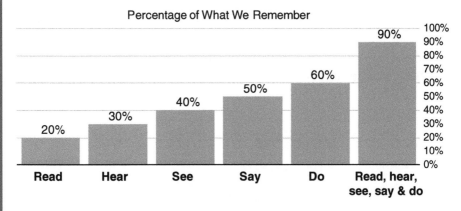

Figure 1.1   Visual representation of the staircase of memorisation.

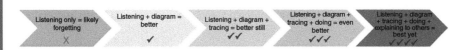

Figure 1.2   Introducing a diagram into the sequence of actions to improve understanding and memorisation.

How is this learning theory relevant to this book?

This book is designed to give you a multi-sensory approach to learning, reinforced by repetition, together with a robust framework on which to 'hang' veterinary facts. The problem-solving framework is based on pathophysiological principles that will lead you to a deeper understanding, enhanced ability to recall information and more reliable diagnoses.

Chapter 2 introduces you to clinical reasoning in general and the logical clinical problem-solving (LCPS) process in particular. It uses case studies to illustrate the strengths and challenges of different clinical reasoning approaches.

The subsequent chapters use particular clinical problems to illustrate and further explain how to use LCPS for common clinical signs. Each of the four steps is consistently colour coded so you can associate the colour to the step. The case scenarios in many chapters will help you visualise how LCPS is applied to real-life cases.

Every chapter opens with an orientating introduction and ends with a key points recap. Figure 1.3 illustrates how the structure of the chapters leads to understanding and memorisation. Take a moment to follow the flow step-by-step.

You can perhaps see what is 'going on' here. The book is designed to help you remember and learn more effectively by providing a

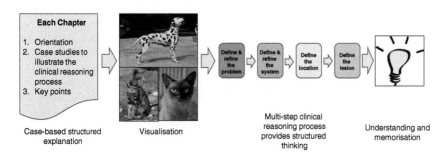

Figure 1.3 How the structure of the chapters leads to understanding and memorisation.

process, scenario-based text, graphics, colour and repetition – many of the elements in the staircase to memorisation. You can add further elements, such as talking through to yourself (subvocalising; see Figure 1.4) each step of the LCPS process for each scenario and perhaps teaching each of the scenarios within the clinical reasoning process to a colleague (a learning buddy; see Figure 1.5).

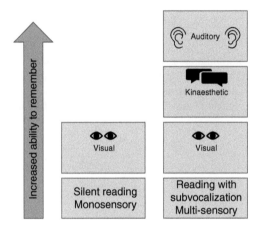

Figure 1.4   Memorisation benefit through subvocalisation.

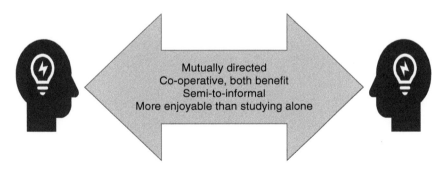

Figure 1.5   Benefits of having a learning buddy.

Key points – learning more effectively

- Make your learning multisensory. The more senses you use, the better you remember.
- Create and use frameworks on which to 'hang' your knowledge; they are powerful tools to help you remember and learn.
- The logical clinical reasoning process, the framework at the heart of this book, is specifically designed to help you become a more effective veterinarian, especially when faced with the unexpected.

References

Ebbinghaus, H. 1885. Memory: A Contribution to Experimental Psychology (translated: Ruger, H. A., and Clara E. Bussenius, 1913). http://nwkpsych.rutgers.edu/~jose/courses/578_mem_learn/2012/readings/Ebbinghaus_1885.pdf.

Flanagan, K. 1996. *Maximum Points, Minimum Panic: The Essential Guide to Surviving Exams.* Dublin: Marino Books.

CHAPTER 2

Introduction to logical clinical problem-solving

Jill E. Maddison[1] and Holger A. Volk[2]

[1]Department of Clinical Science and Services, The Royal Veterinary College, London, UK

[2]Department of Small Animal Medicine and Surgery, University of Veterinary Medicine Hannover, Hannover, Germany

The why

- The aim of this book is to assist you to develop a structured and pathophysiologically sound approach to the diagnosis of common clinical problems in small animal practice.
- The development of a sound basis for clinical problem-solving provides you, a current or future veterinarian, with the foundation and scaffolding to allow you to potentially reach a diagnosis regardless of whether you have seen the disorder before.
- Furthermore, the method presented in this book will help you avoid being stuck trying to remember long differential lists and hence free your thinking skills to solve complex medical cases.
- The aim of the book is *not* to bombard you with details of different diseases – there are many excellent textbooks and other resources that can fulfil this need. What we want to provide you with is a framework by which you can solve clinical problems and place your veterinary knowledge into an appropriate problem-solving context.

Introduction to clinical reasoning

We all remember our first driving lessons, which may have been quite challenging – for us and/or our instructors! We had to think actively about many factors to ensure we drove safely. The more experienced

Clinical Reasoning in Veterinary Practice: Problem Solved!, Second Edition.
Edited by Jill E. Maddison, Holger A. Volk and David B. Church.
© 2022 John Wiley & Sons Ltd. Published 2022 by John Wiley & Sons Ltd.

we became at driving, the more non-driving-associated tasks, such as talking to our passengers, listening to the radio and changing the radio channels, we were able to do while driving. If we had attempted any of these tasks at the beginning of our driver training, we might have had an accident. As we become more experienced at a task, we need to think less about it, as we move to what is known as unconscious competence (Figure 2.1).

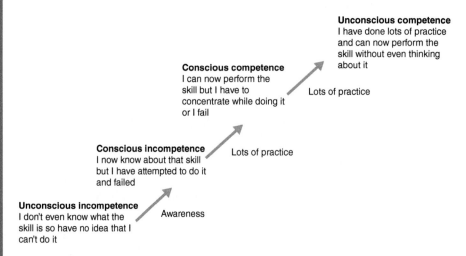

Figure 2.1   Skill acquisition pathway. (This pathway can apply to the acquisition of any skill.)

We see a similar process in clinical education. During the progression from veterinary student to experienced clinician, knowledge and skills are initially learnt in a conscious and structured way. Veterinary undergraduate education in most universities is therefore based on systems teaching, discipline teaching, species teaching or a mixture of all three. These are excellent approaches to help develop a sound knowledge base and understanding of disease processes and treatments.

However, when an animal or group of animals becomes unwell, the clinical signs they exhibit can be caused by a number of disorders of a range of different body systems – the list may seem endless. They do not present to the veterinarian with labels on their heads stating the disease they have (more's the pity!). Therefore, for veterinarians to fully access their knowledge bank about disorders and their treatment, they need to have a robust method of clinical reasoning they can rely on. This method allows them to consolidate and relate their knowledge to the clinical case and progress to a rational assessment of the likely differential diagnoses. This makes it easier to determine appropriate diagnostic and/or management options for the patient. Because you have a clear path, communication with the client becomes easier.

The next part of the journey to becoming an experienced clinician is that clinical judgement and decision-making processes become unconscious or intuitive. The rapid, unconscious process of clinical decision-making by experienced clinicians is referred to in medical literature as intuition or the 'art' of medicine. The conscious thinking process is often referred to as 'science' (evidence based) or analytic. Intuition is context-sensitive, influenced by the level of the clinician's experience, context-dependent and has no obvious cause-and-effect logic. Why is this important? We have all thought 'I just know that the animal has . . .' The unconscious mind will pretend to the conscious mind that the clinical decision was based on logical assumptions or causal relationships. This is not a problem as long the intuition or 'pattern recognition' has resulted in a correct diagnosis. However, when it does not, we need to understand why it failed and have a system in place to rationally progress our clinical decision-making.

This book will provide you with the tools and thinking framework needed to unravel any clinical riddle, unleashing the potential of your unconscious mind rather than blocking your working memory as you try to recall all of the facts you may have once known.

Why are some cases frustrating instead of fun?
Reflect on a medical case that you have recently dealt with that frustrated you or seemed difficult to diagnose and manage. Can you identify why the case was difficult?

There can be a multitude of reasons why complex medical cases are frustrating instead of fun.
- Was it due to the client (e.g. having unreal expectations that you could fix the problem at no cost to themselves? Unwilling or unable to pay for the diagnostic tests needed to reach a diagnosis? Unable to give a coherent history?)

- Was the case complex and didn't seem to fit any recognisable pattern?
- Were you unable to recall all of the facts about a disease, and this biased your thinking?
- Did the signalment, especially breed and age, cloud your clinical reasoning, resulting in an incorrect differential list?
- Did the case seem to fit a pattern, but subsequent testing proved your initial diagnosis wrong?
- Did you seem to spend a lot of the client's money on tests that weren't particularly illuminating?

Can you add any other factors that have contributed to frustrations and difficulties you may have experienced with medical cases?

Apart from the client issues (and as discussed later, we may be able to help a little bit here as well), we hope that by the end of this book, we will have gone some way towards removing the common barriers to correct, quick and efficient diagnosis of medical cases and have made unravelling medical riddles fun rather than frustrating.

Solving clinical cases

When a patient presents with one or more clinical problems, there are various methods we can use to solve the case and formulate a list of differential diagnoses. One method involves pattern recognition – looking at the pattern of clinical signs and trying to match that pattern to known diagnoses. This is also referred to as developing an illness script. Another method can involve relying on blood tests to tell us what is wrong with the patient – also referred to as the minimum database. Or we can use problem-based clinical reasoning. Often, we may use all three methods.

Let's consider three cases. Each of these will trigger thoughts and ideas about possible diagnoses depending on your knowledge and experience.

Case 1: 'Sundance'
Sundance is a 17-year-old female (neutered) domestic short-haired cat with a 1-month history of increased appetite (polyphagia) and increased drinking (polydipsia). Obvious weight loss had been noted by owner over this period of time. Sundance has seemed more agitated and demanding of food and attention.

On physical examination she was obviously thin with a body condition score (BCS) 3/9 and an elevated heart rate (tachycardia) of 240 beats per minute (bpm). There were no other significant findings.

Case 2: 'Brutus'
Brutus is a 10-year-old male neutered Dalmatian with a 3-day history of vomiting bile and excessive urinating and drinking (polyuria/polydipsia) for 10 days. His appetite has been much reduced for about 10 days as well. On physical examination he was found to be depressed and dehydrated with no other significant abnormalities noted.

Case 3: 'Erroll'
Erroll is a 4-year-old neutered male Burmese cat. He has a 2-week history of intermittently vomiting bile-stained material. Over the last 4–5 days he has become progressively anorexic and depressed. 24 hours prior to presentation he had started straining to urinate, and the urine was blood stained. No diarrhoea had been noted by the owners. His water intake was normal until the past 24 hours, when it may have been reduced.

On physical examination he was noted to be very depressed and dehydrated. His rectal temperature was normal (38.1°C). Heart rate was elevated at 220 bpm. Mucous membrane colour was poor and the capillary refill time (CRT) was greater than 3 seconds. Abdominal palpation was unremarkable – the kidneys felt normal and were not painful. The bladder contained some urine but felt normal and could be easily expressed.

So – can we solve all of these cases in the same way? Do we need to? What are the challenges? Let's consider the tools we use to clinically reason.

Pattern recognition
Pattern recognition involves trying to remember all diseases that fit the 'pattern' of clinical signs/pathological abnormalities that the animal presents with. This may be relatively simple (but can also lead to errors of omission) and works best:
- For common disorders with typical presentations
- If a disorder has a unique pattern of clinical signs

- When all clinical signs have been recognised and considered, and the differential list is not just based on one cardinal clinical sign and the signalment of the patient presented
- If there are only a few diagnostic possibilities that are
  o easily remembered or
  o can easily be ruled in or out by routine tests
- If the vet has extensive experience, is well read and up-to-date, reflects on all of the diagnoses made regularly and critically *and* has an excellent memory.

Pattern recognition works well for many common disorders and has the advantage of being quick and cost-effective. . .provided the diagnosis is correct. The vet appears competent to the client because the vet has acted decisively and confidently. . .provided the diagnosis is correct.

An example of a case where pattern recognition will invariably be used by most vets and will be successful (most of the time) is Sundance. The differential diagnoses for the pattern of clinical signs – weight loss despite polyphagia associated with polydipsia, altered behaviour and tachycardia – are very limited with hyperthyroidism being the explanation in the vast majority of cases. Score 10 out of 10 for pattern recognition!

However, pattern recognition can be flawed and unsatisfactory when the clinician is inexperienced (and therefore has seen very few patterns) or only considers or recognises a small number of factors (and is not aware that this process is mainly driven by unconscious processes that might need to be reflected upon if they fail). Or even if the clinician is experienced, it can be flawed for uncommon diseases or common diseases presenting atypically, when the patient is exhibiting multiple clinical signs that are not immediately recognisable as a specific disease, or if the pattern of clinical signs is suggestive of certain disorders but not specific for them.

The pattern of clinical signs that Brutus is showing has a much larger range of causes, but it is likely that an experienced veterinarian will recognise several possibilities though often not all. An inexperienced clinician will consider fewer potential differentials.

Differentials diagnoses that experienced vets will consider for Brutus include liver disease, renal failure, hypoadrenocorticism, hypercalcaemia and diabetes mellitus. Routine blood work will be very helpful (provided it is interpreted correctly). Even if the veterinarian hasn't given a lot of thought to potential differentials (which may hinder discussion with the owner, however), sufficient information may be gained from suitably comprehensive testing (sometimes called 'going fishing').

For Brutus the liver enzymes were substantially increased, hypercalcaemia was noted and the final diagnosis was hypercalcaemia associated with hepatic lymphoma (confirmed on ultrasound-guided biopsy).

The pattern of clinical signs that Erroll is showing are just downright weird, involving different body systems over a period of time and with no 'obvious' single explanation for all of the signs even for very experienced clinicians. His bloodwork only showed an inflammatory leukogram. The final diagnosis was a pancreatic abscess and peritonitis from which *E. coli* was cultured and a urinary tract infection – from which *E. coli* was cultured.

In addition, for the experienced clinician, the success of pattern recognition relies on a correct diagnosis for the pattern observed previously being reached *and* not assuming that similar patterns must equal the same diagnosis. Pattern recognition can lead to dangerous tunnel vision where the clinician pursues his/her initial diagnostic hunch based on pattern spotting to the exclusion of other diagnostic possibilities. Several types or indeed combinations of diagnostic bias can result – some examples are shown in Table 2.1.

Table 2.1   Diagnostic biases in clinical medicine.

Availability bias	A tendency to favour a diagnosis because of a case the clinician has seen recently.
Anchoring bias	Where a prior diagnosis is favoured but is misleading. The clinician persists with the initial diagnosis and is unwilling to change his/her mind.
Framing bias	Features that do not fit with the favoured diagnosis are ignored.
Confirmation bias	When information is selectively chosen to confirm, not refute, a hypothesis. The clinician only seeks or takes note of information that will confirm his/her diagnosis and does not seek or ignores information that will challenge it.
Premature closure	Failing to look for additional information after reaching a potential diagnosis and, as a result, narrowing the choice of diagnostic hypotheses too early.

And finally, the disadvantage of relying entirely on pattern recognition to solve clinical problems means that should the clinician realise subsequently that his/her pattern recognition was incorrect, there is no logical intellectual framework to help reassess the patient. Thus, pattern-based assessment of clinical cases can result at best in a speedy, correct, 'good value' diagnosis but at worst in wasted time and money and, sometimes, it endangers the patient's life.

I'll do bloods!

Routine diagnostic tests such as haematology, biochemistry and urinalysis can be enormously useful in progressing the understanding of a patient's clinical condition. However, relying on blood tests (often called a minimum database) to give us more information about the patient before we form *any* assessment of possible diagnoses can be useful for disorders of some body systems but totally unhelpful for others.

Serious, even life-threatening, disorders of the gut, brain, nerves, muscles, pancreas (in cats) and heart, for example, rarely cause significant changes in haematological and biochemical parameters that are measured on routine tests performed in practice. Over-reliance on blood tests to steer us in the right clinical direction can also be problematical when the results do not clearly confirm a diagnosis. The veterinarian can waste much time and the client's money searching without much direction for clues as to what is wrong with the patient. And of course, the financial implications of non-discriminatory blood testing can be considerable, and many clients are unable or unwilling to pay for comprehensive testing. Using blood testing to 'screen' for diagnoses can be misleading, as the sensitivity and specificity of any test are very much influenced by the precision of the test and the prevalence of a disorder in the population.

For experienced veterinarians, pattern recognition combined with 'fishing expeditions' (i.e. 'I have no idea what's going on so I'll just do bloods and hopefully something will come up!') can result in a successful diagnostic or therapeutic outcome in many medical cases in first-opinion practice. However, there are *always* cases that do not yield their secrets so readily using these approaches, and it is these cases that frustrate veterinarians, prolong animal suffering, impair communication, damage the trust relationship with clients and on the whole make veterinary practice less pleasant than it should be.

You also have to know about *and* remember lots of diagnoses for this approach to be effective. This is problematical if the veterinarian does not recognise or remember potential diagnoses (e.g. for Brutus) or if, as discussed previously, the pattern of clinical signs doesn't suggest many feasible differentials (e.g. for Erroll). It is also less useful for inexperienced veterinarians or veterinarians returning to practice after a career break or changing their area of practice.

It is for all of these reasons that we hope this book will enhance your problem-solving skills as well as build your knowledge base about key pathophysiological principles. We want to assist you to develop a framework for a structured approach to clinical problems that is easy to remember, robust and can be applied in principle to a wide range of clinical problems. The formal term for this is *problem-based inductive clinical reasoning*.

Problem-based inductive clinical reasoning
In problem-based inductive clinical reasoning, each significant clinicopathological problem is assessed in a structured way before being related to the other problems that the patient may present with. Using this approach, the pathophysiological basis and key questions (see the following sections) for the most specific clinical signs the patient is exhibiting are considered before a pattern is sought. This ensures that one's mind remains more open to other diagnostic possibilities than what might appear to be initially the most obvious and thus helps prevent pattern-based tunnel vision.

If there are multiple clinical signs – for example, vomiting, polydipsia and a pulse deficit – each problem is considered separately and then in relation to the other problems to determine if there is a disorder (or disorders) that could explain all of the clinical signs present. In this way, the clinician should be able to easily assess the potential differentials for each problem and then relate them rather than trying to remember every disease process that could cause that pattern of particular signs. It is important that the signalment of the patient is seen as a risk factor, but this should not blind the clinician to potential diagnoses beyond what is common for that age, breed and sex.

Thus, we do look for patterns but not until we have put in place an intellectual framework that helps prevent tunnel vision too early in the diagnostic process.

Figure 2.2 shows the steps in the clinical reasoning flow. As each step is explained you will see the numbered keys to help you understand where you are in the diagnostic process. We use these steps, their colours and numbered keys throughout the book to help 'anchor' the process for you through the repetition shown in Figure 2.1. Colour bars or shading are also used to identify introductory concepts (blue), diagnostic approach and steps (brown) and key introductory and summary points (purple).

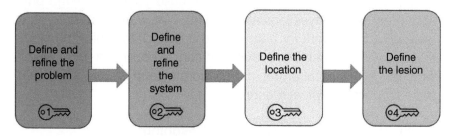

Figure 2.2   Clinical reasoning step-by-step.

Essential components of problem-based clinical reasoning

The problem list
The initial step in logical clinical problem-solving is to clarify and articulate the clinical problems the patient has presented with. This is best achieved by constructing a problem list – either in your head or, in more complex cases, on paper or the computer.

For example, for Erroll the problem list in the order the problems are reported would be:

1 Vomiting
2 Anorexia
3 Depression
4 Dysuria and haematuria.

Why is constructing a problem list helpful?
- It helps make the clinical signs explicit to our current level of understanding.
- It transforms the vague to the more specific.

- It helps the clinician determine which are the key clinical problems ('hard findings') and which are the 'background noise' ('soft findings') that may inform the assessment of the key problems but do not require specific assessment.
- And most importantly, it helps prevent overlooking less obvious but nevertheless crucial clinical signs.

Prioritising the problems
Having identified the presenting problems, you then need to assign them some sort of priority on the basis of their specific nature.
- For example, anorexia, depression and lethargy are all fairly non-specific clinical problems that do not suggest involvement of any particular body system and can be clinical signs associated with a vast number of disease processes.
- However, clinical signs such as vomiting, polydipsia/polyuria, seizures, jaundice, diarrhoea, pale mucous membranes, weakness, bleeding, coughing and dyspnoea are more specific clinical signs that give the clinician a 'diagnostic hook' he/she can use as a basis for the case assessment.

As the clinician increases understanding of the clinical status of the patient, the overall aim is to seek information that allows them to define each problem more specifically (i.e. narrow down the diagnostic options) until a specific diagnosis is reached.

For example, for Erroll the prioritised problem list would be:
1 Vomiting
2 Dysuria and haematuria
3 Anorexia
4 Depression.

This is because vomiting and dysuria/haematuria are specific problems, and their assessment will hopefully assist in reaching a diagnosis – they are our 'diagnostic hooks'. Anorexia and depression will be explained by the underlying disorder and are important to note but are not 'diagnostic hooks' for this case – they are the 'background information'.

Specificity is relative!
The relative specificity of a problem will, however, vary depending on the context.

- For example, for a dog that presents with intermittent vomiting and lethargy, vomiting is the most specific problem, as in all likelihood the cause or consequences of the vomiting will also explain the lethargy.
- In contrast, for the dog that presents with intermittent vomiting and lethargy *and* is found to be jaundiced on physical examination, jaundice is the most specific clinical problem. This is because:
    - The majority of causes of jaundice can also cause vomiting, but the reverse is not true, that is, there are many causes of vomiting that do not cause jaundice.
    - Thus, there is little value in assessing the vomiting as the 'diagnostic hook', as it will mean that many unlikely diagnoses are considered, and time and diagnostic resources may be wasted.
- In this case, assessment of jaundice will lead more quickly to a diagnosis than that of vomiting, as the diagnostic options for jaundice are more limited than those for vomiting.

In other words, although you identify and consider each problem to a certain degree, you try to focus your diagnostic or therapeutic plans on the most specific problem/s (the 'diagnostic hook/s') if (*and this is important*) you are comfortable that the other clinical signs are most likely related. If you are *not* convinced that they are all related to a single diagnosis, then you need to keep your problems separate and assess them thoroughly as separate entities, keeping in mind they may or may not be related.

In emergency cases, the problems at the top of your problem list are those that would immediately endanger the patient and must be immediately addressed – remember your ABC of triaging (airway, breathing, circulation). They may then be followed by the problems that act as the diagnostic hooks to reach the final diagnosis/management plan.

Key concept	
Create problem list	Summarise the clinical problems the patient has presented with.
Prioritise the problem list	Identify which of the problems are specific – those that are 'diagnostic hooks' +/- those that must be addressed immediately as the patient's life is at risk.

The reasons that might make one suspect that the clinical signs are related to more than one problem include the following:

- The chronology of clinical signs is very different, raising the possibility that there is more than one disorder present. It could be one progressive disorder, but it could also be two different disorders.
- The problems don't fit together easily, for example, different body systems appear to be involved in an unrecognisable pattern, for example, as for Erroll.
- Other clues that may be relevant to the case. For example, some clinical signs resolved with symptomatic treatment but others did not.

How do I decide what problems are specific?
As indicated previously, specificity is a relative term and will vary with each patient. There are a few clues that you can look for when trying to decide the most specific problems the animal has:

Is there a clearly defined diagnostic pathway for the problem with a limited number of systems or differential diagnoses that could be involved?

For example: vomiting vs. inappetence

- The problem of vomiting has a very clearly defined diagnostic pathway (discussed in Chapter 3), whereas there is almost an endless set of diagnostic possibilities for causes of inappetence, and there is no well-defined diagnostic approach (Chapter 5).
- Hence, vomiting is a more specific and appropriate 'diagnostic hook' than inappetence.

Could one problem be explained by all of the other problems but not vice versa, or does the differential diagnosis list for one problem include many diagnoses that would explain the other problems but not vice versa?

For example: vomiting vs. jaundice

- As mentioned earlier, jaundice is the more specific problem because most causes of jaundice could also conceivably cause vomiting, but there are many causes of vomiting that do not cause jaundice.
- Hence, the diagnostic pathway for jaundice is more clearly defined (discussed in Chapter 11), and there are a more limited number of possible diagnoses.

As mentioned earlier – are there clinical signs that indicate this patient is at immediate risk, so they must be addressed prior to the other problems?

• For example: severe dyspnoea, shock, severe haemorrhage.

But don't forget to relate each problem to the whole animal.

Once you have narrowed down your diagnostic options for the most specific problems, you use these to direct your diagnostic or therapeutic plans, but don't forget to consider the less specific problems in relation to your differential diagnosis.

For example, your *specific problem* may be polyuria/polydipsia (PU/PD) associated with a urine specific gravity of 1.002 (hyposthenuria), and your non-specific problem may be anorexia. Hence, when considering the potential differential diagnoses for PU/PD associated with hyposthenuria (Chapter 13), those diagnoses for which anorexia is *not* usually a feature, for example, psychogenic polydipsia, diabetes insipidus and hyperadrenocorticism, are much less likely than those diagnoses where anorexia *is* common, such as hypercalcaemia, pyometra and liver disease. It is not always necessary to 'rule out' the former diagnoses, but they have a lower priority in your investigation than the latter group.

Thus, the thinking goes: '*the causes of hyposthenuria are . . ., . . ., . . ., . . ., . . ., . . . (Chapter 13) and in this patient the most likely causes are . . ., . . ., . . ., . . . (because of the other clinical signs or clinical pathology present).*'

In other words, you use the non-specific problems to refine the assessment of the specific problems. One could claim that this is pattern recognition, and indeed it is to a certain extent. However, the step of clarifying the problem list (and thus not overlooking minor signs) and assessing the specific problems in this manner allows the clinician's mind to be receptive to differentials other than the supposedly blindingly obvious one that uncritical pattern recognition may suggest (such as thinking every cat with PU/PD must have renal failure). And as we discuss later in this chapter, the particular steps you take in assessing the specific problems also decrease the risk of pattern-based tunnel vision and confirmation bias.

How likely is a diagnosis?

Priority is also influenced by the relative likelihood of a diagnosis. Common things occur commonly. Therefore, although you shouldn't dismiss the possibility of an unusual diagnosis by any means, the *priority* for the assessment is usually to consider the most likely diagnoses first, provided they are consistent with the data available.

The problem-based approach

Problem-based approach means different things to different people, and you may have already read about or been to courses where it was discussed. Some regard the problem-based approach as meaning '*write a problem list, then list every differential possible for every problem.*' Not a feasible task unless you have an amazing factual memory and endless time! Others view the problem-based approach as meaning '*write a problem list, then list your differentials.*' This is really just a form of pattern recognition, but at least it makes a good start by formulating a problem list.

The basis of this book is the concept of logical clinical problem-solving (LCPS). This approach provides steps to bridge the gap between the problem list and the list of differential diagnoses via a structured format. The problems should be investigated by rigorous use of the following questions as illustrated in Figure 2.2:

- What is the problem? (*Define +/- refine the problem* – some problems do not need to be refined, others do.)
- What system is involved, and *how is it involved? (Define and refine the system.*)
- Where within the system is the problem located? (*Define the location.*)
- What is the lesion? (*Define the lesion* – the differential list.)

The answers to these questions or the pursuit of the answers will determine the appropriate questions to ask in the history. They may alert you to pay particular attention to aspects of the physical examination, and/or they may indicate the most appropriate diagnostic test to use to find the answers as well as prepare you intellectually to assess the results of diagnostic procedures.

Define and refine the problem

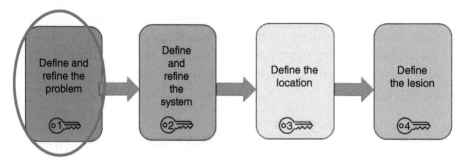

Figure 2.3   Clinical reasoning step-by-step: define and refine the problem.

Example: the owner reports that the dog is vomiting. Is the animal really vomiting or regurgitating – or perhaps even coughing or experiencing reflux?

When considering the important clinical signs the patient is exhibiting, it is essential to try to define the problem as accurately as possible. *A problem well defined is a problem half solved* is a good maxim to work from.

The first question to ask is, *Is there another clinical sign that this problem could be confused with?* This is a vital step, and failure to define the problem correctly has often derailed a clinical investigation that might otherwise have been relatively straightforward.

Other examples include the following:
- The owner says the dog is having fits – is it having seizures, episodes of syncope or vestibular attacks or other strange episodes? (Chapter 8)
- The owner says the dog has red urine – is it blood, haemoglobin or myoglobin? (Chapter 12)

Refine the problem
Some (but not all) problems require further refining to clarify the best diagnostic approach.

Examples include the following:
- Weight loss – is this because of inappetence or despite a normal appetite? (Chapter 5)
- Collapse – with or without loss of consciousness? (Chapters 7 and 8)

Why is it so important to define and refine the problem?

The range of diagnoses to consider, diagnostic tools used and potential treatment or management options for clinical problems that may be perceived by the owner to be the same and present similarly to the veterinarian can be very different. Or the owner might perceive the presenting signs to be attributable to one problem, but in reality, the signs indicate another problem to the veterinarian.

Failure to appropriately define and/or refine the problem can often lead to wasted time and money, as the wrong problem is investigated or treated.

This may:

- Delay reaching a feasible diagnosis
- Delay treatment
- Prolong the disease
- Prolong the patient's suffering
- Sometimes potentially endanger the life of the patient
- Unnecessarily increase the costs to the client
- Frustrate the veterinarian *and* client
- Potentially impair the client–veterinarian relationship.

 Define and refine the system

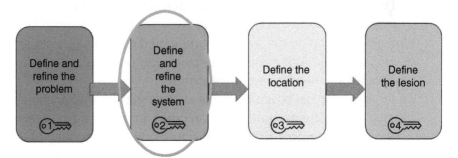

Figure 2.4 Clinical reasoning step-by-step: define and refine the system.

Once the problem is defined, the next step is usually to consider the system involved (Figure 2.4). For every clinical sign, there is a system(s) that *must* be involved, that is it 'creates' the clinical sign – this is what is meant by *defining* the system. However, the really important question is, *How is it involved?* This is *refining* the system. The key questions in this case are *What system is involved in causing this clinical sign?*

(define the system), and *Do I have a primary, that is, structural problem of a body system, or a secondary problem, that is, functional problem where the system involved is affected by other factors?* (refine the system).

Key concept	
Define the system	For every clinical sign, identify the system that must be involved.
Refine the system	For every defined system, determine how the system is affected – primary (structural) or secondary (functional) or, for some problems, local vs systemic.

Examples include the following:
- The body system *always* involved when a patient vomits is the gastrointestinal (GI) system (define the system).
  - However, it may be directly involved due to primary pathology of the gut, such as parasites, inflammation, neoplasia and foreign body. The system is thus refined as *primary (structural)* GI disease.
  - Or vomiting may be occurring due to dysfunction of non-GI organs, such as the liver, kidney, adrenal glands and/or pancreas. The system is thus refined as *secondary (functional)* GI disease.
- The body system that is *always* involved when a patient has generalised weakness is the neurological/neuromuscular system (define the system).
  - However, in refining the system, it may be directly involved due to *primary* neurological/neuromuscular pathology (e.g. inflammation, toxins, neoplasia and infection).
  - Or the neurological/neuromuscular system may be malfunctioning due to the effect of pathology on other organs, causing metabolic derangements that impair neurological/neuromuscular function, such as hypoglycaemia, anaemia, hypoxia and electrolyte disturbances. This is thus refined as *secondary* neurological/neuromuscular disease.

Why is it so important to define and refine the system?
The range of diagnoses to consider, diagnostic tools used and potential treatment or management options for primary, structural problems of a body system are often very different compared to those relevant to secondary, functional problems of that system.

Investigation of primary, structural problems often involves imaging the system in some manner (radiology, ultrasound, advanced trans-sectional imaging, endoscopy and surgery) and/or biopsy. Routine haematology, biochemistry and urinalysis are often of little diagnostic value. For secondary, functional disorders, on the other hand, haematology and biochemistry are often critically important in progressing our understanding of the case and reaching a diagnosis.

Failure to consider what body system is involved (*define the system*) and how it is involved (*refine the system*) can often lead to wasted time and money. This can delay treatment, prolong the disease, prolong the patient's suffering, sometimes potentially endanger the life of the patient, and may increase unnecessarily the costs to the client, frustrate the vet and client and potentially impair the relationship between vet and client. (Notice a recurring theme here?)

In fact, if you do nothing else when assessing a case before seeking the diagnostic 'pattern', ask yourself for each of the specific problems, *What system could be involved* (i.e. define the system), *and how – primarily or secondarily?* (i.e. refine the system). This simple question will immediately open your mind to diagnostic possibilities you may never have contemplated if you were just focusing on the 'pattern'.

Other examples include the following:
- Chronic cough – cardiac or respiratory system? (Chapter 9)
- Jaundice – due to a haemopoietic (haemolysis) or hepatobiliary disorder? (Chapter 11)
- Cardiac arrhythmia – is it due to primary (structural) cardiac disease – for example, dilated cardiomyopathy? Or extra-cardiac disease – for example, gastric dilation and volvulus, splenic pathology? (Chapter 7)
- PU/PD – is it due to primary polydipsia (the patient *wants* to drink) or primary polyuria (the patient *has* to drink)?
  - If due to primary polyuria – is this because of primary (structural) renal disease (e.g. chronic kidney disease) or extra-renal dysfunction, for example, diabetes mellitus, hypercalcaemia and hypoadrenocorticism? (Chapter 13)

An alternative, although closely related, question for some problems is, *Is the problem local or systemic?*
- Epistaxis – due to local nasal disease or systemic disease – for example, coagulopathy and hyperviscosity? (Chapter 12)

- Melaena – GI bleeding due to local disease (ulceration – which in turn may be due to primary or secondary GI disease) or systemic disease, for example, coagulopathy? (Chapter 12)
- Seizures – due to local brain disease, for example, neoplasia, infection/inflammation or systemic disease, for example, electrolyte disturbances or intoxication? (Chapter 8)

How to differentiate primary from secondary system involvement?
There are often clues from the history and/or clinical examination that help you define and refine the body system involved. Or you may not be able to answer this question until further diagnostic tests are performed. But just asking the question ensures that you remember that body systems can malfunction due to direct pathology of that system, for example, inflammation, neoplasia, degeneration, infection or due to functional problems where factors not directly related to the body system can impact on its function.

Define the location

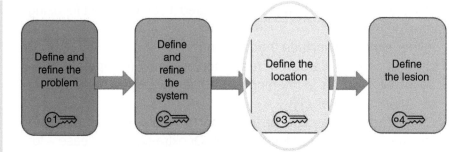

Figure 2.5   Clinical reasoning step-by-step: define the location.

Define the location is the step which may or may not be needed during your problem-based assessment. For some problems it is very important. For others, the *Define the location* question is addressed as part of the *Define the system* assessment. This will become evident in some of the case examples provided later in the book.

Example: having determined that vomiting is due to primary GI disease, where in the GI tract is the lesion located (*define the location*)?

In this example, by asking this question, you will select the most appropriate method either to answer the question or to move on to the next step.

For example, if you believe that your history and physical examination and other ancillary data indicate a lower small intestinal lesion, endoscopy may not be an appropriate method of visualising the area or obtaining biopsies as the scope will not reach the ileum. However, if all of the information you have suggests a gastric or duodenal lesion, endoscopy may be appropriate if available.

Other examples include the following:

- Vomiting due to secondary GI disease – liver, kidney, adrenals and pancreas? (Chapter 3).
  - Brutus is an example of secondary GI disease due to liver pathology.
- Hind limb weakness is due to neurological dysfunction – is the lesion in the spinal cord (and where), peripheral nerves, muscles or brain? (Chapter 7)
- Haematuria – from urethra, prostate, bladder or kidneys? (Chapter 12).
  - Errol is an example of haematuria due to bladder pathology.

 Define the lesion

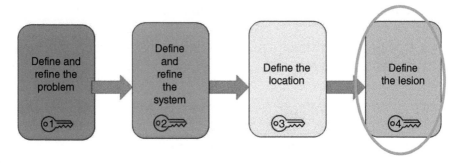

Figure 2.6   Clinical reasoning step-by-step: define the lesion.

Once the location of a problem within a body system is determined, usually the next key question is, *What is it?* You need to identify the pathology – *define the lesion*. This is now your differential list. It can be helpful to remember the types of pathology that can occur in broad terms – for example, degeneration, anomaly, metabolic, neoplasia, nutritional, infection, inflammation, idiopathic ('genetic'), trauma, toxic and vascular (DAMNIT-V).

Which type of pathology is most likely going to depend on the body system or organ involved, the signalment of the patient (species, breed, age, sex etc.), the clinical onset and course of the clinical signs, the geographic location of the patient and what disorders are common in that population.

This assessment can be influenced by whether the patient is in a general clinic or a referral hospital. Common things occur commonly or 'the hoof beats in the night are much more likely to be due to a horse than a zebra' (unless you are on safari, of course!). This doesn't mean that uncommon diagnoses should not be considered (and they will of course be more common in specialist hospitals). It's just that common disorders usually receive diagnostic priority at the beginning of a clinical investigation in general practice.

Example: the patient has a gastric lesion – is it a tumour, foreign body or ulcer?

This question will require visualisation and/or biopsy to answer, but it would have been a waste of time asking the question until you had arrived at the right location.

Other examples include the following:
- Spinal cord pathology identified based on a neurological examination – is it inflammation, infection or a neoplasm?
- Haematuria is due to lower urinary tract disease – infection, calculi or neoplasia?
- Large bowel diarrhoea – parasites, infection, ulceration, stricture, neoplasia or diet related?

Putting it all together

What do I need to do to define the problem, system, location or lesion?
- The diagnostic methods used to define the problem, the system, where appropriate the anatomical location and the lesion will vary depending on the problem.
  - For example, clinical pathology may be needed in some cases to define the problem (e.g. is red urine due to blood or haemoglobin?), but in many cases, the problem will be definable on the basis of history (onset and course of the disease) and clinical examination findings.
- Similarly, diagnostic tests or procedures may be required to define and refine the body system involved in some cases, and for other

problems, the system involved will be evident from clues from the history and/or the clinical examination.

- In some cases, once the problem is defined, for example, regurgitation, the body system is immediately apparent and the anatomical location identified (upper GI tract – oesophagus or pharynx).
- For neurological problems, clinical and neurological examination will often define the problem, system and location, leaving only the lesion needing to be defined by diagnostic testing.

Are the steps always in the same order?

The order in which the problem, system, location and lesion are defined may change for some problems.

- For example, when assessing coughing and diarrhoea, identifying the location occurs before identifying the system, as location identification helps identify the system (discussed in more detail in Chapters 4 and 9).
- For some problems, for example, pruritus (Chapter 15), you might go straight from problem definition to seeking to define the lesion.
- However, for almost all clinical problems, answering *some or all* of the four questions – *What is the problem? What system is involved and how? What is the location of the lesion?* and *What is the lesion?* – will provide a framework to guide your clinical reasoning and diagnostic and therapeutic decisions.

Thus, instead of thinking when faced with a vomiting patient, 'I wonder if it has a gastric foreign body or renal failure or a liver tumour?', your initial energies are directed at defining the problem and system, which will help make your list of differentials (which are usually the location and/or lesion) logical, appropriate and given appropriate priority. In this way, the diagnosis is made thoughtfully, and during the process, all diagnostic options can be considered as the need arises.

But does pattern recognition have a place?

It is important to reiterate that pattern recognition for many cases is *appropriate and justifie*d – depending on your level of experience, knowledge, skill base and mindset. For example, if a pot-bellied elderly terrier with bilaterally symmetrical alopecia, hyperpigmentation and comedones walked into your consulting room and the owner reported that the dog was drinking lots of water, was ravenously hungry and appeared to be panting excessively, then hyperadrenocorticism is the most obvious diagnosis, and going through the motions of assessing each specific problem would be ridiculous (but not if you had never seen a dog with hyperadrenocorticism before!).

However, it is important to be aware that pattern recognition is only foolproof if:

- The pattern is virtually unique to the disease
- You consider a sufficient number of factors in your pattern
- You carefully evaluate that your pattern *does* explain all of the clinical problems (and don't ignore those that don't)
- Or there are a very limited number of diagnostic options.

The value and effectiveness of pattern recognition is very dependent on the clinician's experience, depth of knowledge, understanding and ability to sort data quickly and efficiently.

Of course, once you have considered each individual problem, you do in fact look for a pattern in the clinical signs. However, the insertion of that initial step of considering each specific problem individually and *then* relating it to the other problems present should ensure that you don't miss the less obvious possible diagnoses.

In addition, the process of developing a sound problem-based approach can enhance your ability to pattern recognise because you have a greater understanding of the reasons *why* you believe certain patterns are suggestive of some disorders more than others.

Combinations of clinical signs

There are some combinations/patterns of clinical signs that make the diagnostic options very limited, and it is entirely appropriate to consider them together; for example, the patient with PU/PD who is also polyphagic. If the PU/PD and polyphagia have been present for the same length of time, then they are almost certainly due to the same disorder, and it is quite appropriate to assess them together. There are very few conditions that will cause this pattern of clinical signs (e.g. diabetes mellitus, hyperthyroidism and hyperadrenocorticism), so it is quite appropriate to concentrate on these first.

Does this make sense?

Always ask yourself, particularly when assessing clinical pathology or results of other diagnostic procedures in light of particular problems, *Does this make sense – does this clinicopathological abnormality explain the problem that the animal has?* Good clinicians are good detectives!

Example 1

- A dog is depressed, anorectic, vomiting and polydipsic.
- Its blood glucose is 12 mmol/L (just above the reference range).
- It has 3+ glucosuria and no ketones in the urine.

Does this mean that diabetes mellitus explains all of the dog's clinical signs? No – usually uncomplicated diabetes does not result in depression, anorexia and vomiting. There must be another reason for these clinical signs. Diabetic ketoacidosis might have been an explanation, but it has been ruled out by your urinalysis. Hence, you must look further for an explanation for the vomiting, anorexia and depression.

Example 2

An unwell dog (anorectic, vomiting and depressed) is found to have clinicopathological changes consistent with hyperadrenocorticism. Does this explain all of the dog's clinical signs? No – dogs with uncomplicated hyperadrenocorticism are not metabolically unwell, so there must be some other explanation for the dog's malaise that you will need to identify and resolve before definitive testing for hyperadrenocorticism is possible (because concurrent disease has a significant impact on dynamic adrenal testing).

Think pathophysiologically

Another essential element is to think pathophysiologically. Understanding physiology and pathophysiology is essential to understand medicine.

For example, an animal has profound hypokalaemia. Rather than trying to remember all of the diseases that may cause hypokalaemia, review how the body might lose potassium or fail to acquire it or even 'use it up'. By getting into the habit of thinking in this manner, you can potentially diagnose disorders you may never have heard of (or that may never have been described before!). It will also stimulate you to seek more knowledge about the pathophysiology of disease processes, which will lead to a greater understanding of internal medicine and ultimately to a better retention of knowledge.

It may appear tedious at times!
You may feel at times that being asked to assess each individual's specific problem is a tedious exercise when the diagnosis is obvious, because you think you recognise the pattern of clinical signs. In some, indeed many, cases, depending on your level of experience, this will be absolutely true, whereas in other cases, you will be misled. However, the most important point that we will try to get across is that if you don't 'practice' this structured problem-based approach on relatively simple clinical cases, when you are faced with the complex cases, which you may be feeling frustrated and stressed about at present, you will not be able to apply problem-based principles and as such will be still left floundering as pattern recognition and/or going fishing fail you.

It is also important to recognise that pattern recognition is a process of thinking that doesn't require explicit teaching – it happens naturally, whereas developing a robust structured inductive approach does require explicit articulation and practice of the steps involved.

It is useful to remember that medical diagnoses are often based on the 'balance of probabilities' rather than having to be proved 'beyond reasonable doubt'. Striking the right balance between the diagnostic possibilities and judging what is important or likely and what is less important or less likely can be challenging and, of course, is very influenced by experience but also understanding and knowledge.

Ancillary benefits
The aim of a structured and thorough approach to diagnosis is to reach the answer as quickly as possible and to get the best value from your 'diagnostic dollar/pathology pound/enabling euro' – that is, not to waste the client's money on unnecessary tests and procedures. An additional advantage of following this approach is that you should have a very good idea *why* you are advising doing blood tests or taking radiographs or prescribing a particular medication. And because you know *why*, you can explain your reasons to the client clearly, and they are much more likely to agree to follow your suggestions. Client compliance is positively influenced by the degree to which they understand the reasons for diagnostic or treatment recommendations.

You are also in a much better position to explain the implications of 'normal results' rather than being sent into a panic because you were hoping the blood tests would show something ('because the dog looks really sick, so it must have an abnormal blood test! – but. . .its blood results are absolutely normal! – HELP! – what do I do now?').

Time waster or time saver?

It is common when first faced with the process of problem-based inductive clinical reasoning to feel that it is an academic exercise that there simply isn't time to apply in the context of a busy clinic, 10–15-minute consultation slots and the many conflicting demands on your time. However, if you are able to put in the hard work initially *and* if you discipline yourself to think in this way, it will become second nature, subconscious (thus you have reached unconscious competence) and certainly not as laborious as it may appear at the beginning.

In fact, acquisition of these problem-solving skills will ultimately save time, as it will help you quickly eliminate extraneous background noise and focus on what is important for *this* patient and client. An analogy is the process of learning a new language. To do so, you initially need to learn some vocabulary and grammar (framework), but once you have a basic understanding *and* if you use the new language on a daily basis, further progression to fluency aka unconscious competence comes naturally. But without the basic framework and constant practice, fluency is an unfulfilled dream.

Comments from participants in courses based on this approach include:

- 'I developed a more systemic approach to medicine, which *saved a lot of time* in a busy practice'.
- 'It made me *think more efficiently* in a busy practice'.

Hopefully, this will be your experience too. As with all skills, it takes time to develop the knowledge base and mental discipline required for this form of clinical reasoning, but once developed, it will provide a firm base for the future and, most importantly, will not 'go out of date', no matter how many new diseases/disorders are discovered.

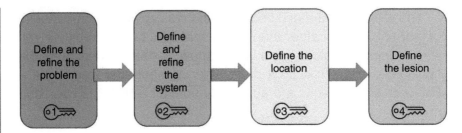

Figure 2.7   Clinical reasoning step-by-step: recap.

Key points

As a result of reading this chapter we hope that you appreciate that:
Problem-based inductive clinical reasoning. . .
- Is much more than just listing problems, then listing differentials for each problem (a common misconception about problem-based medicine)
- Has 'rules' that are easy to remember and can be applied to most clinical problems animals present with
- Has a structured approach to clinical problems centred on four main steps (Figure 2.7) as follows:
  o Define +/- refine the problem
  o Define and refine the system
  o Define the location (where appropriate)
  o Define the lesion
- Provides an intellectual and visual framework to hang your knowledge on, allowing you to recognise and retrieve more easily the information you need
- Reduces the need to remember a long list of differentials (see the first point)
- Helps prevent getting trapped by a perceived 'obvious' diagnosis – it helps avoid diagnostic bias
- Provides memory triggers to ensure an appropriate history is taken and a thorough clinical examination performed
- Provides a clear rationale for choosing diagnostic tests or treatments that can be communicated to the owner
- Helps turn a terrifying case into a manageable one!

CHAPTER 3

Vomiting, regurgitation and reflux

Jill E. Maddison

Department of Clinical Science and Services, The Royal Veterinary College, London, UK

The why

- Veterinarians in general practice frequently assess animals whose owners report they are vomiting.
- The causes and consequences of vomiting can range from clinically inconsequential to life threatening.
- In contrast, regurgitation is a much less common clinical sign. Almost invariably, the patient who is truly regurgitating as their primary clinical problem will have serious disease.
- Gastric reflux can also be confused with vomiting and has different implications for the animal that need to be recognised.
- It is therefore essential that the clinician has a robust and rapid way to assess patients during the initial consultation so that rational decisions can be made about appropriate diagnostic and/or therapeutic plans.

Pathophysiology

The main function of vomiting is to protect the animal from ingested toxins. Dogs in particular have a propensity to eating disgusting things and have a very well-developed vomiting reflex.

To develop a rational approach to the patient who is reported to be vomiting, it is important to appreciate the pathophysiology of vomiting and regurgitation.

Vomiting or emesis is the forceful expulsion of gastric contents through the oesophagus, mouth and, sometimes, nostrils. It is a neurologically complex process resulting from the synchronised

Clinical Reasoning in Veterinary Practice: Problem Solved!, Second Edition.
Edited by Jill E. Maddison, Holger A. Volk and David B. Church.
© 2022 John Wiley & Sons Ltd. Published 2022 by John Wiley & Sons Ltd.

activity of a number of abdominal, pharyngeal and thoracic structures. The act of vomiting is coordinated in the medulla oblongata and cannot occur without a functional vomiting centre. In contrast, regurgitation is a passive process, which involves the retrograde movement of food and fluid from the oesophagus, pharynx and oral cavity without the initiation of reflex neural pathways other than the gag reflex.

The essential neurological components of the emetic reflex are the following:
- Visceral receptors
- Vagal and sympathetic afferent neurons
- Chemoreceptor trigger zone (CRTZ)
- Vomiting centre within the reticular formation of the medulla oblongata.

It is important to understand the stages that occur in the act of vomition, as they contribute to the clinical manifestation of vomiting, and this also assists the clinician to differentiate vomiting from regurgitation.

The first stage of vomiting is *nausea*. In this stage, gastric tone is reduced, duodenal and proximal jejunal tone is increased and duodenal contents reflux into the stomach. The patient often appears depressed, hypersalivates and as a result may exhibit repeated swallowing and/or lip-licking behaviour.

As an aside, while most patients who vomit will also be nauseous, it is important to recognise that the neural pathways involved in nausea and vomiting are not the same. Indeed, the neural pathways involved in nausea are still not well understood. The clinical relevance of this is that drugs that are effective anti-emetics may not be effective at reducing nausea. If signs of nausea and food aversion persist once vomiting is controlled, consider adding a drug that has good efficacy against nausea such as ondansetron to the patent's management. Noting, of course, that the persistence of nausea may also reflect progress of the underlying disease.

The nauseous stage is followed by *retching* (an unproductive effort to vomit, also known as 'dry heaves') and then *vomiting*. When the animal vomits, the epiglottis is closed and the soft palate presses up against the nasopharynx. The abdominal muscles and the diaphragm contract. The contraction of the abdominal muscles is usually visible to an observant owner. The cardia then opens, the pyloric stomach contracts and vomiting occurs. Reverse peristalsis, cardiac rhythm disturbances and increased colonic motility may also occur during the vomiting process.

The closure of the epiglottis and pressing of the soft palate up against the nasopharynx protect against aspiration of gastric contents. In contrast, during regurgitation, which is a passive process without neurological coordination, these actions do not occur. As a result, aspiration pneumonia is a common sequela to disorders that cause regurgitation and less likely in vomiting unless the animal is obtund.

Initiation and the process of vomiting

Vomiting is essentially initiated by either humoral or neural pathways. The *humoral pathway* involves stimulation of the CRTZ within the medulla oblongata by blood-borne substances. The *neural pathway* is through activation of the vomiting centre.

Vomiting centre

All animal species that vomit have a brainstem 'vomiting centre', which is a group of several nuclei that act in concert to coordinate the somatomotor events involved in expelling gastric contents. Non-vomiting species such as horses, rodents and rabbits also have the brainstem nuclei and motor systems necessary for emesis but lack the complex synaptic interaction between the nuclei and viscera required for a coordinated reflex.

There does not appear to be a discrete vomiting centre within the reticular formation of the medulla oblongata. Rather, there is an 'emetic complex' that refers to groups of loosely organised neurons distributed throughout the medulla, which are sequentially activated and play a role in emesis. This complex will be referred to in this chapter as the vomiting centre, however, as conceptually this assists the understanding of the physiology and pathophysiology involved.

The vomiting centre receives input from vagal and sympathetic neurons, the CRTZ, the vestibular apparatus and the cerebral cortex. It may also be stimulated directly by blood-borne toxins that can cross the blood–brain barrier (BBB).

Central stimulation

Central stimulation of the vomiting centre occurs via higher centres in the central nervous system (CNS). Stimuli include nervousness, unpleasant odours, pain and psychogenic factors. Opioids and benzo-diazepine receptors have been implicated in centrally initiated vomit-ing, but their exact mode of action has not been well characterised pharmacologically. Centrally induced vomiting may also occur due to direct stimulation of the emetic centre by elevated cerebrospinal fluid pressure or CNS inflammation or neoplasia.

Vestibular apparatus
Labyrinthine dysfunction associated with motion sickness and middle/inner ear infection also has input into the vomiting centre via neural pathways arising from the vestibular system. The CRTZ is involved in this pathway in the dog but not the cat.

Chemoreceptor trigger zone
The CRTZ is located in the area postrema in the floor of the 4th ven-tricle. It has no BBB, therefore allowing toxins and chemicals that would normally be excluded from the CNS access to the brain. The CRTZ is stimulated by endogenous toxic substances produced in acute infectious diseases or metabolic disorders such as uraemia or diabetic ketoacidosis as well as by drugs and exogenous toxins.

Peripheral receptors
Peripheral receptors are located mainly in the gastrointestinal (GI) tract, particularly the duodenum, but also in the biliary tract, perito-neum and urinary organs. The receptors may be stimulated by disten-sion, irritation, inflammation or changes in osmolarity. There are a few receptors in the lower bowel, which explains why patients with inflam-matory lower bowel disease may occasionally vomit.

Assessment of the patient reported to be vomiting

 Define the problem

It's important to differentiate vomiting from regurgitation, which involves the retrograde movement of food and fluid from the oesoph-agus, pharynx and oral cavity without initiation of reflex neural path-ways other than the gag reflex.

It's also important to differentiate vomiting from gastric reflux, which involves retrograde movement of food and fluid from the stomach into the oesophagus. This material may then travel some or all of the way to the pharynx and nasopharynx and may be inhaled, causing acid damage to mucosae it contacts. The severity ranges from subclinical to severe and life threatening. Many patients present for the respiratory consequences of 'silent reflux', but in this chapter we will focus on the presentation that can be confused with vomiting because material from the stomach comes out of the mouth.

It is also important to differentiate vomiting from coughing followed by gagging, which is often confused by owners with vomiting. Cat owners in particular may confuse vomiting and coughing in their pets.

Owners are often unable to differentiate vomiting, regurgitating, refluxing and gagging, and therefore it is important to ask specific questions to elicit appropriate information, for example, amount of effort involved, character of vomitus, etc. If still uncertain, the veterinarian may need to observe the animal. Even with veterinary observation, it is difficult and sometimes impossible to differentiate reflux and regurgitation without fluoroscopy. Without fluoroscopy, the concurrent problems need to be considered to reach a reasonable conclusion. Patients with nausea, vomiting and gastric dysmotility are predisposed to reflux, as are brachycephalic breeds.

Why is it important to differentiate vomiting from regurgitation, reflux and coughing?
The differential diagnoses, appropriate diagnostic tools and management strategies are completely different for patients who are truly vomiting compared with patients who are regurgitating, gagging or coughing. There is much in common in the treatment of vomiting and reflux because diseases that lead to vomiting may subsequently lead to reflux. It is important to appreciate this so that a gastric antacid can be prescribed to reduce the risk of reflux oesophagitis, which can be the reason a patient with an acute vomiting disorder does not recover as expected and which can contribute significantly to patient morbidity and mortality.

Patients who are vomiting (due to primary GI or secondary GI disease) may be treated symptomatically or investigated, depending on the case, using a variety of diagnostic tools, including clinical pathology, diagnostic imaging, endoscopy and exploratory laparotomy.

When regurgitation is the predominant clinical sign, it will usually be due to oesophageal disease (very occasionally pharyngeal) and usually carries a poor or guarded prognosis due to the type of lesion – for example, foreign body, stricture or megaoesophagus. The patient should not be treated symptomatically without diagnostic investigation to define the lesion where possible. In addition, the investigation of regurgitation essentially involves visualising the oesophagus (by endoscopy and/or diagnostic imaging tools) – it is rare for routine clinical pathology to be of diagnostic value in defining the type of lesion (megaoesophagus, foreign body etc.), although it may be of value once megaoesophagus is diagnosed in assessing possible metabolic causes.

Similarly, the patient who is gagging most likely has a lesion in the pharyngeal region or upper oesophagus, and visualising the lesion is the appropriate diagnostic path. Clearly, the animal that is coughing has respiratory or cardiac disease and requires an entirely different diagnostic approach.

Failure to define the problem appropriately can therefore potentially endanger the patient and may lead to wasted time and money and impair the veterinarian–client relationship and trust.

Clues to help differentiation of vomiting, regurgitation and reflux

The associated behaviour of patients who vomit differs from those who regurgitate or reflux. As discussed, vomiting is a neurologically coordinated activity with defined stages and physical manifestations. The patient will exhibit abdominal effort prior to bringing up material, and vomiting is often preceded by hypersalivation – manifested by licking of lips and repeated swallowing. The vomiting may be projectile.

In contrast, regurgitation and reflux are passive processes – there are no coordinated movements. Regurgitation is often induced or exacerbated by alterations in food consistency and exercise and facilitated by gravity when the head and neck are held down and extended. Patients who regurgitate will often gag as material accumulates in the pharynx. Reflux is often watery and low in volume but acidic, and patients may exhibit behaviour indicating local irritation.

The character of the vomitus may also give the clinician clues. While undigested food may be brought up by vomiting or regurgitation, if the food is partially digested and/or contains bile, the patient is vomiting and/or refluxing, *not* regurgitating. The pH of the vomitus is occasionally, but not always, useful. Acidic material strongly suggests vomiting or reflux, but pH-neutral material may be the product of vomiting, reflux or regurgitation.

As mentioned, because the epiglottis does not close, regurgitating patients are at considerable risk of aspirating gastric contents. Thus, if an owner reports that his/her animal developed a cough at the same time it started 'vomiting', the clinician should be alert to the possibility that aspiration has occurred and that this is more likely to occur with regurgitation than vomiting.

There is a caveat, however, which should be kept in mind. Patients who have experienced serious vomiting of acidic gastric contents may develop a secondary oesophagitis and present with signs suggestive of both vomiting *and* regurgitation or reflux. Usually, vomiting will have been the first sign noted. Animals that ingest caustic or irritant material causing oesophagitis and gastritis may also present with signs of both vomiting and regurgitation.

Haematemesis
Patients may vomit fresh blood or digested blood. Digested blood has the appearance of coffee grounds and is often not recognised by the owner as blood (understandably). Owners are usually extremely concerned if fresh blood is observed in vomitus, though this may not be of great clinical consequence if it has resulted simply from the physical effect of intense vomiting rupturing a small superficial blood vessel.

Nausea
While most patients who vomit will also be nauseous, it is important to recognise, as mentioned earlier, that the neural pathways involved in nausea and vomiting are not the same. Indeed, the neural pathways involved in nausea are still not well understood.

Define and refine the system

Primary vs. secondary gastrointestinal disorders

Reviewing the physiology of vomiting as discussed in the previous section and as shown in Figure 3.1, it is apparent that vomiting may occur due to primary GI disease or from secondary or non-GI disease.

In contrast, regurgitation is almost always due to primary oesophageal disease (Table 3.1).

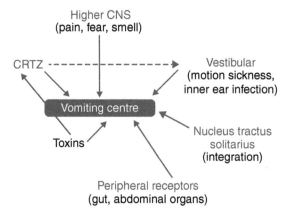

Figure 3.1 The relationship between the elements of the emetic reflex.

Primary GI diseases are those where there is specific primary GI pathology such as gut disturbance due to dietary indiscretion, inflammation, infection, parasites, obstruction or neoplasia. There may be metabolic consequences of the GI disease, but the *primary pathology is in the GI tract*.

Secondary GI disease is where the vomiting or regurgitation has occurred due to *pathology elsewhere in the body* – the gut is just the 'messenger'. Abnormalities of other body systems may indirectly cause vomiting either due to the action of toxins on the CRTZ, vomiting centre and vestibular system or by stimulation of peripheral non-GI-associated vomiting receptors.

Examples would include renal failure, liver disease, ketoacidosis, pancreatitis, hypercalcaemia, hypoadrenocorticism and other metabolic disorders. In most cases, there is no pathology identifiable in the gut, or where there is, for example, ulceration secondary to liver disease, uraemia or hypoadrenocorticism, the primary cause is the metabolic disorder. While symptomatic management strategies might be directed at the gut pathology in these cases (such as the use of anti-ulcer drugs), there is no diagnostic benefit to imaging the gut, for example, by endoscopy.

Why is it important to differentiate primary from secondary GI disease?

It is important to determine whether primary or secondary GI disease is occurring in the vomiting or regurgitating animal, as much time and money can be wasted if the wrong system is investigated. As discussed in Chapter 2, the range of diagnoses to consider, diagnostic tools used and potential treatment or management options for primary, structural problems of a body system such as the GI tract are often very different compared to those relevant to secondary, functional problems of that system. Investigation of primary GI disease often involves some form of imaging modality (radiology, ultrasound, endoscopy and surgery) and/or biopsy. Routine haematology and biochemistry are often of little diagnostic value in GI disease, although they may give clues about the clinical status of the patient. In contrast, for secondary GI disorders, haematology, biochemistry and other tests are often critically important in progressing towards a diagnosis.

It is also important to appreciate that there are cases of primary GI disease causing vomiting, such as gastroenteritis caused by dietary indiscretion or other irritants, that can be safely treated symptomatically, as the cause is transient and will resolve within days without specific treatment. Symptomatic management such as withholding food, antiemetic treatment and/or dietary change is appropriate for these patients. However, there are few, if any, secondary GI causes of vomiting (such as liver disease, renal failure, hypoadrenocorticism and hypercalcaemia) where the cause is transient, which will respond to symptomatic treatment and/or will resolve without specific therapeutic intervention.

The uncommon secondary GI causes of regurgitation all cause megaesophagus (Table 3.2), so the clinical decision pathway leading to their diagnosis begins with the diagnosis of megaoesphagus by endoscopy or diagnostic imaging and *then* the search for a metabolic cause. As mentioned, symptomatic treatment of regurgitation without establishing the cause is not prudent.

Thus, the clinician's clinical reasoning, *in the consultation room*, about whether primary or secondary GI disease is likely to be present is a crucial component of the rational management of patients reported to be vomiting or regurgitating and of clear communication with the client.

What are the clues that the patient has primary or secondary GI disease causing vomiting?

Primary GI disease should be strongly suspected if:

- An abnormality is palpable in the gut, for example, foreign body and intussusception
- The vomiting is associated with significant and concurrent diarrhoea
- The patient is clinically and historically normal in all other respects
- The onset of vomiting significantly preceded any development of signs of malaise – depression and/or anorexia
- The vomiting is consistently related in time to eating (although this can also occur with pancreatitis).

It is important to note, however, that primary GI disease cannot be ruled out even if none of the aforementioned features are present. For example, vomiting may be delayed for some hours (up to 24 hours) in animals with non-inflammatory gastric disorders. Animals with foreign bodies or secretory disorders of the bowel often vomit despite not eating. In lower bowel disorders, vomiting more commonly occurs at variable times after eating.

Animals with primary GI may also be depressed and inappetant due to the lesion (there are neural inputs to the satiety centre in the hypothalamus from the gut) or due to the secondary effects of prolonged vomiting with dehydration or electrolyte disturbances. Usually, the malaise will occur at the same time or after the onset of vomiting.

Thus, the features in the aforementioned bulleted list are strong clues that primary GI disease is present, but their absence does not preclude it.

Animals with secondary GI disease are vomiting due to the effect of toxins on the vomiting centre or CRTZ or because of the stimulation of non-GI-associated peripheral receptors. The vomiting is usually unrelated to eating – *except pancreatitis in dogs*.

With secondary GI disease:

- Animals will often have evidence from the history and/or clinical examination of abnormalities affecting other organ systems, for example, jaundice, polyuria/polydipsia (PU/PD).
- Vomiting is usually intermittent, unrelated to eating and may often occur subsequent to the onset of other signs of malaise.
- In general, animals that are vomiting due to extra-GI disease are metabolically ill and are not usually bright, alert and happy.
- If a patient has been metabolically ill (depressed and inappetant) for a significant period *before* vomiting was observed, then secondary GI disease is more likely.

Secondary GI causes of regurgitation will frequently have other systemic signs such as generalised weakness or metabolic malaise. It is usually only patients with megaoesophagus due to focal myasthenia gravis who present with regurgitation as their only clinical sign.

Exceptions to the 'rules'
The exception to these generalisations about the features of secondary GI disease is pancreatitis in dogs. Canine pancreatitis behaves similarly to a primary GI disease in that it causes acute-onset vomiting in an initially often otherwise well dog and often subsequent to an episode of dietary indiscretion. The vomiting often occurs immediately after eating, and decreased appetite and depression may not precede the onset of vomiting.

Pancreatitis in cats, however, usually behaves similarly to a secondary GI disease. Cats with hyperthyroidism may also vomit intermittently over a prolonged period and seem otherwise well (although, of course, they may also have other clinical signs suggestive of hyperthyroidism).

 Define the location

If primary GI disease is determined to be present, the temporal relationship of vomiting to eating and the character of the vomitus should be used to assess where the lesion is likely to be – the upper or lower GI tract.

Diagnostic tools such as contrast radiography may be appropriate to localise the lesion. An assessment of the likely location of the lesion is important, as this may determine what further diagnostic procedures are suitable. For example, endoscopy would be appropriate for examining the stomach and possibly duodenum but will be of little use if lower small bowel disease is suspected.

Defining the location for secondary GI disease usually involves routine clinical pathology and dynamic or function tests +/− imaging to localise the organ affected, for example, liver, kidney, pancreas and adrenals.

The location of the problem for patients who are regurgitating is almost always the oesophagus (occasionally the pharynx), whether the cause is primary or secondary GI. Thus, regurgitation is a clinical sign where location is considered first, and then the question is asked, *Is this a primary or secondary GI lesion?*

 ## Define the lesion

Primary GI diseases causing vomiting
Once the lesion has been located within the GI tract, it must now be identified. Biopsy may be appropriate or the type of lesion may be evident by visual inspection (e.g. foreign body).

In the GI tract, as elsewhere, neoplasia and inflammation often look grossly identical, and biopsies should always be taken even if the GI tract looks grossly normal.

Diseases of the stomach
- Gastritis
  - Dietary indiscretion
  - Drug induced, for example, non-steroidal anti-inflammatory drugs (NSAIDs)
  - Immune-mediated inflammatory disease
  - Infection, for example, *Helicobacter pylori*
    - Rarely clinically significant
- Gastric foreign bodies
- Gastric ulceration (see section below discussing haematemesis)
- Gastric neoplasia
- Disorders of the pylorus
  - Pylorospasm
  - Pyloric obstruction
  - Congenital pyloric stenosis
  - Chronic hypertrophic gastropathy
- Abnormal gastric motility

Intestinal disease

Those intestinal diseases for which vomiting is a predominate clinical feature include the following:

- Infectious enteritis, for example, parvovirus, corona virus (diarrhoea will usually also be present)
- Dietary indiscretion (diarrhoea often present)
- Intestinal obstruction – foreign body and intussusception
- Inflammatory bowel disease especially in cats (dogs tend to more commonly present with diarrhoea as the major clinical sign).

The closer the obstruction is to the pylorus, the more frequent and severe the vomiting.

Secondary GI diseases causing vomiting

A large number of secondary GI disorders can cause vomiting. However, most of these can be eliminated with relatively few tests – at least in dogs. Cats are more problematic, especially in the diagnosis of pancreatic and hepatic disease. In Table 3.1, the most important secondary GI disorders are listed with tests that are useful in their diagnosis.

Table 3.1 Secondary gastrointestinal causes of vomiting in cats and dogs.

Disorder	Clinical pathology that may be useful
Pancreatitis	Pancreatic lipase immunoreactivity (PLI), amylase (not in cats), lipase (not in cats), white blood cell (WBC) count, ALP, presence of lipaemic serum
Hepatic disease	ALT, ALP, GGT, bile acids, bilirubin, albumin, urea, glucose
Renal disease	Urea, creatinine, phosphate, SDMA, urine specific gravity (SG)
Hypoadrenocorticism	Na^+,K^+, urea, cortisol, calcium, glucose
Diabetic ketoacidosis	Blood and urine glucose, ketones
Toxaemia due to infection	WBC count
Hypercalcaemia	Serum Ca^{2+} (total and ionised)
Hypokalaemia/ hyperkalaemia	Serum K^+
CNS disease	Cerebrospinal fluid (CSF) analysis (possibly)
Dirofilariasis (cats)	Heartworm antigen tests (often negative), eosinophil count
Lead toxicity	Blood lead and/or urinary delta-aminolevulinic acid (δ-ALA)
Hyperthyroidism (cats)	Thyroxine (T4)

You should consult other textbooks to read about specific details of primary and secondary GI diseases causing vomiting and regurgitation.

Haematemesis
Persistent vomiting of fresh blood or vomiting of digested blood (coffee grounds) can be of significant clinical concern. The cause may be primary GI disease or secondary GI disease. Contrary to popular belief, most patients that are vomiting do *not* have gastric ulceration and do not need to be treated with an anti-ulcer drug. However, there may be a role for use of drugs that suppress gastric acid secretion (preferably proton-pump inhibitors) to prevent secondary oesophagitis.

Haematemesis may be the only sign of gastric bleeding, but concurrent melaena is common (see Chapter 12).

Primary GI causes of haematemesis include:
- Neoplasia
  o Lymphoma, adenocarcinoma, leiomyoma and leiomyosarcoma
- Gastric foreign body
- Severe inflammatory disease.

Secondary GI causes of haematemesis include:
- Coagulopathy
- Secondary GI diseases causing gastric ulceration
  o NSAIDs
  o Hepatic disease
  o Hypoadrenocorticism
  o Gastrinoma
  o Mast cell tumour (non-GI location)
  o Trauma
  o Renal failure
  o Systemic inflammation
    ▪ For example, pancreatitis, sepsis
  o Extreme exercise
    ▪ For example, sled dog racing.

Causes of regurgitation

Table 3.2 Oesphageal disorders causing regurgitation.

Megaoesophagus	• Congenital • Acquired – primary GI • Acquired – secondary GI	• Idiopathic • Polymyositis • Myasthenia gravis • Polyneuritis • Hypothyroidism • Hypoadrenocorticism • Neoplastic neuromyopathy • Lead toxicity • Tick paralysis (*Ioxodes holycyclus*)
External compression	• Persistent right aortic arch • Mediastinal lymphoma • Thyroid tumours • Hiatal hernia	
Internal obstruction – physical or functional	• Foreign body • Oesophagitis • Stricture	
Intra-mural lesions	• Neoplasm • Abscess • Granuloma	• For example, *Spirocerca lupi* in endemic areas

Diagnostic approach to the patient reported to be vomiting

It is imperative to carefully evaluate the history and physical examination findings for any clues that indicate whether the patient is vomiting or regurgitating and may suggest secondary or primary GI disease. You cannot always determine from the history and physical examination whether primary or secondary GI disease is most likely, but it is important that you ask yourself these questions: *Is this patient vomiting or regurgitating?* and *Does this patient have primary or secondary GI disease or I can't tell?,* as this will assist in directing your history taking and physical examination as you search for clues to enable you to answer these key questions.

In some vomiting cases, it will be obvious that primary GI disease is most probable (e.g. the bright, happy dog that, for several days, has been vomiting consistently half an hour after eating and has no other systemic signs). Or it may be clear that secondary GI disease is most likely (e.g. the cat that has been intermittently vomiting for a week, inappetant for 4 weeks and is also polydipsic). However, often, you cannot be sure based on the history and physical, so your diagnostic procedures will be aimed initially at answering the question, *What system is involved and how?* You won't always be able to answer the question initially, but it is essential that you ask it.

If indicated by the history and/or physical examination, investigate secondary GI disease with appropriate diagnostic tools such as biochemistry, haematology and urinalysis. Only a proportion of vomiting animals will require a diagnostic work-up, but it is still important to consider whether primary or secondary GI disease is likely, as this will influence your symptomatic treatment.

As discussed earlier, the most common causes of primary GI disease, such as gastritis due to dietary indiscretion, will usually respond satisfactorily to symptomatic treatment (which should rarely, if ever, include antibiotics). However, most secondary GI disease will not, and further information is required for management and prognosis.

When is clinical pathology useful?

In general, clinical pathology is most useful for progressing our understanding about secondary GI diseases causing vomiting. In contrast, for most primary GI disease, clinical pathology tests may provide information about the systemic effects of vomiting but *not* about the aetiology of the gut disorder.

Even if primary GI disease is strongly suspected, it may be helpful to perform appropriate tests to assess the patient's hydration and electrolyte/acid–base status, as prolonged and severe vomiting may cause biochemical derangements such as alkalosis or acidosis, prerenal azotaemia, hypokalaemia, hyponatraemia and hypochloraemia. Noting, however, that diagnostic procedures aimed at visualising the GI tract such as plain and/or contrast radiographs or endoscopy are more diagnostically useful in primary GI disease. Ultrasonography or exploratory laparotomy can be useful diagnostically for both primary and secondary GI disorders.

If you are unable to determine from the history and physical examination whether the animal has primary or secondary GI disease, it is cheaper, less invasive and usually quicker to investigate secondary GI disease first with appropriate tests and *then* investigate primary GI disease as needed if clinical pathology is normal. If there is any risk that the patient has an intestinal obstruction, then plain abdominal radiographs +/– ultrasonography should be performed as soon as possible. And if the patient has a concurrent cough, then this requires urgent investigation, as a serious disorder causing regurgitation is very possible.

When is a fuller work-up rather than symptomatic therapy indicated?

In general practice, we obviously do not investigate every vomiting patient presented to us. Symptomatic treatment is quite appropriate if you have made an assessment that the patient is vomiting, not regurgitating and probably has primary GI disease of a transient nature such as dietary indiscretion or food intolerance. A fuller work-up involving clinical pathology (either for diagnostic information or to assess the systemic effects of vomiting) +/– imaging is indicated if:

- The patient is regurgitating
- There has been no response to symptomatic therapy
- Vomiting is persistent and severe
- Other systemic signs are present indicating secondary GI disease, such as PU/PD and icterus
- There is inappetance and/or depression that commenced well before the onset of vomiting
- The patient is severely depressed
- There is a palpable abnormality in the abdomen.

In conclusion

Vomiting is a common clinical sign in small animal practice. Causes range from being relatively clinically innocuous and transitory to being an indication of serious primary or secondary GI disease.

A logical approach to assessing the patient that presents with the problem of vomiting is important to ensure that the problem and system are defined correctly so that diagnostic and treatment plans are rational and justifiable.

Clinical pathology will often progress understanding of secondary GI disorders but is not usually particularly helpful in primary GI disorders where imaging of the GI tract is often more diagnostically useful.

Key points

As a result of reading this chapter you should be able to:
- Appreciate the importance of differentiating regurgitating, reflux and vomiting
- Understand what initiates vomiting and, hence, how different disorders cause vomiting
- Appreciate the importance of determining whether vomiting is due to primary or secondary gastrointestinal disease
- Develop a rational diagnostic approach to the vomiting patient and to appreciate when a diagnostic work-up vs. symptomatic therapy is appropriate
- Understand the secondary gastrointestinal causes of vomiting and the most appropriate methods of diagnosis
- Review primary gastrointestinal disease processes that cause vomiting
- Understand the causes and consequences of disorders of the oesophagus
- Recognise the patient at risk of reflux and its consequences.

Questions for review

- When is a fuller work-up of a vomiting patient indicated as opposed to symptomatic treatment?
- What clinical features of a patient would strongly suggest to you that it was vomiting because of *primary* gastrointestinal disease?
- What clinical features of a patient would strongly suggest to you that it was vomiting because of *secondary* gastrointestinal disease?

Case example

'Muriel' is a 7-year-old Labrador (neutered) dog who presented with a 3–4-week history of reduced appetite and depression. She started to intermittently vomit bile-stained material about 2 weeks ago, and the vomiting has become much more frequent over the past week. The vomiting occurs unrelated to eating, and abdominal effort is obvious when she vomits. Prior to vomiting she appears restless and frequently licks her lips. No diarrhoea has been noted. Water intake is normal.

On physical examination she is thin (body condition score 3/9). There is no evidence of abdominal discomfort. Rectal temperature is normal. Heart rate and respiratory rate are within normal limits, pulses are strong and synchronous.

Define the problem

Is Muriel vomiting or regurgitating or refluxing?

She is vomiting as evidenced by abdominal effort observed, lip licking indicating hypersalivation and bile in the vomitus.

Define the system

Does Muriel have primary or secondary GI disease?

Most indicators in this case suggest that the vomiting is due to secondary GI disease because:

- The vomiting was *preceded* by 1–2 weeks of depression and reduced appetite.
- The vomiting is usually intermittent and unrelated to feeding (although of
- increasing frequency latterly).

This does not preclude primary GI disease but is more typical of secondary GI disease. Primary GI disease is less likely (although it cannot be completely excluded just yet).

Define the location

Where is the problem in the secondary GI system?

Secondary GI causes of vomiting of most relevance for Muriel include:
- Hepatic disease
- Hypoadrenocorticism
- Chronic (but not acute) pancreatitis
- Electrolyte perturbations due to various disorders (calcium, potassium).

Because polyuria and polydipsia are not features in this case (assuming the owner's history is correct), other conditions, which are less likely (but not excluded yet), would be:
- Renal disease
- Diabetic ketoacidosis.

Primary GI disease is less likely (although it cannot be completely excluded just yet) and will be investigated if there is no evidence for secondary GI disease. GI neoplasia or inflammatory bowel disease would be the most likely differentials if primary GI disease is present.

Define the lesion

This will be determined when the location is identified.

Case outcome

The diagnostics planned assessed the differentials considered for secondary GI disease (define the location +/- lesion). Biochemistry results were consistent with presence of a significant hepatopathy, ultrasound examination supported diffuse parenchymal disease and histopathology on an ultrasound-guided biopsy confirmed hepatocellular carcinoma.

CHAPTER 4

Diarrhoea

Jill E. Maddison[1] and Lucy McMahon[2]

[1]Department of Clinical Science and Services, The Royal Veterinary College, London, UK

[2]Anderson Moores Veterinary Specialists, Winchester, UK

The why

- Veterinarians frequently assess animals with diarrhoea in general veterinary practice.
- Many cases will be transient and respond to symptomatic management.
- Those cases that are chronic can be a source of great frustration for all concerned.
- A structured approach to diarrhoea, including classification of the type of diarrhoea, and a judicious mix of diagnostic tests and therapeutic trials can greatly improve the outcome.

Introduction and classification

Diarrhoea is a common clinical sign in animals presented to veterinarians in small animal practice. Similar to vomiting, the clinical consequences can range from insignificant to life threatening, although the latter is less common than the former. Many acute cases require little diagnostic intervention and resolve with or without symptomatic treatment. Chronic diarrhoea, however, can be a diagnostic challenge and the source of much frustration for the client and veterinarian. It is defined as diarrhoea that lasts for more than three weeks or intermittent diarrhoea over a period of one month or more. Animals can have chronic diarrhoea for months to years. Often, the animal may not be particularly unwell, and the diarrhoea may be chronic but intermittent and may respond partially but not entirely to different therapeutic interventions.

Clinical Reasoning in Veterinary Practice: Problem Solved!, Second Edition.
Edited by Jill E. Maddison, Holger A. Volk and David B. Church.
© 2022 John Wiley & Sons Ltd. Published 2022 by John Wiley & Sons Ltd.

Diagnostic investigation of chronic diarrhoea can involve various procedures that range from the inexpensive to the expensive and the non-invasive to the invasive. Unlike many clinical problems, therapeutic trials often play an important role in helping the clinician reach a probable diagnosis. However, trials need to be conducted logically and the outcomes reviewed critically.

The temptation to give multiple treatments aimed at different aetiologies in the hope that something will work is understandable. However, even if there is a positive response to multi-modal therapy, if the diarrhoea recurs once treatment stops (as it often does), the clinician is no wiser about the underlying cause and how to manage the patient long term. Patience is needed by all parties, and excellent communication between the veterinarian and the client is imperative. The clinician needs to have a rational diagnostic and therapeutic approach to chronic diarrhoea in the dog and cat, and this will be dependent on the classification of the type of diarrhoea that is present and its potential causes.

Pathophysiology

Diarrhoea can be due to osmotic or secretory mechanisms, increased gut permeability or altered gut motility. Although many types of diarrhoea are due to more than one mechanism, an understanding of the mechanisms of diarrhoea facilitates a rational approach to its diagnosis and treatment.

In general, osmotic and secretory mechanisms occur with small bowel disorders, whereas increased permeability and altered motility can relate to both small and large bowel disorders. Altered motility occurs in most diarrhoeal diseases. However, primary motility disorders are very uncommon in dogs and cats.

Classification of diarrhoea

Although symptomatic therapy (or no therapy!) is appropriate for the majority of animals with acute diarrhoea, chronic diarrhoea does not usually respond to non-specific symptomatic treatment and will often present the veterinarian with a diagnostic challenge where the more routine laboratory aids are not useful.

The diagnostic work-up, differential diagnoses and therapy for small and large bowel diarrhoea may differ, although there are some causes common to both. Therefore, it is of utmost importance that before embarking on invasive diagnostic procedures or extensive therapy, an assessment is made as to whether the diarrhoea is:

- Acute or chronic
- Relatively mild or more severe, with the presence of secondary systemic effects
- Small bowel or large bowel origin, or mixed
- Due to primary or secondary gastrointestinal (GI) disease.

Failure to elicit sufficient information from the client about the characteristics of the diarrhoea, so as to allow appropriate classification as small bowel, large bowel or mixed, may result in inappropriate diagnostic procedures or therapeutic trials with increased expense to the client and frustration of the veterinarian and client.

Define the problem

Diarrhoea is defined as an alteration in the normal pattern of defaecation, resulting in the passage of soft, unformed stools with increased faecal water content and/or increased frequency of defecation. It is important to consider the animal's previous pattern of defecation, as the frequency of defaecation and the nature of faeces vary between individuals.

There are a few uncommon situations where it may not be obvious to the owner that his/her animal has diarrhoea. Occasionally, the owner may mistake anal or vaginal discharges for diarrhoea, or see vomitus on the floor and think it is diarrhoea. The patient with constipation may pass small amounts of liquid faeces, which the owner thinks is diarrhoea. Conversely, the patient who is straining to defaecate and attempting to defaecate frequently because of large bowel disease may be interpreted by the owner as being constipated. Therefore, it is important that the clinician is cognisant of these issues and aims to define the problem as a first priority in the consultation.

Define the location

In cases of diarrhoea, the problem-based system we discussed in Chapter 2 is applied, but in a slightly different order. Identification of the location occurs *first*, which *then* assists in defining the system. This is because, almost always, large bowel diarrhoea reflects primary GI disease, whereas small bowel diarrhoea can occur with either primary or secondary GI disease. Thus, defining the location first aids in defining the system.

A thorough history is essential to differentiate small from large bowel disease. It is important to carefully question the owner as to the character of the faeces and to elicit information regarding consistency, colour, frequency and presence of blood or mucus. Related abnormalities should also be assessed, such as whether there has been significant weight loss, loss of appetite or vomiting. The characteristics of small and large bowel diarrhoea are detailed in Table 4.1.

Because large bowel diarrhoea has fewer and more specific characteristics than small bowel diarrhoea, it is often easiest to note if there is any fresh blood, mucus and small amounts of faeces passed frequently. If the diarrhoea has none of these characteristics, then the patient has small bowel diarrhoea. Note also that diarrhoea may have features of both small and large bowel, which indicates either primary small bowel with secondary effects on the lower bowel or diffuse disease involving both the small and large intestine.

Table 4.1   Characteristics of small and large bowel diarrhoea.

	Small bowel diarrhoea	Large bowel diarrhoea
Consistency, volume and pattern	Faecal volume and/or water content is increased. Diarrhoea may be projectile and does not usually involve significant tenesmus or urgency.	Small amounts of faecal material are passed frequently. Tenesmus and urgency are often present, particularly if the lower colon or the rectum is involved.
Blood	If blood is present, it is usually digested (melaena) or, in acute diarrhoea, reddish-brown.	If blood is present, it will be undigested (haematochezia).
Appearance	Colour may be grey if large amounts of undigested fat are present. A yellow-green coloration is common and due to malabsorbed bile salts.	Mucus is often present either on the surface (indicating the lesion is in the lower colon or rectum) or throughout the faeces (indicating a lesion in the higher colon).
Weight loss	Chronic small bowel diarrhoea is often (but not always) associated with weight loss.	Usually there is no weight loss caused by large bowel diarrhoea per se but there may be as a result of the pathology such as severe inflammation or neoplasia.

Table 4.1 (Continued)

	Small bowel diarrhoea	Large bowel diarrhoea
Vomiting	• Vomiting may also be present (but need not be). Relationship to eating can be variable depending on the location of the lesion.	Vomiting can occur occasionally but is infrequent and is unrelated to eating.
Borborygmus and flatulence	Gas commonly occurs with small bowel diarrhoea, as malabsorbed carbohydrates are fermented by colonic bacteria producing CO_2 and H_2S.	Uncommon.
Appetite	Appetite may be variable depending on the underlying aetiology.	Usually, the appetite is unaffected.
Water balance	If the diarrhoea is severe, the animal may be dehydrated. If the diarrhoea is very watery, the patient may have an increased water intake.	Large bowel diarrhoea per se does not usually adversely affect water balance.
Physical examination	Physical examination may reveal increased gas or thickened loops of bowel but is often unrewarding. Always do a rectal examination to check for melaena or large bowel signs such as mucus and fresh blood about which the owner may not be aware.	Physical examination is often unremarkable, but it is imperative to do a rectal examination if possible to check for strictures, masses or thickened mucosa.

Define and refine the system

Diarrhoea can be due to primary disorders of the small bowel and/or large bowel or due to other systemic, secondary GI disorders such as hepatic disease, exocrine pancreatic insufficiency, pancreatitis, hyperthyroidism or hypoadrenocorticism. As discussed earlier, large bowel diarrhoea is almost always due to primary GI disease, whereas small bowel diarrhoea may occur with either primary or secondary GI disease.

Severe systemic diseases such as sepsis and uraemia can cause large bowel diarrhoea, but this will be a very minor clinical sign in relation to the patient's other systemic clinical signs. Thus, secondary disorders are not usually likely differentials when considering the work-up of a patient whose primary problem is large bowel diarrhoea.

Diarrhoea due to primary GI disease is more common than diarrhoea due to secondary GI disease. In animals with secondary GI disease, with the exception of exocrine pancreatic insufficiency and some dogs with hypoadrenocorticism, diarrhoea is not usually the primary presenting complaint.

 ## Define the lesion

The following tables summarise the causes of acute and chronic small and large bowel diarrhoea (Tables 4.2–4.4).

Table 4.2   Causes of acute small bowel diarrhoea in dogs and cats.

Cause	Examples	Comments
Diet related	• Overeating (especially puppies) • Dietary change • Spoiled food • Dietary indiscretion	• Including change to food that causes allergy/hypersensitivity.

Parasites/protozoa	• Parasites
	  ○ Most commonly ascarids (*Toxocara* and *Toxascaris* spp., also hookworms *Ancylostoma* and *Uncinaria* spp.)
	• Protozoa
	  ○ *Giardia* spp.
	  ○ Coccidia, for example *Cystisospora* spp. (formerly called *Isospora*)
	  ○ *Cryptosporidium* spp.
		• Zinc sulphate flotation is a sensitive test for Giardia cysts, provided three faecal samples collected over 5 days are examined (~95% sensitive).
		• The ELISA test can identify Giardia antigen in faeces. The test is reported to be about 90% sensitive and is probably more sensitive than performing zinc sulphate flotation examination on a single faecal sample.
		• Faecal IFA and PCR are also available.
		• A negative result does not necessarily exclude Giardia infection, and some clinicians will treat with metronidazole or fenbendazole regardless and proceed with further investigations only if the diarrhoea persists.

Table 4.2   (Continued)

Cause	Examples	Comments

Infection (bacterial/ viral)	• Viral enteritis
	  ○ Parvovirus/ panleukopenia
	  ○ Coronavirus
	  ○ Distemper
	  ○ Feline immunodeficiency virus (FIV)/ Feline leukaemia virus (FeLV)
	  ○ Other viruses (e.g. adenovirus, norovirus, torovirus)
	• Bacterial enteritis
	  ○ *Campylobacter* spp.
	  ○ *Salmonella* spp.
	  ○ *E. coli*
	  ○ *Clostridium* spp.
		• Microbial culture of faeces is often unrewarding due to the abundant normal flora in the gut and the predominance of anaerobes.
		• *E. coli* is frequently, and *Salmonella* is sometimes, isolated from faeces of normal animals, and therefore their presence does not necessarily imply that they are the cause of the diarrhoea. *Campylobacter* spp. and *Clostridium* spp. are also found in animals with and without diarrhoea, which makes interpretation of results quite difficult.
		• *Clostridium perfringens* and *Clostridium difficile* have equal prevalence in dogs with and without diarrhoea. However, there is a correlation between the presence of diarrhoea and the detection of toxins that are produced by these bacteria, although enterotoxin can also be found in healthy dogs.
		• Identification of an overgrowth of *Clostridia* or Clostridial spores on faecal smears means nothing diagnostically and will occur in many situations when gut flora is disturbed by a variety of GI disorders.

Toxins	• Toxins
	  ○ Lead
	  ○ Organophosphates
	  ○ Plants
	  *Ingestion of many toxins can cause acute diarrhoea sometimes in combination with other systemic signs
		• Plants that may cause diarrhoea if ingested (as well as other clinical signs) include:
		  ○ Lily of the valley
		  ○ Daffodil bulbs
		  ○ Aloe vera
		  ○ Asparagus fern
		  ○ Chrysanthemums
		  ○ Cyclamens.

(Continued)

Table 4.2 (Continued)

Cause	Examples	Comments
Unknown	• Acute haemorrhagic diarrhoea syndrome (AHDS)	• Previously called haemorrhagic gastroenteritis (HGE). This is a syndrome causing acute onset of vomiting and bloody diarrhoea. • Characteristically the patient will have significant haemoconcentration (increased packed cell volume [PCV]) with a normal or low plasma protein due to protein loss into the bowel. It is typically described in small breed dogs but any size/breed can be affected. • It is now believed that the cause may be novel necrotising toxin produced by Type A *Clostridia perfringens*. • However, antimicrobial therapy does not improve outcome unless the patient is septic.
Secondary GI disease	• Acute pancreatitis • Severe systemic disease	• See previous comments regarding presence of other clinical signs.

Table 4.3 Causes of chronic small bowel diarrhoea in dogs and cats.

Cause	Examples	Comments
Diet related	• Diet-responsive disease or food-responsive enteropathy (FRE)	• Food intolerance is a non-immunological reaction to a component of food, for example, gluten, preservative, bony material and other irritants. • Food allergy/hypersensitivity is an immunological reaction to a component of food, for example, beef, chicken and dairy. • Diagnosis of dietary allergy or intolerance is usually a process of trial and error by using elimination diets, as there is no sensitive or specific diagnostic test. • Current evidence would suggest that blood tests for anti-food antibodies are not specific and not clinically useful for dogs and cats with FRE.

Table 4.3 (Continued)

Cause	Examples	Comments
Parasites/ protozoa	• Intestinal parasites (as previously mentioned) • Protozoa (as previously mentioned)	See comment in Table 4.2.
'Infection'/ bacterial/viral	• *Campylobacter/ Salmonella* • Feline infectious peritonitis	Note comments in Table 4.2 in relation to bacterial causes of diarrhoea.
Antibiotic responsive	• Antibiotic-responsive diarrhoea (ARD) • Secondary small intestinal bacterial overgrowth (SIBO)	• ARD: small intestinal diarrhoea that is responsive to antibacterials but no underlying cause can be identified. • SIBO: secondary to an underlying problem such as exocrine pancreatic insufficiency, inflammatory bowel disease, partial obstruction or motility disorders.

Infiltrative	• Immunosuppressive-responsive or non-responsive chronic enteropathy (IRE and NRE) – also termed inflammatory bowel disease (IBD), for example,
	  ○ Lymphocytic-plasmacytic enteritis
	  ○ Eosinophilic enteritis
	• Diffuse or focal lymphoma
	• Adenocarcinoma/ adenoma
	• Mast cell tumour (feline)
	• Smooth muscle/stromal cell tumours (canine)
		• Diarrhoea is the most common clinical signs of IBD in dogs.
		• Vomiting is the more common clinical sign in cats.
		• Intestinal biopsy is primarily required to characterise infiltrative inflammatory gut disease (IBD vs. neoplasia) and/or protein-losing enteropathy.

Miscellaneous	• Lymphangiectasia • Inherited selective cobalamin deficiency • Chronic intussusception • Chronic partial obstruction	• Lymphangiectasia is usually secondary to IBD but primary forms exist.

(Continued)

Table 4.3   (Continued)

Cause	Examples	Comments
Secondary GI (not an exhaustive list)	• Hypoadrenocorticism –dogs • Hyperthyroidism – cats • Exocrine pancreatic insufficiency • Chronic pancreatitis • Liver disease (hepato-cellular failure, choles-tasis, portal hypertension) • Severe systemic disease	

Table 4.4   Causes of acute and chronic large bowel diarrhoea in dogs and cats.

Parasites/protozoa	• *Giardia* spp. (more commonly small bowel but can also cause large bowel diarrhoea • *Tritrichomonas foetus* (cats) • *Entamoeba* spp. • *Trichuris vulpis* (whipworm) • *Ancylostoma caninum* (hookworm)
Infection (bacterial/viral)	• *Campylobacter spp.* (interpret positive results with caution) • *Clostridium perfringens; Clostridium difficile** • *Salmonella spp.** • *Yersinia enterocolitica** • Feline infectious peritonitis (FIP) • Granulomatous colitis (boxers, French bulldogs) – caused by invasive and adherent *E. coli* **These bacteria are rarely identified as causal agents in canine chronic diarrhoea; they may be more commonly identified in faecal samples from raw-fed pets, but raw food is not currently proven to cause diarrhoea more often than commercial pet food.*
Diet related	• Food-responsive enteropathy (FRE) • Passing foreign material • Fibre-deficient diet

Table 4.4   (Continued)

Inflammatory	• Immunosuppressive-responsive or non-responsive enteropathy = inflammatory bowel disease (IBD), for example, ○ Lymphocytic-plasmacytic enteritis (colitis) ○ Eosinophilic enteritis (colitis)
Neoplasia	• Diffuse or focal lymphoma • Adenocarcinoma/adenoma • Mast cell tumour (feline) • Smooth muscle/stromal cell tumours (canine)
Miscellaneous	• Stress-induced colitis can occur relatively commonly in hospitalised or newly kenneled dogs, which may be due to an overgrowth of *Clostridium perfringens* • Structural disease such as caecocolic intussusception (rare)

Diagnostic approach to the patient with diarrhoea

Small bowel diarrhoea
Acute vs. chronic

It is important to ascertain the duration the diarrhoea has been present. Acute diarrhoea that is not severe, fulminating and potentially life threatening does not usually require extensive diagnostic investigation and will usually respond to non-specific therapy. Fulminating acute diarrhoea, for example, viral and acute haemorrhagic diarrhoea syndrome (AHDS), may not require extensive diagnostic testing but will require intense supportive therapy and should not be treated on an outpatient basis if at all possible. In contrast, chronic diarrhoea persisting for weeks to months indicates that a structured approach to therapeutic trial and investigation is required.

When to investigate?

If diarrhoea persists despite symptomatic treatment or is chronic, severe and associated with significant weight loss and/or evidence of hypoproteinaemia, dehydration or systemic illness, then a more detailed investigation is indicated. Only a small proportion of diarrhoea cases require investigation as chronic disorders. An animal presenting with intermittent but repetitive episodes of diarrhoea over many months should also be considered for investigation unless there is a proven cause (e.g. regular garbage bin raiding).

The following is a general outline that can be used to approach stable cases of diarrhoea in adult dogs and cats in general practice. More severely affected animals and very young animals will require investigation and/or more intensive supportive treatment earlier in the course of their disease. *Every case should be considered individually, and client factors such as budget must be taken into account.*

1 Take a detailed history to assess for trigger factors (bin raiding, extra table scraps from the roast dinner, inappropriate diet or snacks, hunting etc). Perform a thorough physical examination to look for relevant abnormalities (e.g. palpable bowel lesion, dehydration, weight loss).

2 Ensure anthelmintic history is up to date, and if in doubt treat with an appropriate anthelmintic (usually more appropriate in young animals).

3 Recommend highly digestible food until diarrhoea resolves. If animal is not eating, monitor the situation in case intervention is needed (e.g. recheck in appropriate time period between 24 and 72 hours).

4 Antibiotic treatment is *rarely indicated* in acute diarrhoea unless the animal is systemically unwell, and even then it may not be warranted.

5 Consider faecal culture:
   • If the animal is systemically unwell
   • When diarrhoea is acute and haemorrhagic
   • If the diarrhoea is very severe
   • In multiple animals in a crowded environment such as a kennel environment
   • If the owner or the pet is immunocompromised or if the owner is also affected with diarrhoea.

Overall, most dogs and cats with chronic diarrhoea do not require faecal culture; it rarely adds to the clinical picture, and it increases the overall cost of investigation.

Treat with antibiotics if bacterial cause is strongly suspected but culture is not possible. Select antibiotics following appropriate rational antibiotic therapy guidelines.

6 The majority of acute diarrhoea cases will resolve or improve within 24–48 hours. However, if the problem becomes chronic. . .

7 Consider the merits of faecal parasitology and *Giardia* testing depending on age of animal and previous treatments/response to fenbendazole treatment. Note that some dogs with *Giardia* infection will respond to fenbendazole but relapse afterwards.

8 Recommend a diet trial (commercial or homemade, novel protein source or hydrolysed).

- Use the animal's diet history to choose a 'novel' protein-source diet or choose a hydrolysed diet if many different foods have been given.
- The diet must be fed for 2–3 weeks initially by which time some response is expected and up to 12 weeks if successful before other foods are introduced.
- No other foods, chews, supplements or drinks other than water should be given. Diet trials are important as food-responsive chronic enteropathy is common, and the next diagnostic step is often invasive and costly (gut biopsy).
- If the diarrhoea is large bowel in origin in a dog, diets can be similar to those mentioned above or a fibre-enriched diet can be trialled – commercial high-fibre diets or psyllium/bran added to a balanced diet can be used. Bran should not be given if gluten sensitivity is suspected. However, gluten sensitivity in dogs is very uncommon and has only been identified in a handful of breeds e.g. Irish Setters, Wheaten terriers and Border terries.
- Care must be used if fibre is given to underweight animals as overall calorie intake tends to become reduced especially if appetite is low.
- Diet trial alone is rarely appropriate in significantly underweight, anorexic, hypoproteinaemic or systemically unwell animals.

9 Before any invasive, costly or extensive diagnostic plans, ensure that seconordary GI disease is not present, for example, exocrine

pancreatic insufficiency (EPI), hyperthyroidism in cats, hepatic disease hypoadrenocorticism in dogs, by performing routine haematology and biochemistry +/- total T4 (cats), basal cortisol/ACTH stimulation test (dogs), trypsin-like immunoreactivity (TLI). Secondary disease is more likely if diarrhoea is small bowel or mixed in origin.

- Even if the electrolytes are normal, if a dog is systemically unwell and does *not* have a stress leukogram, consider doing a basal cortisol/ACTH stimulation test to rule out hypoadrenocorticism before any invasive tests, for example, biopsy.
- Measurement of serum cobalamin is routinely done at this point to assess whether supplementation is needed. Low serum cobalamin is seen with distal SI disease but normal levels don't rule it out.

10 Test for *Tritrichomonas* with PCR if it is a cat with large bowel signs (may do this earlier in the process if it is a purebred cat or from a multi-cat household or shelter).

11 Perform an abdominal ultrasound to assess for structural bowel lesions that may occur with chronic diarrhoea (e.g. hyperechoic mucosal speckles/striations; intestinal wall thickening, intestinal masses, lymph node enlargement in neoplasia) and for other disorders that may cause diarrhoea, for example, abdominal neoplasia, intussusception. Ultrasound is indicated sooner if there is a palpable abnormality in the abdomen or if diarrhoea is severe and accompanied by weight loss or severe vomiting.

12 Assuming that secondary GI disease has been ruled out, if small bowel diarrhoea persists after points 1–10 for more than a month or so and, depending on the severity, species and breed (German shepherd/young large breed dog), the animal's clinical condition and owner concerns, consider treating for antibiotic-responsive diarrhoea with metronidazole (10 mg/kg PO BID) or tylosin (5–10 mg/kg PO SID).

- Four to six weeks of therapy is usually the recommended treatment. The most appropriate drug has not been determined by controlled clinical trials.

- Relapse following the treatment course is common.
- The role of pre/probiotics in cases of idiopathic ARD has yet to be determined.
- Relapses <u>may</u> be reduced or less severe in patients fed a high-fibre diet.

13 If all the above fails *or* if the patient is hypoproteinaemic *or* significantly underweight *or* if neoplasia is suspected on physical examination or imaging, biopsy is indicated.

- Endoscopic biopsy is preferred if appropriate expertise and facilities are available.
  - o Whilst there are some limitations with this technique, surgical biopsy may be overly invasive for many cats and dogs with chronic diarrhoea.
- Exploratory laparotomy may be required:
  - o If endoscopic equipment and expertise are not available
  - o Diagnostics have indicated that the disease is a focal lesion that may be unreachable with an endoscope, for example, a jejunal mass.
- If possible, consult a medicine specialist prior to biopsy if you are unsure.

14 If biopsy is not an option for cost reasons or lack of access to appropriate facilities/expertise, following careful client discussion of the risks of misdiagnosis and inappropriate treatment. . .

- Treat with prednisolone 2-3 mg/kg once daily and observe response.
- Large dogs should have no more than 40 mg/m^2 once daily.
- If good response is seen, taper the prednisolone dose by 20–25% every 4 weeks.
- Consider a second immunosuppressive drug (e.g. azathioprine, ciclosporin, chlorambucil, mycophenolate or leflunomide) if steroid side effects are moderate to severe to allow more rapid tapering of prednisolone. Chlorambucil or ciclosporin are the most commonly used second-line drugs in cats.

Summary

Acute and chronic diarrhoea are common clinical signs in small animal practice. Cats and dogs with mild chronic diarrhoea can usually undergo dietary or anthelmintic trials before costly investigation. Further investigation may be appropriate due to the severity of diarrhoea, concurrent clinical signs such as weight loss or a lack of response to therapeutic trials.

Clinical pathology is frequently normal in dogs and cats with diarrhoea, but it is an important step during investigation to rule out non-GI disorders.

Intestinal biopsy is usually the final step during investigation of diarrhoea and is not necessary in many cases. Inflammatory change on intestinal biopsy is non-specific and may be seen in FRE, ARD and IRE. Treatment trials are still required to differentiate between these causes.

Key points

As a result of reading this chapter you should be able to:
- Recognise the importance of differentiating small and large bowel diarrhoea
- Develop a rational approach to the investigation of small bowel diarrhoea
- Develop a rational approach to the investigation of large bowel diarrhoea
- Identify the causes of small bowel diarrhoea
- Identify the causes of large bowel diarrhoea
- Differentiate when symptomatic therapy vs. a diagnostic work-up is indicated
- Understand how to perform a dietary trial properly.

Questions for review

- Compare and contrast the characteristics of small and large bowel diarrhoea.
- List at least five causes of acute small bowel diarrhoea.
- List at least five causes of chronic small bowel diarrhoea.
- List at least five causes of large bowel diarrhoea.
- When is faecal bacterial culture indicated?
- How should a dietary trial should be performed?
- When is intestinal biopsy indicated in cases of chronic diarrhoea?

Case example

'Colin' is a 10-month-old male neutered British shorthair cat. He presents with a 3-month history of waxing and waning diarrhoea. He is otherwise lively and well, and his appetite is normal. Vomiting has not been observed. Diarrhoea is semi-formed to liquid, passed frequently in small volumes, sometimes with tenesmus. Mucus and blood are occasionally seen.

Colin is an indoor-only cat and is up to date with routine vaccinations and parasite control. He is fed a commercial balanced diet suitable for his age. He was rehomed from a multi-cat household, and his previous owner reported that some of the other cats had suffered with diarrhoea in the past.

Physical examination is unremarkable. Colin is in good body condition and palpation of his abdomen is normal.

Define the problem

Colin has semi-formed to liquid faeces passed in small volumes, frequently. This is compatible with diarrhoea, and this cannot be easily confused with anything else.

Define the location

When the problem is diarrhoea, we define the location first, as this helps us to confirm the affected body system. Colin has semi-formed to liquid faeces, increased frequency of defaecation, small faecal volume, tenesmus, mucus and blood. These are all seen with large bowel diarrhoea.

Define the system

Colin has large bowel diarrhoea with no signs of small bowel diarrhoea (e.g. weight loss, appetite changes). It is therefore very likely that Colin has a primary GI cause of his diarrhoea.

Define the lesion

Large bowel diarrhoea in young cats is most commonly caused by parasitic or protozoal infection. Feline infectious peritonitis and food-responsive enteropathy are other possible differentials in this age group. Neoplasia is less likely, although lymphoma can sometimes affect cats under a year of age.

Case outcome

Colin's diarrhoea did not improve during a properly performed diet trial of a 'novel' protein-source diet. His owners had a limited budget and were keen to perform a step-by-step investigation of his diarrhoea. Faecal testing was performed initially due to the increased chance of infectious diarrhoea at his age and also with the knowledge that he was originally from a multi-cat household where other cats have had diarrhoea in the past.

Faecal parasitology, Zn sulphate flotation for Giardia cysts and *Tritrichomonas* PCR were performed. Only the *Tritrichomonas* PCR was positive.

Treatment was discussed with Colin's owners. Some cats with *Tritrichomonas* infection do not require treatment if their diarrhoea is relatively mild as the disease usually resolves over time. However, resolution may take many months, and cats may continue to excrete the organism even once diarrhoea has resolved. Colin's owners were keen to treat him, and he was given ronidazole at a dose of 25 mg/kg once daily for 2 weeks. His diarrhoea resolved and did not recur.

Ronidazole should be used with caution and with informed owner consent as it may cause neurological and GI side effects. It is not licensed in most small animal markets and may not be readily available in formulations suitable for cats without the use of a licensed compounding pharmacy.

CHAPTER 5

Weight loss

Jill E. Maddison

Department of Clinical Science and Services, The Royal Veterinary College, London, UK

The why

- Weight loss or failure to gain weight is a relatively common problem in small animal practice.
- Weight loss may be clinically inconsequential or an indication of disease.
- Depending on other clinical signs, it may be a non-specific problem, which will be explained when the more specific problems are assessed.
- Or it may be the 'diagnostic hook' that forms the core of your clinical assessment and reasoning.
- It is therefore essential to have a logical, pathophysiologically based approach to the patient who has lost weight or failed to gain weight (or grow).
- The key questions relating to defining the problem, system, location and lesion are important but may occur in a variable order rather than strictly sequential.

 ## Define the problem

The first step when an animal is presented for weight loss is to *ensure that the caloric intake and palatability of the diet are adequate* for the animal's needs. Owners of large and giant breed dogs

Clinical Reasoning in Veterinary Practice: Problem Solved!, Second Edition.
Edited by Jill E. Maddison, Holger A. Volk and David B. Church.
© 2022 John Wiley & Sons Ltd. Published 2022 by John Wiley & Sons Ltd.

particularly may inadvertently underestimate the dog's caloric requirement, especially if the dog is growing or is very active. The normal caloric requirement of a normally active dog or cat can be calculated using the following formula:

$$\left[\left(30 \times \text{weight in kg}\right) + 70\right] \times 1.2 \text{ kcal}$$

This can probably be doubled for a growing dog, a very active animal or one that is pregnant or lactating. An easier formula to remember during a short consultation (though it is a much more rough guide not favoured by nutritionists) is 40–70 kcals/kg – bottom of the range for large dogs and at the top of the range for small dogs or cats.

As a rough guideline, 1 cup of standard dry food is approximately 400 kcals and 400 g of wet food approximately 360 kcals (best though to check product information provided).

Only if the diet and caloric intake are adequate for the animal's life stage and style can weight loss be regarded as a clinical problem.

It can sometimes be difficult to distinguish general weight loss from severe muscle wasting that is resulting in loss of body weight and the appearance of emaciation. Therefore, while all of the following diagnostic approaches are appropriate for loss of body weight with a normal or increased appetite, keep in mind that very occasionally one may be dealing with muscle atrophy for which the system involved (neuromuscular – see Chapters 7 and 8) and type of disorders (infectious, immune mediated etc.) are very different. It is probably worthwhile, therefore, to at least check serum markers of muscle damage – CK and AST enzymes in all patients who appear to have lost weight despite a normal or increased appetite.

Refine the problem

A crucial step in assessing the patient who has lost weight is to consider the weight loss in the context of the animal's appetite. Weight loss conditions are divided into the following:
- Those associated with a decreased appetite
- Those where the appetite is normal or increased.

WEIGHT LOSS DUE TO DECREASED APPETITE

 Refine the problem

Can't eat or won't eat?
If the owner reports that an animal is not eating, the first key question is, *Is it because the animal can't eat or won't eat?* It is important to ensure that the animal does not have any condition causing difficulties in prehension or mastication or a swallowing defect – dysphagia ('can't eat').

True loss of appetite ('won't eat') may occur in many disease conditions. Loss of appetite is a frequent presenting complaint, as owners will usually be aware of the amount of food eaten by their pet, as feeding is an important part of the pet-owner interaction and bond, and it is often the first indication to an owner that there is something wrong.

Appetite is controlled by feeding-satiety centres of the hypothalamus, and many factors will directly or indirectly influence this centre. For example:
- Blood glucose levels
- Body temperature
- Metabolic products
- Electrolyte balance
- Blood calcium levels
- Neural input from the gastrointestinal (GI) tract
- Substances released by neoplasia
- Neurobehavioural factors (e.g. stress and fear)
- Loss of the sense of smell
  - May cause anorexia particularly in cats, hence nasal disorders may need to be investigated.

Can't eat
Prehension and mastication
Animals with prehension or mastication difficulties can appear hungry and interested in food. They are either unable to pick food up properly, show evidence of pain when trying to eat or drop food from their mouth when chewing.

Dysphagia
Difficulty in swallowing (dysphagia) is indicated by excessive, forceful attempts to swallow or by regurgitation of food from the mouth or nostrils.

Define the lesion

Prehension and mastication difficulties are most often associated with disorders of the mouth and pharynx.

Local disorders of the mouth include the following:
- Inflammation
- Ulceration
- Foreign bodies
- Dental disease
- Neoplasms.

Less commonly, impaired prehension or mastication may be due to inflammation of the muscles of mastication (myositis) or neuro-muscular lesions resulting in paralysis of the muscles of the jaw or tongue. The muscles of mastication are innervated by cranial nerve V (trigeminal) and the tongue by cranial nerve XII (hypoglossal).

Dysphagia can be due to the following:
- Local disorders of the tongue or pharynx such as inflammation, foreign bodies, trauma or neoplasia
- Palatine abnormalities
- Rarely, neurological disorders involving cranial nerve IX (glos-sopharyngeal), cranial nerve X (vagus) or cranial nerve XII (hypoglossal)
- Cricopharyngeal achalasia, which is a rare congenital disorder of young animals in which the cricopharyngeal sphincter fails to relax when the animal swallows. Its aetiology is unknown, but it is surgi-cally correctable by a cricopharyngeal myotomy.

Assessment of inflammation
Local pathology
Inflammation of the lips, gums, tongue, gingival or oropharyngeal structures may cause problems with prehension, mastication or swallowing. Inflammation can be due to local disease or systemic disease.

Systemic pathology
Systemic disorders include the following:
- Uraemia due to renal failure
- Viral infections in cats (tongue)

- Immune-mediated disorders (e.g. pemphigus)
- Neutropenia
  - Drug dyscrasias, for example, phenylbutazone and phenobarbitone
  - Bone marrow failure, for example, feline leukaemia virus (FeLV) associated
  - Immune-mediated neutropenia.

  Local disorders include the following:
- Irritants (plant and chemical)
- Foreign bodies (may be wedged across the hard palate)
- Dental disease
- Eosinophilic complex (most commonly seen in cats, occasionally in dogs)
- Lymphocytic/plasmacytic stomatitis
- Neoplasms
  - Benign
    - Papillomas
    - Epulis
  - Malignant – unfortunately, the majority of oral tumours are malignant. The most common ones are:
    - Malignant melanoma
    - Squamous cell carcinoma
    - Fibrosarcoma.

 ## Define the problem

Won't eat

For an animal that has not eaten for 24–48 hours and is in good bodily condition with no evidence of malaise, it may be most appropriate to adopt a 'wait and see' approach – to advise the owner that if the cause of the loss of appetite is serious, the animal is most likely to develop other clinical signs such as vomiting or diarrhoea that may help localise the problem.

It is important in these cases to determine whether the diet has been changed recently or whether there are environmental conditions that may be responsible, for example, very hot weather, absent owner, new pet or baby in the house and change of ownership or house.

Define the lesion

When an animal is presented because of anorexia or inappetance with no other clinical abnormalities, in many cases, a thorough physical examination will reveal more specific abnormalities that can be investigated, for example, pyrexia, masses, severe constipation, severe heart disease, anaemia and icterus.

In some cases, an underlying cause cannot be found on physical examination alone. In these cases, the diagnostic approach is partly dependent on the duration the animal has been anorectic and the degree of weight loss that has been sustained.

If the anorexia is prolonged and/or the animal has lost significant weight and/or is exhibiting signs of non-specific malaise, then further diagnostic procedures are indicated. As a plethora of disease processes can cause anorexia, for example, liver disease, renal failure, neoplasia, infection, electrolyte imbalance, endocrine abnormalities, anaemia and toxins, it can appear a daunting task to determine the cause.

Causes of anorexia/hyporexia that are particularly relevant in hospitalised patients include pain and nausea. The latter should be considered in the patient who may have been vomiting and has been treated with an anti-emetic agent that has controlled the vomiting well, but the animal still remains food averse. Not all anti-emetic drugs are effective anti-nausea drugs, so it is important that the clinician is cognisant of this when managing vomiting patients.

Diagnostic procedures should be directed at trying to determine the system involved and should, if possible, start with non-invasive or more cost-efficient tests and then proceed to more invasive or more expensive infectious procedures if indicated.

Appropriate tests to evaluate inflammation/infection, serum protein, liver and renal function, electrolytes and calcium levels should be performed. In cats, viral infections such as FeLV and, more commonly, feline peritonitis (FIP) should be considered. In an older animal, a more rigorous search for neoplasia (e.g. abdominal and thoracic imaging) may be indicated.

Disorders to consider if there are no or only vague, non-specific concurrent clinical signs and minimal or no changes in routine haematology and biochemistry include primary GI disease, atypical hypoadrenocorticism (dogs), pancreatitis (cats), pyelonephritis, lead toxicity (cats), neoplasia, hepatic disease and primary central nervous system disease.

WEIGHT LOSS WITH NORMAL OR INCREASED APPETITE

Define the system

The 'system definition' question for the problem defined as weight loss despite a normal or increased appetite is, *Is the weight loss due to maldigestion, malabsorption and/or malutilisation?* While strictly speaking these are not 'body systems', this classification provides a clear clinical reasoning framework that is based on sound pathophysiological principles. But first some physiology.

Normal physiology
There are three phases of assimilation of nutrients – any phase may be perturbed, resulting in malassimilation.
Luminal:
- Enzyme *secretion* (primarily pancreatic) into the gut lumen
- *Digestive activity* within the gut lumen
Mucosal:
- Digestive activity of the mucosal cell surface
- Absorption of nutrients into the mucosal cell
- Any processing of nutrients within the mucosal cell
Delivery:
- Transfer of nutrients from the mucosal cell into the blood.

Pathophysiology
Maldigestion occurs when there is a deficiency or dysfunction of pancreatic enzymes or mucosal enzymes.

Malabsorption may occur if the mucosal and/or transport phase of assimilation is impaired.

An example of an abnormal *luminal* condition is dysmotility in hyperthyroidism resulting in rapid intestinal transit.

Abnormal *mucosal* function may involve the following:
- Deficiency of brush border protein transport. This may be congenital as in inherited selective cobalamin deficiency or acquired secondary to diffuse intestinal disease.
- Enterocyte defects that may occur, for example, in inflammatory bowel disease or villus atrophy.

The *transport* phase may be abnormal due to the following:
- Lymphatic obstruction
  o Primary due to lymphangiectasia
  o Secondary due to obstruction caused by neoplasia, infection or inflammation
- Vascular compromise
  o Vasculitis, for example, due to infection or immune-mediated disease
  o Portal hypertension caused by a hepatopathy or right-sided heart failure.

Once the nutrients reach the systemic circulation, they will be delivered to where they are needed. If the nutrients are consumed excessively or are lost, then this is defined as *malutilisation*.
- *Malassimilation* of nutrients
  o Maldigestion
    ▪ Animals with maldigestion will usually present with grossly abnormal faeces and significant weight loss, despite a normal or often greatly increased appetite.
  o Malabsorption
    ▪ Diarrhoea is usually present in animals with malabsorption but it may be subtle, and occasionally faeces may seem relatively normal.
- *Malutilisation* – nutrients are digested and absorbed normally but are utilised abnormally by the body.
  o Diarrhoea is usually not a predominant feature, although it may occur with other clinical signs in some disorders such as hyperthyroidism and liver disease.

Maldigestion

 Define the lesion

The most common cause of maldigestion as the primary reason for weight loss is exocrine pancreatic insufficiency (EPI) – other disorders occur infrequently or are just one component of a disease's pathophysiology.

Animals with EPI invariably have diarrhoea, and it is an important differential in the patient with chronic small bowel diarrhoea. Occasionally, animals with EPI may also develop large bowel diarrhoea. This may be due to the irritant effects of malassimilated fats on colonic mucosa and/or bacterial overgrowth.

Examples of other disorders where maldigestion occurs include the following:
- Secondary enzyme deficiency resulting when luminal conditions are not optimal for enzyme function
  - For example, inactivation of pancreatic enzymes due to gastric acid hypersecretion
- Loss of or impaired bile salt activity due to ileal or liver disease
- Brush border enzyme deficiency
  - Congenital
    - Trehalase (cats)
    - Aminopeptidase N (beagles)
  - Acquired enzyme loss
    - Relative lactose deficiency.

Malabsorption

 Define and refine the system

Malabsorption may be due to primary or secondary GI disease.

 Define the lesion

Primary GI diseases causing malabsorption
Primary GI causes of malabsorption are driven by infiltrative disease of the small bowel causing extensive damage to the intestinal wall.

Determination of the aetiology of primary GI causes of malabsorption usually requires a gut biopsy. Structural gut disease may also impact on digestion, as there are digestive enzymes in the mucosa.

Primary GI causes of malabsorption include the following:
- Parasitic disease
- Inflammatory bowel disease
- Infiltrative neoplasia, for example, lymphosarcoma and mast cell tumour
- Diet-responsive chronic enteropathy
- Granulomatous feline infectious peritonitis
- Lymphangiectasia
- Deep mycoses (in appropriate geographical areas)
- Occasionally, severe small intestinal bacterial overgrowth (SIBO) or antibiotic-responsive enteropathy will cause clinically significant malabsorption.

Secondary GI diseases causing malabsorption

The most notable secondary GI disorders that will cause malabsorption are hyperthyroidism and hepatic disease.
- Hyperthyroidism causes increased faecal bulk secondary to increased food intake and a rapid gut transit time, which decreases the time available to absorb nutrients.
- Hepatic disease can result in maldigestion and malabsorption as a result of decreased bile salt excretion and malabsorption due to portal hypertension. In the vast majority of cases of liver disease, other clinical signs will predominate, but weight loss may appear excessive in relation to the change in appetite.

Malutilisation

 Define the lesion

Examples of disorders that cause malutilisation include the following:
- Diabetes mellitus
- Congestive heart failure (also a component of malabsorption involved)

- Dirofilariasis (in endemic areas)
- Neoplasia
- Hyperthyroidism
- Liver disease
  - Animals with liver disease will usually have a reduced appetite, but it can be relatively normal and occasionally increased if the patient is not nauseous. It has been demonstrated that people with acute liver disease can become highly catabolic with marked increases in energy expenditure and therefore experience significant weight loss if increased calories are not consumed. Significant alterations in metabolism leading to early recruitment of alternate fuel sources and accelerated catabolism are reported in people, as well as a shift to muscle protein and adipose tissue utilisation.
  - While the metabolism of animals with liver disease has not been studied as thoroughly, significant weight loss greater than that expected for the nutrient intake is often clinically observed in these patients. Patients with hepatic neoplasia or lymphocytic cholangitis (cats) seem most likely to have weight loss despite an excellent or increased appetite. Concurrent malabsorption may be a contributing factor.
- Renal disease
  - Animals with glomerular renal disease may lose weight due to protein loss in the urine, although this needs to be marked and is usually accompanied by systemic signs of hypoproteinaemia. Most animals with tubular renal disease lose weight because of a *reduced* appetite, but the diagnosis should be considered in a patient with weight loss despite an apparently normal appetite, as the appetite may decline so gradually and subtly that the owner does not really notice and considers that the pet is eating relatively normally. Or the pet is in a multi-pet household where it is difficult to keep track of who is eating what. Combined with the catabolic effect of renal protein loss and skeletal muscle wasting, these patients can present with significant weight loss (but will *not* have an *increased* appetite).

Concurrent clinical signs and the history will usually assist you to narrowing the focus for diagnostic procedures. Note that some disorders cause true polyphagia (diabetes mellitus, hyperthyroidism). Occasionally liver disease and neoplasia can be associated with an increase in appetite (the exception rather than the rule). Other disorders do not increase appetite; rather, they are associated with weight loss despite a normal appetite (e.g. heart failure, heartworm disease, neoplasia [usually], liver disease [usually] and renal disease). They all may also cause a reduced appetite, in which case the degree of weight loss can be more marked than expected for the degree of inappetence.

Summary

Weight loss is a relatively common clinical sign that may be the prime focus of the case assessment, or it may be a consequence of other more specific problems. It is essential to assess whether the weight loss occurred *because* of a reduced appetite or *despite* a normal or increased appetite.

If the weight loss has occurred because of a reduced appetite the key question is "Can't eat or won't eat?"

Remember that if diarrhoea is an important clinical feature, incorporate the diagnostic approaches discussed in Chapter 4 as appropriate.

A history of persistent diarrhoea will usually indicate that maldigestion or malabsorption is most likely. However, in cats particularly, consider hyperthyroidism. The only practically relevant cause of maldigestion in isolation (not associated with other clinical signs) is EPI, which can be diagnosed by determining plasma trypsin-like immunoreactivity (TLI) levels. Remember that hyperthyroidism and hepatic disease can cause a degree of malabsorption and hence increased faecal fat content.

Serum biochemistry and haematology may give peripheral information about the type of primary GI pathology causing malabsorption but cannot provide a specific tissue diagnosis. Blood tests, however, may be useful to rule out causes of malutilisation – always consider hyperthyroidism in cats and request a T4 when appropriate. And of course, serum biochemistry and haematology may reveal the reason for weight loss in a patient with a decreased appetite.

In the patient with weight loss despite a normal or increased appetite (or in the patient where the degree of appetite loss is not sufficient to explain the degree of weight loss), if maldigestion, malutilisation and secondary GI causes of malabsorption have been ruled out, malabsorption due to primary GI disease must be occurring. Therefore a gut biopsy (via endoscopy or laparotomy) is usually now needed to establish the diagnosis.

Key points

As a result of reading this chapter you should be able to:
- Develop a pathophysiologically sound diagnostic approach to the problem of weight loss in cats and dogs
- Recognise the importance of relating appetite to weight loss
- Recognise that weight loss despite a normal or increased appetite is an important diagnostic hook
- Appreciate the importance of differentiating between maldigestion, malabsorption and malutilisation.

Questions for review

- What are the key questions you need to ask to define and refine the problem in a patient that presents with the problem of weight loss?
- If a patient has lost weight because it is not eating, what is the next key question you need to ask?
- Malabsorption can be due to primary or secondary GI disease. List as many causes of primary GI disorders causing weight loss that you can remember. What are the secondary GI disorders that can cause malabsorption?

Case example

'Mabel' is an 11-year-old female neutered cocker spaniel who presented for her annual vaccination. The owner had no concerns with Mabel at home.

Mabel's weight was usually stable at around 15 kg, but when weighed on arrival at the clinic she was 13.2 kg. The owner had not noted any changes in appetite or the amount of food or water ingested at home, and there had been no change in exercise frequency or diet. Her faeces were reported to be normal and vomiting had not been observed. The owner was surprised that she had lost weight.

On physical examination, a firm circular lump under her left forelimb which was not attached to any underlying structures was identified. It was approximately 6 cm in diameter. There was evidence of hepatomegaly on abdominal palpation. No other physical abnormalities were detected.

Define the problem

Mabel's problem list is:
1. Weight loss
2. Forelimb mass
3. Hepatomegaly.
   Refine the problem and further assessment:
   The weight loss has occurred despite a normal appetite.

Define the system:

Mabel has no diarrhoea, thus malutilisation as the reason for the weight loss is most likely. The forelimb mass and hepatomegaly may or may not be related.

Define the lesion

Weight loss due to malutilisation
   Causes of malutilisation are:
• Diabetes mellitus
• Congestive heart failure

- Dirofilariasis
- Neoplasia
- Hyperthyroidism
- Liver disease
- Renal disease.
  Forelimb mass
- May be neoplastic, fibrosis, inflammation.
  Hepatomegaly
  Could be due to congestion (right-sided heart failure), infiltration (inflammatory, neoplastic), endocrine (e.g. hyperadrenocorticism, diabetes mellitus), increased activity (e.g. immune-mediated disease).
  Further assessment
  Mabel had no clinical signs indicating congestive heart failure, and she did not live in an endemic area for *Dirofilaria*. She did not have a palpable thyroid mass, which in dogs makes hyperthyroidism extremely unlikely (almost always associated with a substantial thyroid mass).
  It was decided to delay the booster vaccination and start investigations. Haematology and biochemistry were performed to assess the other possible causes of malutilisation. A fine-needle sample was taken from the mass.

Case outcome

Blood results revealed a moderate (packed cell volume [PCV] 27%) non-regenerative anaemia, normal ALT level and significantly increased ALP level (1500 U/L).

Fine-needle aspirate (FNA) results showed a population of epithelial cells with poor morphology, possibly neoplastic. The pathologist's comment was that this was possibly mammary tissue and there were signs of malignancy.

An ultrasound scan was recommended prior to considering biopsy/lump removal.

The ultrasound scan revealed multiple masses throughout right and left lung fields, multiple well-demarcated liver masses and a left adrenal gland mass.

No further investigations were taken at this stage. The likely diagnosis was mammary carcinoma under the left foreleg and secondary metastatic disease in lungs/liver. Thus causing weight loss due to malutilisation caused by neoplasia.

CHAPTER 6

Abdominal enlargement

Jill E. Maddison

Department of Clinical Science and Services, The Royal Veterinary College, London, UK

The why

- An enlarged abdomen may be an obvious clinical sign and the reason the animal is presented to the veterinarian.
- Or it may be a finding during the clinical examination.
- As with many clinical signs, the causes of abdominal enlargement range from clinically innocuous to life threatening.
- A robust structured approach to its assessment is crucial – this will involve elements of the logical clinical problem-solving approach, but the process is adapted to ensure it is relevant to the range of causes of abdominal enlargement. The approach primarily focuses on defining and refining the problem and lesion.

 ## Define the problem

Abdominal enlargement may be due to the intra-abdominal presence of fluid but can also be due to gas or solid material or to weakness of the abdominal musculature causing apparent enlargement. It is essential to clarify this as the first step.

Remembering the five Fs is a good starting point:
- Fluid
- Fat
- Flatus – for example, gastric torsion
- Faeces
- Foetus.

Clinical Reasoning in Veterinary Practice: Problem Solved!, Second Edition.
Edited by Jill E. Maddison, Holger A. Volk and David B. Church.
© 2022 John Wiley & Sons Ltd. Published 2022 by John Wiley & Sons Ltd.

In addition, significant enlargement of intra-abdominal organs (spleen and liver) or the presence of tumour masses may also cause abdominal enlargement.

A 'pot-bellied' appearance is common in dogs with hyperadrenocorticism due to a combination of factors – abdominal muscle weakness, redistribution of fat and hepatomegaly.

The presence of an abdominal effusion *per se* rarely disrupts organ function. This is in contrast to pleural effusion, which will usually cause significant and sometimes life-threatening disruption of respiratory function as the normal expansion of the lungs is restricted.

Diagnostic procedures to identify the cause of the abdominal enlargement might include abdominal imaging and abdominocentesis. Once the problem is defined, that is, the substance causing abdominal enlargement has been identified, then the diagnostic approach to progress to a diagnosis is usually reasonably clear.

We will now concentrate on the problem of abdominal enlargement caused by fluid accumulation, as it is here that certain steps are important to further refine the problem and go on to define the system involved and lesion. Patients with abdominal effusion will often have noticeable (to the owner and/or veterinarian) abdominal enlargement and a detectable 'fluid wave'. Frequently, however, such enlargement is automatically assessed to be due to 'ascites' and therapy initiated without further identification of the cause.

If the cause of the abdominal enlargement is confirmed as being due to the presence of intra-abdominal fluid, then characterisation of the fluid is crucial in guiding further diagnostic steps.

Diagnostic tools needed to classify fluids are relatively simple. They include gross examination, measurement of protein content and examination of a stained smear (can be done in-house or at a laboratory depending on the tools and expertise available). Some texts will provide information on the specific gravity (SG) of effusions. However, refractometers used to measure SG have only been validated for urine so shouldn't be used for other body fluids.

The first step in establishing a diagnosis is to classify the type of fluid present – it is not always an exact science, but more often than not it will assist in narrowing down the list of diagnostic possibilities.

Fluid characterisation
Abdominal fluid may be broadly classified as follows:
- Haemorrhagic
- Urine
- Transudate
- Modified transudate
- Exudate
- Eosinophilic
- Chyle
- Cystic fluid (if a cystic structure is sampled)
- Bile.

 Define the location

The distribution of the fluid may be useful in narrowing down the possible causes:
- The presence of both abdominal and pleural effusion suggests generalised disease, for example, heart failure, hypoproteinaemia, coagulopathy and feline infectious peritonitis (FIP).
- Fluid confined to one cavity could be due to any of the reasons mentioned above as well as more localised pathology.
- If subcutaneous oedema is also present, hypoproteinaemia is most probable.

 Refine the problem: Ascites – transudate/modified transudate

Ascites
Ascites is defined as the abnormal accumulation of transudate or modified transudate in the peritoneal cavity.

Pure transudate
- Low cellularity (<0.5–1.0 × 10^9 cells/L)
- Primary cell type is mononuclear cells with some mesothelial cells
- Protein <25–30 g/L.

Modified transudate
- Higher cellularity (up to 5.0×10^9 cells/L)
- Increased numbers of neutrophils
- Protein up to 35 g/L
- The fluid may appear serosanguinous (i.e. contains some red blood cells).

A modified transudate is, as the name suggests, a transudate the characteristics of which have been modified by time within the abdominal cavity, and thus the causes are the same as a transudate.

 ## Define the lesion: Ascites – transudate/modified transudate

Portal hypertension (due to various causes) is the most common cause of ascites.

Portal hypertension
Portal hypertension can be classified based on the location of portal blood flow restriction into the following:
- Pre-hepatic hypertension
- Intra-hepatic pre-sinusoidal portal hypertension
- Post-hepatic obstruction.

Pre-hepatic hypertension
Pre-hepatic hypertension is an uncommon cause of ascites, because if the portal vein is obstructed, lymph flow from the bowel dramatically increases and compensates for obstructed portal vein drainage. In addition, collateral communications open up between the portal system and the caudal vena cava.
   Causes include:
- Blockage to portal vein flow by stenosis
- Portal vein thrombosis
- Extrinsic compression of the portal vein by abscesses, neoplasms or enlarged lymph nodes in the porta hepatis.

Liver size is usually normal, and the ascites has a low protein content (<25 g/L).

Intra-hepatic portal hypertension

Intra-hepatic portal hypertension can occur in the following conditions:

- End-stage chronic hepatitis
  - Results in fibrosis and cirrhosis
- Intra-hepatic neoplasia
- Hepatic arteriovenous fistulas
  - Uninhibited inflow of arterial blood into the portal system increases blood flow through the liver and elevates the hydro-static portal vein pressure.

The liver size can be normal, increased or decreased, and the protein content of the ascites is variable.

Post-hepatic obstruction

This is the most common type of portal hypertension.

Causes include the following:

- Right heart failure
- Pericardial disease
- Right atrial neoplasms
- Thrombosis or extrinsic compression of the caudal vena cava or hepatic veins, for example, by neoplasms.

Because the pressure in the caudal vena cava is elevated at the same time as portal vein pressure, there is no gradient between the two systems, and no collaterals form to decompress the elevated portal pressure.

The ascitic fluid in these cases has a relatively high protein content (>25 g/L), because it is derived from protein-rich hepatic lymph. The total protein concentration of the ascitic fluid usually approximates the serum albumin concentration.

Usually, the liver size is increased, and ascites and pleural effusion are often present concurrently, contrary to the isolated ascites that occurs with intra-hepatic or pre-hepatic portal hypertension.

Hypoproteinaemia

Hypoproteinaemia alone is rarely the sole cause of ascites. Sinusoidal epithelial cells in the liver form an extremely porous membrane, which is almost completely permeable to macromolecules, including plasma proteins. In contrast, splanchnic capillaries have a pore size 50–100 times less than that of the hepatic sinuosoids. As a consequence, the trans-sinusoidal oncotic pressure gradient in the liver is virtually zero, while it is 0.8–0.9 (80–90% of maximum) in the splanchnic circulation.

Oncotic pressure gradients at such extreme ends of the spectrum minimise any effect the changes in plasma albumin concentration may have on trans-microvascular fluid exchange. Therefore, the old concept that ascites is formed secondary to decreased oncotic pressure is false, and plasma albumin concentrations have little influence on the rate of ascites formation. In patients with liver disease, portal hypertension rather than hypoalbuminaemia is critical to the development of ascites, and ascites rarely develops in patients with a wedged hepatic venous portal gradient of less than 12 mmHg.

When hypoproteinaemia occurs as a result of chronic liver disease or glomerular disease, avid sodium retention occurs via an undefined mechanism. Avid sodium retention results in fluid retention and hence ascites. The mechanism may involve:

- Activation of the renin-angiotensin-aldosterone system
- Deficiency of atrial natiuretic factor
- Changes in intrarenal blood flow under the regulation of intrarenal prostaglandins
- In addition, in the case of hepatic cirrhosis, hepatic venous outflow obstruction causes a rise in portal venous pressure and hepatic sinusoidal perfusion pressure.

Ascites as a result of hypoproteinaemia alone usually does not occur until the albumin concentration is less than 15 g/L and usually less than 10 g/L. Thus, if ascites is present in a hypoproteinaemic animal but the albumin concentration is greater than 15 g/L, hepatic or glomerular disease is more probable than protein-losing enteropathy, as avid sodium retention (and thus fluid) occurs in both glomerular and hepatic disease but not in protein-losing enteropathy.

Lymphatic obstruction
Obstruction of lymphatic flow, for example, by intra-abdominal neoplasia, abdominal organ torsion or a diaphragmatic hernia, can cause ascites.

Refine the problem: Exudates

Characteristics
- Exudates usually have high cellularity (>5.0 × 10⁹ cells/L).
  - However, some exudates may have only moderate cellularity (e.g. FIP exudates and neoplastic exudates).
- The cell type present is neutrophils and mononuclear cells.
  - In *non-septic exudates,* the neutrophils are non-degenerative, and there is no evidence of organisms. The fluid may appear serosanguinous (i.e. contains some red blood cells).
  - In *septic exudates*, the nucleated cell count is extremely high, degenerate neutrophils are the predominant cells and bacteria can often be observed within neutrophils and macrophages.
  - Neoplastic cells may be seen in neoplastic effusion, which can be non-septic or septic.
- The protein level is >30 g/L.

  Cystic fluid (e.g. hydronephrosis) may also have the characteristics of a non-septic exudate, that is, high protein and moderate to high cellularity (the cells may be degenerating and look aged).

 Define the lesion: Exudates

Causes of non-septic exudates
- Bile peritonitis
  - Initially non-septic but soon becomes septic if rupture is associated with biliary tract necrosis or bacterial cholecystitis.
  - In traumatic biliary rupture, bile is initially sterile but causes changes in mucosal permeability leading to secondary bacterial infection.
  - The patient will usually be jaundiced, although this may not occur immediately.
- FIP
  - The fluid often contains fibrin strands, and cellularity may or may not be particularly high.
  - The fluid is often but not always high in protein and appears grossly yellow and 'sticky'.
- Neoplasia

- Non-septic peritonitis
    - For example, secondary to pancreatitis
- Chronic inflammatory hepatopathies such as lymphocytic cholangitis in cats; this is less common in dogs
- Diaphragmatic hernia
- Steatitis
- Urine peritonitis (assuming the urine is sterile).

Causes of septic exudates
- Peritonitis
    - Penetrating abdominal wound
    - Bowel perforation
    - Bile peritonitis
    - Ruptured intra-abdominal abscess, for example, pancreatic, renal, hepatic
    - Ruptured intestinal neoplasia.

 ## Refine the problem: Eosinophilic effusions

Eosinophilic effusions have the characteristics of either a transudate or exudate, but in addition, greater than 10% of the cells are eosinophils.

Define the lesion: Eosinophilic effusions

Causes
- Aberrant larval migrans
- Mast cell tumour
- Lymphoma
- Fungal disease
- Disseminated eosinophilic granulomatosis.

 ## Refine the problem: Blood

To confirm that blood obtained by abdomino- or thoracocentesis has not come from a 'normal' vessel or the heart, check to see if the sample clots after withdrawal. If it does not (and the animal does not have a bleeding disorder), then the blood has been free in the abdomen or thorax for sufficient time to defibrinate (usually >1 h). If the blood clots, then you have probably inadvertently tapped a vascular organ or blood vessel.

Haemorrhagic effusions initially have a similar cellular distribution to peripheral blood, although neutrophils and macrophages will increase in number with time. Erythrophagocytosis is often present, which can also assist in distinguishing true haemorrhagic effusion from traumatic collection.

Animals with intra-abdominal haemorrhage as a result of a ruptured neoplastic spleen will often be polydipsic (and polyuric with a urine SG of any value).

 ## Define the lesion: Blood

Haemoabdomen can be due to intra-abdominal disease (e.g. bleeding neoplasm such as splenic haemangiosarcoma, fracture of the liver or spleen, avulsion of renal arteries or iatrogenic postoperatively) or systemic disorders such as a coagulopathy (discussed in Chapter 12). Bleeding may also occur retroperitoneally, for example, due to renal tumours, which will not result in free fluid in the abdomen.

 ## Refine the problem: Urine

The presence of urine throughout the abdomen can be due to the bladder being large and flaccid or a ruptured bladder or avulsed ureter.

If uncertain about whether fluid obtained from an abdominal tap is urine or an effusion (very dilute urine can grossly look the same as a transudate), measure the urea or creatinine concentration.

- If it is urine, the urea or creatinine concentration should be substantially higher than the plasma concentration.
- If it is an effusion, the urea or creatinine concentration will be about the same as plasma.
- However, this is usually useful only during the first 24 hours after bladder rupture. After this time, equilibrium develops between the peritoneal fluid and serum, thus reducing the diagnostic value of measuring urea or creatinine.

Refine the problem: Chyle

Chyle is triglyceride-rich fluid that leaks into the thoracic or peritoneal cavity from the thoracic duct or intestinal lymphatics.

Characteristics
- It remains opaque when centrifuged.
- The protein concentration is 20–60 g/L.
- Cellularity – cell numbers range from 0.4–10.0 × 10^9 cells/L.
- Cell type
  - Early in the disease, predominantly small lymphocytes with few neutrophils.
  - Later, non-degenerate neutrophils become more predominant, there are fewer lymphocytes, macrophages increase in number and plasma cells may be present.
- The fluid clears when ether is added (which dissolves the chylomicrons).
- The triglyceride concentration is greater than that in serum, and the cholesterol concentration is less than that in serum.
- Cholesterol: triglyceride ratio < 1.
- Sudanophilic fat globules are present.

Pseudochylous effusion looks similar to chyle but does not have the last four characteristics listed above. The relevance of differentiating pseudochylous from chylous effusion is questionable – as they are both caused by a similar range of pathologies, differentiation does not assist in narrowing down the list of possible causes.

 Define the lesion: Chyle

Causes of chyle and pseudochyle include:
- Lymphangiectasia
- Obstruction or rupture of lymphatics due to neoplasia
- Right-sided heart failure.

In conclusion

The key to assessing the patient with abdominal enlargement is to first confirm what is causing the enlargement. If fluid is detected, then it is relatively easy to classify the type of fluid present, which then permits generation of a rational differential list.

But remember, there are overlapping differentials, and as often in clinical medicine, the picture isn't always clear cut. All information gathered from the history, clinical examination, fluid analysis, laboratory tests and diagnostic imaging is valuable in helping reach a diagnosis, noting that there are disorders such as idiopathic chylothorax where the aetiology remains frustratingly elusive.

Key points

As a result of reading this chapter you should be able to:
- Recognise the importance of first defining why the abdomen is enlarged
- If abdominal enlargement is due to a fluid effusion, know the different types of fluid that may be present
- Understand the differences between transudates, modified transudates, non-septic exudates and septic exudates
- Appreciate the different causes for the different types of effusion.

Questions for review

- Compare and contrast the characteristics of a transudate, modified transudate and exudate.
- Why is hypoproteinaemia alone rarely the sole cause of ascites?
- What other mechanisms contribute to the development of ascites in patients with hepatic or glomerular disease?
- When do high-protein transudates (protein > 25 g/L) most commonly occur?

Case example

'Blossom' is a 13-year-old female neutered domestic shorthair cat. Owner had noticed the cat's stomach getting gradually bigger over the last week or so, and today she is unable to jump or move around easily. Her appetite has remained normal, and there has been no increase in drinking or urination and no vomiting, diarrhoea, coughing or difficulty breathing at home.

On physical examination the abnormalities noted were that Blossom was underweight with a body condition score of 2/9. Her BCS had been recorded as 5/9 12 months previously. Marked abdominal distension was present, with an obvious fluid wave. She was bright and responsive and all vital signs were normal.

Define the problem

Blossom's problems are abdominal enlargement and abdominal fluid – further definition will require fluid analysis.

The fluid characteristics were: clear, straw coloured, protein 35 g/L, low cellularity. The bilirubin concentration was 3 μmol/L (serum bilirubin = 6 μmol/L).

Cytology report: The smears contain a background of thick basophilic fluid and a small amount of blood along with a low number of moderately preserved cells. The cells seen are a mixed population of neutrophils, macrophages and small lymphocytes. Occasional reactive mesothelial cells are also seen. The macrophages often have an increased amount of cytoplasm. All cells are morphologically normal and no infectious organisms are seen.

This was assessed as a high-protein modified transudate or, less likely, a low-cellularity non-septic exudate.

Weight loss is refined as weight loss despite a normal appetite. It is not clear yet whether both problems are related, but it is likely that they are.

Define the system

Weight loss: In the absence of noted faecal changes weight loss is most likely due to malutilisation.

Define the lesion

Modified transudate: The protein at the high end of the reference range indicates intra- or post-hepatic portal hypertension. Causes of intra-hepatic portal hypertension include hepatic fibrosis, chronic hepatitis, hepatic neoplasia, chronic cholangitis. Causes of post-hepatic portal hypertension in a cat include right-sided heart failure, pericardial disease, thrombosis or extrinsic compression of the caudal vena cava or hepatic veins, for example, by neoplasms.

Non-septic exudate (less likely due to the low cellularity): Causes relevant for this cat include FIP, inflammatory hepatopathy and abdominal neoplasia.

Causes of malutilisation include diabetes mellitus, hyperthyroidism, neoplasia.

Diagnostics

Haematology and biochemistry results were all within reference ranges.

Thoracic radiology revealed no abnormal findings. This does not completely rule out heart disease as a cause of the abdominal effusion, but in the absence of other signs of cardiac failure such as tachycardia and pleural effusion, it becomes a less likely differential.

Next steps were to assess the abdomen via abdominal ultrasound, and if no abnormalities were found, to assess the heart further by echocardiography.

Case outcome

Abdominal ultrasound revealed a large, dense, hyperechoic mass extending from the right lateral lobe of the liver through to the left medial lobe.

Aspirates of this mass were sent for cytology. Clustered round or epithelial cells displaying mild to moderate anisocytosis and anisokaryosis were identified, thought to represent a malignant round or epithelial cell neoplasm.

On exploratory laparotomy the mass was non-resectable. Biopsies confirmed a diagnosis of biliary carcinoma with abundant fibrosis and lymphocytic inflammation.

CHAPTER 7

Weakness

Holger A. Volk[1], David B. Church[2] and Jill E. Maddison[3]

[1] Department of Small Animal Medicine and Surgery, University of Veterinary Medicine Hannover, Hannover, Germany

[2] Department of Clinical Science and Services, The Royal Veterinary College, London, UK

[3] Department of Clinical Science and Services, The Royal Veterinary College, London, UK

The why

- Weakness is a common presenting complaint in general practice.
- True weakness is a sign of central nervous system (CNS) or neuromuscular system dysfunction but may be confused with skeletal dysfunction.
- This chapter provides you with a toolkit to define and refine the system involved as well as refine the potential diagnoses to those that are more common.
- Even if the underlying aetiology is not 100% defined, this can allow you to give the owner some answers about probable causes and prognosis.

Define and refine the problem

When an animal presents with a history of episodic weakness, exercise intolerance or collapse, appropriately defining the problem is essential, although sometimes difficult.

An owner may state that his/her dog is having collapsing episodes, but it is imperative that the clinician defines the problem by gathering the following key information:

- What happens before or after the episode?
- What was observed during the episode?

Clinical Reasoning in Veterinary Practice: Problem Solved!, Second Edition.
Edited by Jill E. Maddison, Holger A. Volk and David B. Church.
© 2022 John Wiley & Sons Ltd. Published 2022 by John Wiley & Sons Ltd.

- Does exercise or other triggers influence the episode?
- Does the animal lose consciousness during the episode (seen in syncope or seizures)?
  This will enable the clinician to ascertain whether:
- The animal loses *consciousness* (indicating syncope or seizures).
- There is *no* evidence of *rhythmic convulsive* activity (more likely syncope than seizures).
- The animal:
  o Is normal in between the episodes (*episodically weak*)
  o exhibits weakness precipitated by exercise (*fatigability*)
  o Is consistently weak (*persistently weak*).
- The animal shows a *spastic* or *flaccid* 'weakness' (reduction [paresis] or absence [plegia] of voluntary movement) associated with or without incoordination (*ataxia*).

Other common presenting complaints that may be seen in the flaccidly weak patient include the following:
- Regurgitation
- Difficulty rising
- Exercise intolerance
- Episodic weakness
- Fatigability
- Altered voice
- Change in musculature
- Stiff, stilted gait
- An inability to lift the head up normally or, especially in cats, a state of persistent cervical ventroflexion.

 ## Define and refine the system

Animals with dysfunction of the CNS or neuromuscular system can present collapsed or weak. The nervous system is divided into the CNS (brain and spinal cord) and the neuromuscular system (peripheral nerves, neuromuscular junction and musculature). The CNS regulates the neuromuscular system.

The cause of weakness either can be a *primary, structural* disorder of the CNS or neuromuscular system or be a *secondary, functional* disorder resulting from the dysfunction of a number of other systems that result in impaired CNS or neuromuscular function.

Secondary, functional disorders resulting in impaired CNS or neuromuscular performance include:
- Reduced delivery of nutrients to the brain, nerves or muscles
  - Glucose
  - Oxygen
- Change in the internal milieu of muscles and nerves that alter their function
  - For example, calcium and potassium imbalances
- Production of endogenous toxins
  - For example, uraemia.

Hence, it is apparent that weakness may be caused by:
- *Primary, structural CNS or neuromuscular disease* involving the following:
  - Brain
  - Spinal cord
  - Peripheral nerves
  - Neuromuscular junction
  - Muscles
- *Secondary, functional CNS and/or neuromuscular disease* caused by:
  - Cardiovascular/haemopoietic disorders
    - Heart, vessels and blood
  - Metabolic disorders
    - Electrolytes
    - Glucose
    - Endogenous toxins
  - Respiratory disorders.

Skeletal disorders
Skeletal disorders involving joint or bone pathology may be confused with weakness due to neurological/neuromuscular disease (also see Chapter 14). Examples would include dogs with bilateral cruciate rupture or lumbosacral disease presented for pelvic limb 'weakness'.

As a result, it is vitally important that before embarking on a diagnostic work-up for a neurological problem (structural or functional), skeletal disorders are considered and ruled out where appropriate. Also keep in mind that a patient may have concurrent skeletal and

CNS or neuromuscular system disorders such as the German shepherd dog with a pelvic limb gait abnormality contributed to by hip-dysplasia-induced degenerative joint disease *and* degenerative myelopathy (also see Chapter 14).

This chapter will discuss the problem of generalised weakness. See Chapter 8 for the detailed clinical reasoning approach for animals presenting with the primary sign of 'collapse' and Chapter 14 for the detailed clinical reasoning approach for animals presenting with the primary complaint of a gait abnormality.

Define the location

In CNS or neuromuscular disorders causing weakness, the clinical and neurological examination is the key in determining the system involved and, when appropriate, what part of the system. The neurological examination can help you define the location of the lesion within the CNS (see Chapters 8 and 14) or neuromuscular system and this in turn can assist in confirming the system involved and whether there is likely to be a structural or functional disorder.

Common neurological examination findings in neuromuscular disorders
- Tetraparesis +/− proprioceptive ataxia
  - Paresis is a sign of motor dysfunction and ataxia of sensory nerve/proprioceptive dysfunction. In general, if you find paresis without ataxia, think 'muscular'
- Muscle atrophy/pain
- Reduced spinal reflexes and muscle tone
- Sensory deficits or self-mutilation
  - In general, evidence for sensory dysfunction strongly suggests a primary neuromuscular problem, as it is unusual for a functional problem to result in predominantly sensory dysfunction.

It is also always important to check for *autonomic dysfunction*, as this can be associated with a range of neuropathies. Autonomic dysfunction can be manifested by changes such as the following:
- Mydriasis or anisocoria
- Decreased tear production

- Hyposalivation
- Bradycardia
- Constipation
- Urinary retention.

Neuroanatomical localisation within the CNS or neuromuscular system

The neurological examination can be divided into two parts (see also Chapter 8).

Hands-off examination – observation
- Mentation and behaviour
- Posture
- Gait
- Identification of abnormal involuntary movements (Chapter 8).

Hands-on examination
- Postural reaction testing
- Cranial nerves assessment
- Spinal reflexes, muscle tone and size
- Sensory evaluation.

Hands-off examination – observation
Mentation and behaviour
The most important part is the hands-off examination. The first thing you always need to assess and ask the owner about is if the animal has developed or shows an abnormal behaviour pattern and has a change in the level of mentation (e.g. obtundation).

If you see changes in behaviour or an altered level of mentation, then consider brain involvement (Chapter 8). Conditions affecting purely the neuromuscular system should not cause an altered mentation or behaviour changes.

Posture and gait
Observe the animal from a distance (from the front or back [walking towards or away from you] and passing by from the side).
- *Ataxia* is a lack of coordination of movement and may occur in conditions affecting sensory (proprioceptive) pathways.
  - Ataxia is best appreciated when the animal is walked slowly.

- *Paresis* is defined as a *decrease* of voluntary movement.
  - o Paresis in neuromuscular conditions can get worse with exercise, so also assess the animal trotting.
  - o Flaccid paresis is an indication of neuromuscular system dysfunction.
    - ▪ Most of the conditions will affect all four limbs.
      - • Pelvic limbs are usually more severely affected, as they have the longer neuromuscular pathways.
    - ▪ Peripheral nerve disorders can cause ataxia and paresis.
      - • Most peripheral nerves are mixed nerves with sensory and motor tracts.
    - ▪ Neuromuscular junction deficits and muscle disease only cause paresis.
      - • This can resemble an orthopaedic lameness.
  - o Spastic (upper motor neuron) paresis can be seen with CNS involvement.
- *Plegia* is characterised by an *absence* of voluntary movement.

Hands-on examination
Postural reactions
Postural reaction tests can be helpful to confirm which limbs you think are affected. They are not so useful in determining which part of the nervous system is affected, as they are more similar to a 'screening test', testing the afferent proprioceptive (sensory) and efferent motor pathways (receptor → peripheral nerve → spinal cord → brain → spinal cord → motor unit; see also Chapter 14).

Cranial nerve examination
CNS or neuromuscular diseases can affect the cranial nerves. It is therefore important to assess cranial nerve function in patients presenting with weakness.

Tests relevant to cranial nerve function include:
- Menace response
- Pupillary light response
- Palpebral reflex
- Gag reflex
- Facial sensation
- Assessment of facial muscle symmetry
- Schirmer tear test.

Spinal reflexes

In assessing spinal reflexes, a standard approach facilitates your capacity to detect abnormalities.

Generally, changes in muscle tone should be assessed first and then the spinal reflexes themselves.

- Muscle tone can be reduced in neuromuscular disorders.
- Reflexes may also be attenuated due to muscle fibrosis or joint contractures.
- They may appear exaggerated if there is a lack of antagonistic muscle tone (pseudohyperreflexia, seen with sciatic nerve lesion).
- Reflexes should be, therefore, interpreted only in light of the rest of the examination (gait, posture and muscle tone).

In neuromuscular conditions, the reflexes are usually decreased in the affected limbs (it can be useful to assess the animal before and after exercise).

- Decreased or absent reflexes are caused by a lesion in the reflex arc (receptor → peripheral nerve → spinal cord → peripheral nerve → neuromuscular junction → muscle).
  - o Decrease in tendon reflexes
    - Patellar reflex (reduced level of stifle extension)
    - Biceps, triceps or gastrocnemius reflex (decrease in muscle contraction of the muscle).
  - o Decreased withdrawal (flexor) reflexes are shown as reduction in the degree of flexion of individual joints
    - Pelvic limbs assessment: reduced → hock flexion (sciatic dysfunction)
    - Thoracic limbs assessment: reduced elbow flexion.

Palpation

Palpation can help you to detect muscle atrophy or hypertrophy, swelling, pain, masses, muscle contractures and muscle tone. Palpation should be done both when the animal is standing and in lateral recumbency.

Sensory evaluation

Assessment of sensation can be helpful if you think the neuromuscular deficits are caused by peripheral nerve dysfunction. It is, however, rare that animals will have severe nociceptive deficits with conditions affecting the neuromuscular system.

Table 7.1 Neuroanatomical localisation within the neuromuscular system. Neurological deficits to be considered with neuromuscular disease.

Neurological examination	Peripheral neuropathy	Polyradiculo-neuropathy (motor)	Junctionopathy	Myopathy
Mentation Posture/gait	Appropriate level and quality Plantigrade stance Flaccid paresis or plegia of affected limb(s) (motor impairment) Ataxia (sensory impairment)	Appropriate level and quality Flaccid paresis or plegia of affected limb(s)	Appropriate level and quality Usually unremarkable (without exercise) Exercise-induced stiff, stilted gait then/or flaccid paresis or plegia of affected limbs (during exercise or for severe phenotype)	Appropriate level and quality Stiff, stilted gait (often aggravates with exercise) Paresis
Postural reactions	Postural reaction deficits on affected limb(s) (sensory and/or motor)	Postural reaction deficits on affected limbs (motor part impaired)	Unaltered to altered depending on severity of disease or exercise level	Usually unaltered Can be altered with severe phenotype or exercise
Spinal reflexes	Decreased to absent on affected limb(s)	Absent to reduced on affected limbs	Unremarkable unless severe phenotype or exercised	Unremarkable
Muscle tone and mass	Reduced to absent muscle tone with moderate to severe muscle atrophy (motor)	Reduced to absent muscle tone with moderate to severe muscle atrophy when chronic (motor)	Usually unremarkable	Atrophy or hypertrophy Reduced tone or contractures (hypertonicity – myotonia)
Sensation	With sensory nerve involvement decreased to absent sensation and nociception	Unremarkable	Unremarkable	Unremarkable
Cranial nerves	Can be involved	Unremarkable	Facial weakness possible	Masticatory muscle atrophy possible
Pain	Paraesthesia, self-mutilation	Spinal pain possible	Unremarkable	Possible muscle pain (e.g. inflammatory/infectious and neoplastic diseases)
Others	Autonomic signs possible			

Neuromuscular system deficits that can be seen with defects in the different parts of the neuromuscular system are shown in Table 7.1.

- If the neurological deficits are asymmetrical, a primary structural CNS or neuromuscular abnormality becomes far more likely (Tables 7.2 and 7.3).
- If the condition is also painful, then there should be an increased index of suspicion for inflammatory, infectious, traumatic or neoplastic conditions.

Secondary functional lesions affect the neuromuscular system diffusely so that the neurological deficits are usually symmetrical in presentation. For these conditions, pain cannot be elicited from structures in the neuromuscular system.

Define the lesion

You have localised the lesion to the CNS or neuromuscular system and potentially to a specific part within this system. It is now time to identify the lesion. What questions might help you to refine your list of possible diagnoses and consider the most appropriate diagnostic pathway to identify which diseases can have a direct (primary) or indirect (secondary) effect on the CNS or neuromuscular system?

- Primary CNS/neuromuscular
  - o Which diseases cause lateralising (asymmetrical) signs or symmetrical signs?
  - o Which disease processes could be associated with pain?
  - o What is the clinical course of the disease (acute vs. chronic onset; improving, static, episodic and/or deteriorating)?
  - o The five-finger rule (Figure 7.1) can help you remember these key questions and narrow down your differential list.
- Secondary disorders
  - o Apart from weakness, what other clinical signs do you recognise that could indicate secondary involvement of the CNS or neuromuscular system?

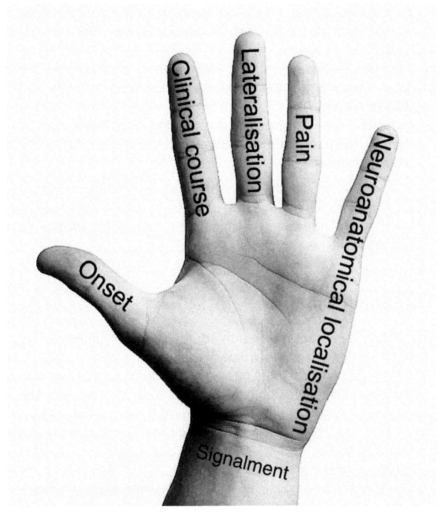

Figure 7.1   The five-finger rule.

- Cardiac disease?
  - For example, arrhythmias, pulse deficits, changes in pulse quality and peripheral blood perfusion problems
- Upper respiratory disease?
  - For example, stridor, respiratory distress and clinical signs of reduced oxygenation

- Lower respiratory disease?
  - For example, abnormal thoracic auscultation (pulmonary? pleural effusion?)
- Endocrinopathy?
  - For example, skin and haircoat changes, changes in body conformation and abdominal wall weakness, hyperglycaemia
- Haematological disorders?
  - For example, changes in mucous membrane colour and heart sounds
- Gastrointestinal changes
  - For example, vomiting vs. regurgitation (Chapter 3)
- Hyperthermia vs. pyrexia?

In addition, the characteristics of the weakness will assist in refining the list of possible diagnoses. As discussed earlier when defining the problem, weakness can present episodically or persistently. Exercise can trigger an episode and aggravate some of the causes of episodic weakness progressing to persistent weakness.

Weakness in cats
Cats, in contrast to dogs, do not tend to present with episodic weakness – they will usually 'self-regulate' their activity and more commonly present with persistent weakness. This is usually manifested by ventral flexion of the neck and lying with their head on their paws, that is, looking really relaxed even in the middle of a consulting room or other strange and stressful environment. Ventral flexion of the head is seen in cats with neuromuscular disease, as they lack a nuchal ligament. Cats also might have elevated (prominent) scapulae when they rest and walk.

Episodic weakness
Episodic weakness without loss of consciousness will usually occur with:
- Secondary functional neuromuscular disorders
  - Cardiovascular dysfunction

- o Metabolic derangements
  - ▪ Energy deprivation (hypoglycaemia)
  - ▪ Electrolyte abnormalities
- Primary structural neuromuscular disorders
  - o Neuromuscular junctionopathies
    - ▪ Myasthenia gravis
  - o Myopathies.

See Table 7.2 for specific examples of disorders causing episodic weakness.

Persistent weakness

Persistent weakness usually occurs with:
- Secondary functional neuromuscular disorders
  - o Derangements in calcium or potassium homeostasis
  - o Endogenous toxaemia
- Primary structural neuromuscular disorders
  - o Primary peripheral nerve dysfunction
  - o Neuromuscular junction abnormalities
  - o Primary muscle dysfunction.

   Persistent weakness *aggravated by exercise* usually occurs with:
- Secondary functional neuromuscular disorders
  - o Cardiovascular system disorders
  - o Metabolic disorders
- Primary structural neuromuscular disorders
  - o Peripheral neuropathy
  - o Junctionopathy
  - o Myopathy.

See Table 7.3 for specific examples of disorders causing persistent weakness.

The direction of your diagnostic procedures will depend on other clinical signs and abnormalities that are present in addition to the presenting complaint of weakness.

Table 7.2   Potential diagnoses for episodic or exercise-induced weakness.

Category	Differentials	Symmetry of neuromuscular deficits	Pain
Secondary (functional) neuromuscular			
Cardiovascular/ haematopoietic	Structural cardiovascular disease	S	–
	Arrhythmias	S	–
	Anaemia	S	–
	Hyperviscosity syndromes	S	–
	Acute haemorrhage	S	–
Respiratory	Heartworm disease	S	–
	Upper respiratory dysfunction (laryngeal paralysis, brachycephalic airway syndrome and tracheal collapse)	S	–
	Pulmonary disease	S	–
Metabolic	Hypoglycaemia (e.g. pancreatic islet tumour and exercise induced)	S	–
	Hyperkalaemia, for example, hypoadrenocorticism	S	–/+
Primary (structural) CNS or neuromuscular			
Neuropathy	Exercise-induced collapse (CNS)	S	–
Junctionopathy	Myasthenia gravis	S	–
Myopathy	Metabolic myopathies (e.g. mitochondrial or lipid storage myopathy); malignant hyperthermia	S	–

S, symmetrical neuromuscular deficits.

Table 7.3 Potential diagnoses for persistent weakness.

Category	Differentials	Symmetry of neuromuscular deficits	Pain
Secondary (functional) neuromuscular			
Cardiovascular/haematopoietic	• Cardiovascular disease	S	–
	• Arrhythmias	S	–
	• Anaemia	S	–
	• Hyperviscosity syndromes	S	–
Metabolic	• Hypokalaemia, for example,	S	–
	○ Primary aldosteronism		
	• Hyperkalaemia, for example,	S	–/+
	○ Hypoadrenocorticism		
	• Hypocalcaemia, for example,	S	–/+
	○ Primary hypoparathyroidism		
	• Hypercalcaemia, for example,	S	–
	○ Primary hyperparathyroidism		
	○ Paraneoplastic syndrome		
	○ Vitamin D toxicity		
	• Hypo-/hypermagnesaemia	S	–
	• Hypoglycaemia, for example,	S	–
	○ Insulinoma		
	○ Hunting dog hypoglycaemia		
	• Hyperadrenocorticism	S	–/+
	• Hypothyroidism	S/AS	–
	• Diabetes mellitus (cats)	S	– .
	• Endogenous toxaemia, for example,	S	–
	○ Sepsis		
	○ Hepatic encephalopathy		

Category	Differentials	Symmetry of neuromuscular deficits	Pain
Neoplasia	• Paraneoplastic, for example, ○ Insulinoma causing neuropathy	S	–
Nutritional	• Vitamin E/selenium deficiency	S	–
Toxic	• Lead (neuropathy)	S	–
	• Organophosphate toxicity		–
	• Spider bite		
	• Tick paralysis		
	• Botulism		
	• Snake envenomation		
Primary (structural) CNS or neuromuscular			
Neuropathy	*Non-inflammatory*		
	• Acquired	AS	+/-
	• Neoplasia (e.g. lymphoma)	S	+/-
	• Inherited	AS	+/-
	• Breed-specific myopathy, for example,	S	+/-
	○ Alaskan Malamute	AS	–
	○ Leonberger		
	Inflammatory		
	• Infectious	AS	–
	• Protozoal	AS	–
	• Immune mediated	AS	–
	• Polyradiculoneuritis	S/AS	–
	• Chronic neuritis	AS	–
Junctionopathy	Myasthenia gravis	S	–

(Continued)

Table 7.3 (Continued)

Category	Differentials	Symmetry of neuromuscular deficits	Pain
Myopathy	*Non-inflammatory*		
	• Acquired		–
	• Exertional rhabdomyolysis	S	+
	• Neoplasia (e.g. lymphoma)	AS	+/–
	• Paraneoplastic inherited	S	–
	• Muscular dystrophy	AS	+
	• Myotonia	S	–
	• Metabolic myopathies	S	–
	• Breed-specific myopathy, for example,	S	–
	○ Great Dane		
	○ Labrador		
	Inflammatory		
	• Infectious		
	• Protozoal	AS	+/–
	• Rickettsial immune mediated	AS	+/–
	• Polymyositis	AS	+/–
	• Dermatomyositis	AS	+/–

AS = asymmetrical neuromuscular deficits; S, symmetrical neuromuscular deficits.

Diagnostic approach to the patient presenting with weakness

Your diagnostic approach will be determined by your problem-solving path. Most of the diagnostics for diseases that affect the neuromuscular system secondarily can be performed in general practice. These include detailed history, complete physical and neurological examination, blood and urine tests, blood pressure measurements, examination of the retina (looking for convoluted and/or dilated blood vessels or bleeding, indicating signs of hypertension) and imaging modalities accessible in first-opinion practice such as radiography and ultrasonography.

   Diagnostic tests can be grouped into
- Clinical pathology
  - Haematology, serum biochemistry and urinalysis
  - Serology
    - Acetylcholine receptor antibodies
    - Tests for *Neospora caninum, Toxoplasma gondii*
  - Endocrine function testing
    - Hypothyroidism
    - Hyperadrenocorticism
    - Hypoadrenocorticism
    - Iatrogenic steroid myopathy
  - Cerebrospinal fluid analysis
  - Genetic testing
    - A number of primary CNS and neuromuscular disorders are brought about by gene abnormalities, and there is an increasing battery of tests that allow the abnormalities to be identified. Most of them are for breed-specific diseases.
- Assessment of structure
  - Diagnostic imaging
  - Biopsy
- Functional assessment
  - Electrophysiology
  - Dynamic testing
    - Edrophonium response test
    - Exercise test.

In conclusion

The patient presenting weak or collapsed can pose a significant diagnostic dilemma. Understanding the pathophysiology underlying weakness can assist the clinician to follow a structured diagnostic pathway and importantly reduces the need to remember long lists of differential diagnoses.

Focus on the key questions – which part of the CNS or neuro-muscular system is involved, and is the involvement due to primary structural or neuromuscular pathology or dysfunction secondary to some other problem resulting in neuromuscular dysfunction? If you follow these steps, you will be able to reach a refined list of possible explanations or even diagnoses rationally and expediently.

Key points

As a result of reading this chapter you should be able to:
- Recognise the importance of clearly defining the problem to dif-ferentiate episodic weakness and persistent weakness
- Recognise that 'thinking pathophysiologically' is essential to rank in appropriate order the body systems under consideration
- Recognise that weakness may be caused by a primary structural CNS or neuromuscular defect or by a functional CNS or neuro-muscular defect
- Recognise that weak cats may present differently to weak dogs.

Questions for review

- What disorders can cause episodic weakness?
- Compare and contrast the neurological examination findings in a patient with a peripheral neuropathy vs. junctionopathy vs. myopathy.

Case example

'Jessie' is a 7-year-old female neutered cross-bred dog. Jessie has been normal until 2 months ago. She is okay in the house, but as soon she exercises she collapses on her back limbs. No other clinical signs have been noted by the owner. Her general physical examination was unremarkable.

Define the problem

Jessie's problem is defined as hind limb weakness and can be further refined as episodic, exercise-induced pelvic limb weakness.

Define the system:

Episodic weakness triggered by exercise can be due to primary or secondary neurological/neuromuscular disease. Differentials to consider and influence plans are:

Primary neurological/neuromuscular disorders
- Narcolepsy, cataplexy (but she does not appear to have lost consciousness)
- Myasthenia gravis
- Metabolic myopathies (such as mitochondrial, hyperthermia or lipid storage myopathies).

Secondary neuromuscular disorders
- Cardiovascular/haemopoietic disorders, for example, intermittent arrhythmias, anaemia (no indication on clinical exam), polycythaemia, hyperviscosity syndrome
- Hypoglycaemia (e.g. insulinoma, hypoadrenocorticism, sepsis)
- Respiratory disease such as laryngeal paralysis (no indication here).
  A neurological examination is important to help assess the system +/- location.

Neurological examination findings:
- Mentation: unremarkable quality and level.
- Posture/gait: paraparetic, which becomes worse on exercise. No ataxia noted.
- Postural reactions: paw positioning and hopping fairly unremarkable.
- Cranial nerves: reduced menace response and palpebral reflex.
- Good facial sensation.
- Spinal reflexes: intact.
- Palpation: unremarkable.
- Nociception: not tested as appears to have good sensation.

Define the location

Assessment of the neurological findings:
- Mentation: unremarkable quality and level – no indication of brain involvement.
- Posture/gait: paraparetic, which becomes worse on exercise. No ataxia noted. Thus no nerve involvement and most likely junctionopathy or muscular (primary or secondary).
- Postural reactions: paw positioning and hopping fairly unremarkable, which is another sign that the dog is not weak and has no loss of sensory input.
- Cranial nerves: reduced menace response and palpebral reflex. Good facial sensation. Facial weakness can be seen with neuromuscular diseases, either generalized lower motor neuron (LMN) disease or junctionopathies.
- Spinal reflexes: intact. This makes a muscular or nerve problem less likely.

Post-synaptic junctionopathies such as myasthenia gravis do usually not affect the myotatic reflexes.

Our neurolocalisation is generalized to that Jessie has a chronic progressive, exercise-induced (episodic), symmetrical, non-painful junctionopathy (neuromuscular).

Define the lesion

The main differential causes for the junctionopathy are:
- Immune mediated – myasthenia gravis
- Paraneoplastic disease
- Toxins (organophosphate poisoning – not likely in this case).

Secondary disorders still needed to be ruled, especially hypoglycaemia and hyperviscosity.

Specific testing for myasthenia gravis is indicated if haematology and biochemistry results are normal.

Thoracic radiographs would be appropriate to assess for lung masses, thymoma and megaoesophagus.

A Tensilon response test could be done, noting that a positive result does not confirm myasthenia gravis as many neuromuscular disorders will partially respond to increased levels of acetylcholine in the neuromuscular junction. The test can help indicate if treatment might be successful.

Case outcome

All haematology and biochemistry results were within the reference ranges.

Thoracic radiographs were unremarkable.

nAChR antibody level: 1.5 nmol/l (normal <0.6 nmol/l) confirming a diagnosis of myasthenia gravis.

Jessie was managed with pyridostigmine and was able to be weaned off medication after 6 months.

CHAPTER 8

Fits and strange episodes

Holger A. Volk

Department of Small Animal Medicine and Surgery, University of Veterinary Medicine Hannover, Hannover, Germany

The why

- Paroxysmal episodes or 'fits' can be challenging for any experienced clinician.
  - Firstly, the patient is usually normal at presentation.
  - Secondly, the identification of the type of episode is dependent on a good description from the person who witnessed the episode.
  - Thirdly, most of these paroxysmal episodes appear unpredictable and uncontrollable for the owner, and therefore, their observation might be heavily biased by an emotionally loaded perception of reality.
- A clear characterisation of the presenting complaint via an in-depth history taken, asking the right questions, and potentially having a video of the episode is pivotal for a successful work-up.
- This chapter will provide you with the toolkit to differentiate syncope, narcolepsy/cataplexy, pain, compulsive behaviour disorders, vestibular attacks, paroxysmal movement disorders, neuromuscular weakness and epileptic seizures.

Define and refine the problem

Paroxysmal episodic disorders can have many presentations affecting posture, muscle tone, uncontrolled movements and alteration in behaviour. Apart from characterising the episode itself, it is important to establish any triggers or clinical signs the animal might show before or shortly after an episode (Table 8.1).

Clinical Reasoning in Veterinary Practice: Problem Solved!, Second Edition.
Edited by Jill E. Maddison, Holger A. Volk and David B. Church.
© 2022 John Wiley & Sons Ltd. Published 2022 by John Wiley & Sons Ltd.

Common episodic events that need to be differentiated are syncope, narcolepsy/cataplexy, behaviour changes, vestibular attacks, movement disorders, neuromuscular weakness (see also Chapter 7) and epileptic seizures.

Syncope

Episodes of syncope are usually characterised by a sudden, short, transient loss of consciousness and postural tone. The animals are flaccid during the episode but can experience a brief myoclonic jerk just before collapsing. We have seen this especially in cats with third-degree atrioventricular block. This can be confused with brief focal seizures. However, most animals with syncopal episodes do not show any pre- or post-episodic signs. Syncopal episodes are commonly associated with exercise or movement rather than occurring at rest. Recovery is usually nearly instant. There can be multiple episodes per day, which can occur shortly after each other and show no improvement on anti-epileptic drugs. In fact, anti-seizure drugs can impair cardiorespiratory function, and therefore, these episodes can get worse with anti-seizure drug treatment.

Narcolepsy

Narcolepsy is a rather rare disorder of the sleep–wake cycle. Cataplectic attacks are common in narcolepsy, which can resemble syncopal collapse and seizures. Cataplectic attacks are usually triggered by food, excitement and stress or pharmacologically (e.g. physostigmine). Following the 'trigger', the affected animal will become flaccid and collapse. Narcoleptic animals experience chronic fatigue, although they do not necessarily sleep more. They can be restless at night and sleepy during the day because of a disturbed and irregular sleep pattern. A history of others affected in the litter or in the breeding line is not uncommon.

Paroxysmal behaviour changes

Pain can be experienced episodically and trigger a behavioural response, which can resemble focal epileptic seizures, for example, nerve root impingement or irritation caused by lateral disc protrusion/extrusion resulting in 'freezing', myoclonic jerks, muscle spasms and/or muscle fasciculations.

Behaviour disorders such as episodes of aggression or compulsive behaviour changes (stereotypic behaviours, e.g. continuous rhythmic pacing, licking and vocalisations) can also look similar to sensory seizures. Dogs and cats are usually normal in between episodes. Compulsive behaviour changes, however, are not associated with changes in muscle tone or in the level of consciousness, and usually, a behavioural trigger can be identified.

Vestibular attacks

Transient vestibular episodes are a rare phenomenon characterised by the same cardinal signs seen with non-intermittent vestibular disease such as head tilt, nystagmus and ataxia. Nystagmus and gait abnormalities can also be seen with seizures, but it is rare that a seizure causes a head tilt. These patients will typically have no altered consciousness during an episode and are fairly normal before and after an episode. These episodes will not respond to standard anti-seizure drug treatment.

Paroxysmal movement disorders

The most common movement disorders that can be seen in practice are idiopathic head tremors or paroxysmal dyskinesias. Differentiating epileptic seizures from paroxysmal dyskinesia is also challenging in people. In contrast to epileptic seizures, they usually are associated with movements, rarely occur at rest or out of sleep, are episodic and involve an increase in muscle tone (dystonia), can be associated with generalized termors and do not affect the level of consciousness or cause autonomous signs such as hypersalivation.

Furthermore, paroxysmal dyskinesias are distinguishable from focal seizures by the lack of secondary generalisation of motor activity as would be seen in a generalised motor seizure. However, the muscle tone is often increased on both sides of the body (e.g. extended and increased muscle tone in two or four limbs), but the consciousness is as aforementioned not impaired as it would be if this would be a seizure affecting both brain hemispheres. They do not respond to first-line anti-seizure drugs.

As a rule of thumb, if you are presented with a purebred dog, which has a paroxysmal episode that does not cause autonomic

Table 8.1 Clinical characteristics of episodic disorders.

Discriminator	Syncope	Narcolepsy/cataplexy	Neuromuscular weakness	Paroxysmal behaviour changes (compulsive disorder)	Vestibular attack	Paroxysmal dyskinesia	Idiopathic head tremor	Epileptic seizure
Between episodes	–	Altered sleep/wake cycle	–/show signs of weakness	–	–	–	–	–(idiopathic epilepsy)/abnormal (structural epilepsy, reactive seizures)
Precipitating event/trigger	Exercise, excitement	Excitement, food, pharmacologically	Exercise, excitement	Behavioural triggers (e.g. fear)	–	–/movement or exercise	–	–/flashing lights
Pre-event changes	–	–	–	–	–	–	–	Pre-ictal behaviour changes (prodrome [hours to days] and/or aura [minutes]) such as staring, freezing, attention seeking, fear
Event description	Brief, sudden collapse and recovery	Sudden collapse	Stiff, stilted gait prior to collapse	For example, pacing, barking, licking, chasing imaginary objects, chewing objects	Head tilt, nystagmus, collapse/fall towards side of head tilt	Dystonia, tremor	Tremor of head in 'yes'/'no' direction	Depending on seizure focus, focal or generalized tonic-clonic movements most common

Level of consciousness	Unconscious	Asleep	–	–/impaired (disorientated)	–	Impaired/unconscious
Autonomic signs	Heart rate/rhythm changes possible	–	–	–	–	Hypersalivation, defaecation, urination
Muscle tone	Flaccid	Flaccid	– to flaccid	Unilateral decrease in extensor muscle tone	Hypertonicity	Tonic (hypertonicity)/tonic-clonic alternating movement (convulsions)
Lateralising signs	–	–	–	Yes	Possible	Asymmetrical seizures (structural epilepsy)
Duration	Seconds	Seconds to minutes	Minutes to hours	Seconds to hours	Minutes to hours	Seconds to minutes/status epilepticus (>10 minutes)
Post-episodic changes	–	–	–	–	Can appear tired	Yes, such as behaviour changes, blindness, gait abnormalities
Further comments	–	–	–	Subtle signs of vestibular disease might persist	Episodes can stop when interrupted	Head/facial muscles often involved

–, normal, none or not shown.
Neuromuscular weakness and syncope – see Chapter 7 for further details.

dysfunction, is normal after the episode, does not look similar to a generalised tonic-clonic seizure, has appropriate mentation during an episode even if changes in muscle activity are bilateral and/or does not respond as well to anti-epileptic drugs, you should consult the relevant internet databases for a breed-specific movement disorder.

In brief, these paroxysmal movement disorders usually lack the following:

- An identifiable precipitating event such as an aura (sensory seizure activity, e.g. behaviour change [attention seeking, sniffing and staring], lasting a couple of minutes just before the motor seizure activity)
- Autonomic signs (e.g. hypersalivation, urination and defaecation)
- Generalisation of increased motor activity (e.g. generalised tonic or tonic-clonic seizure)
- An impairment of consciousness. Dogs with impaired consciousness will not be able to look into the owner's eyes during the event, and this is a good question to ask the owner.

Epileptic seizures
The brain is a 'complex' structure but has only 'simple' (limited) ways of expressing dysfunction. A seizure is a clinical sign caused by forebrain dysfunction – it is not a diagnosis (one specific disease). A plethora of structural and functional causes can result in seizures (see the following section when we talk about defining the lesion). Seizures can have many forms depending on which part of the brain is affected by seizure generation and propagation; for example, a seizure could just affect a specific part of the sensory cortex, and the animal might only have a change in behaviour (staring, freezing, sniffing, etc.) or only one part of the motor cortex is affected and the animal only demonstrates orofacial automatisms.

The location of the 'symptomatogenic' zone (area of the brain causing the observed clinical signs) usually overlays or is close to the epileptogenic zone (area of the brain causing the seizure) and therefore indicates the origin of the seizure. Seizure semiology, using clinical signs of cerebral dysfunctions caused by a seizure, not only helps to confirm that the event is a seizure but also provides information about its origin. It is relatively simple and is clinically cost-effective. Depending on the brain areas or parts being affected by the seizure motor, sensory (including behaviour changes) and vegetative changes and automatisms can be differentiated and help to characterise the seizure event.

Is it an epileptic seizure?
- Increased muscle tone is far more likely in seizures.
  - The most common recognised seizure is a generalised tonic-clonic seizure.
  - Most commonly, the animal first goes stiff (tonic phase), loses proprioception and collapses into lateral recumbency, then the tonic-clonic phase (rhythmic alternating muscle contractions) starts, followed often by running movements (automatisms).
  - Atonic seizures are very uncommon, and a 'floppy' collapse should guide the clinician to 'think' syncope or cataplexy.
- Rhythmic alternating muscle contractions are common in both focal and generalised seizures.
- Seizures often first involve the head and facial muscles (eye or facial muscle twitching).
- Stereotypical – most animals will have only one (or two) type(s) of seizure (seizure onset generalized, focal seizure onset with or without secondary generalisation).
  - Seizures in an animal typically originate from the same epileptic focus and spread following the same brain pathways.
- The ictus (seizure itself) normally lasts 1–2 minutes.
- Most seizures exhibit several stages:
  - Pre-ictal behaviour changes (prodrome [hours to days] and/or aura [minutes])
  - Ictus
  - Post-ictal behaviour or neurological deficits (hours to days).

Apart from the seizure itself, it is the post-ictal changes that are recognised by the owner.
- Common post-ictal dysfunctions are as follows:
  - Behaviour changes such as fear, aggression and disorientation
  - Increased appetite
  - Compulsive pacing
  - Blindness, usually with normal pupillary light reflexes consistent with 'central' blindness
  - Menace response deficits

- o Miosis contralateral to the lesion (if one lesion [secondary to disinhibition of the oculomotor nucleus])
- o Gait abnormalities, especially ataxia and 'conscious' proprioceptive (paw position) deficits.
- Seizures often, but not always, occur at rest or while sleeping.
- Seizures usually impair the consciousness of the animal.
- Most of the seizure disorders will at least initially respond to first-line anti-seizure drugs.

 ## Define and refine the system

Defining the problem appropriately is essential for paroxysmal disorders, as the different problems will guide you to rank the systems involved in order of priority. If the presenting complaint is an epileptic seizure, a vestibular episode, cataplectic/narcoleptic attacks, episodic behaviour changes or a movement disorder, the system that needs to be examined more closely is the brain within the central nervous system (CNS).

The brain can be affected either directly or indirectly. In addition to causing changes in behaviour, seizures or movement disorders will have an effect on the neuromuscular system, but this would be 'ranked' below the CNS in importance. Vestibular disorder can be caused by CNS and peripheral nervous system dysfunction, and a brief discussion of how this occurs can be found in the following section. Other conditions discussed previously (syncope and neuromuscular weakness) also affect the neuromuscular system. A discussion of which other systems might be involved in these clinical presentations and how they can be prioritised can be found in Chapter 7.

 ## Define the location

The neurological examination can assist you to localise the lesion to an exact neuroanatomical location. Despite recent developments in advanced imaging, the neurological examination is still the key to open the drawer to gain access to the most appropriate diagnostics to help you identify the underlying cause of the condition. Especially with seizure disorders, it can be helpful to determine if the lesion is located peripherally (extra-cranial) or centrally (intra-cranial), as this can guide the diagnostic pathway to efficiently establish a diagnosis.

Vestibular attacks

An appreciation of the vestibular system's function is important to help you understand how to localise the lesion correctly and why this is important. The vestibular system's main function is to maintain an animal's equilibrium during movement and orientation against gravity. It is divided into two main sections: the peripheral ('extra-axial', inner ear and vestibulocochlear nerve) and the central ('intra-axial', within brainstem or cerebellum) part.

The vestibular system is responsible for maintaining the position of the eyes, neck, trunk and limbs with reference to the position of the head. The vestibular nuclei communicate with the nuclei of the nerves controlling eye positioning and movement. Other pathways connect the vestibular nuclei with the cerebellum, cerebrum, other brainstem centre (e.g. vomiting centre; Chapter 3) and the spinal cord.

The vestibular system is a unilateral system, which means that the left vestibular system controls the posture of the left side of the animal, and the right one controls the right side. The vestibular nuclei give rise mainly to a pathway that is facilitatory to extensor muscles. However, some fibres inhibit contralateral extensor tone and ipsilateral flexor muscles.

Keeping this in mind, it is logical that a head tilt and a reduced extensor tone of the limbs are towards or on the side of the lesion. 'It looks like the animal is running around a curve'. The jerk nystagmus develops from the dysfunction of the pathways connecting the vestibular nuclei with the cranial nerve nuclei responsible for the eye movement. The slow phase of the jerk nystagmus goes into the direction of the lesion; the fast phase is the compensatory one.

Clinical signs of dysfunction of the vestibular system include (Figure 8.1):
- Loss of balance
- Head tilt
- Leaning towards one side

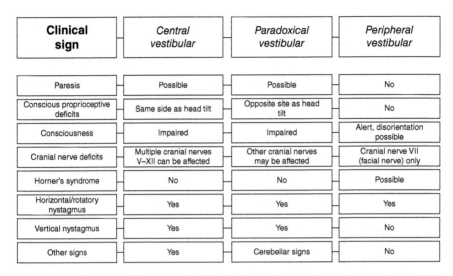

Clinical sign	Central vestibular	Paradoxical vestibular	Peripheral vestibular
Paresis	Possible	Possible	No
Conscious proprioceptive deficits	Same side as head tilt	Opposite site as head tilt	No
Consciousness	Impaired	Impaired	Alert, disorientation possible
Cranial nerve deficits	Multiple cranial nerves V–XII can be affected	Other cranial nerves may be affected	Cranial nerve VII (facial nerve) only
Horner's syndrome	No	No	Possible
Horizontal/rotatory nystagmus	Yes	Yes	Yes
Vertical nystagmus	Yes	Yes	No
Other signs	Yes	Cerebellar signs	No

Figure 8.1 The combination of clinical signs determines the location of the lesion in patients with vestibular signs.

- Rolling
- Circling
- Jerk nystagmus
- Positional strabismus.

If you find in addition to your vestibular dysfunction, signs of brainstem or cerebellar dysfunction think 'central' vestibular syndrome and intra-cranial work-up – reciprocally, if not, think 'peripheral' vestibular syndrome and extra-cranial work-up.

Narcolepsy, paroxysmal behaviour changes and paroxysmal movement disorders

These disorders are caused by a forebrain dysfunction. If you find on your neurological examination signs of lateralisation (asymmetrical neurological deficits) or skull/neck pain, then intra-cranial structural lesions are more likely (see the following sections for more detail).

Seizures

Epileptic seizures = forebrain dysfunction. Your neurological examination will therefore need to centre on assessing forebrain function. But do not ignore the rest of the neurological examination, as identification of multifocal or widespread neurological disease might alter your clinical reasoning.

Epileptic seizures themselves can be the first and the only initial sign of structural brain disease, such as neoplasia in the 'silent areas of the brain' (silent areas are those areas that cannot be examined by the neurological examination, e.g. frontal or olfactory lobe). However, more commonly, the neurological examination might identify the following neurological deficits in dogs with intra-cranial – structural forebrain disease:

- Mentation changes (quality – behaviour changes such as compulsive pacing, head pressing and head turn and/or level – obtundation)
- Postural reaction deficits (such as decreased or absent paw positioning) contralateral to the lesion and/or hemiparesis
- Vision deficits contralateral to the lesion
- Decreased or absent menace response, with normal pupillary light reflex contralateral to the lesion
- Reduced facial sensation and response to nasal septum stimulation contralateral to the lesion
- Ad addendum:
  o Some animals might have neurological deficits affecting both sides equally
  o Focal-onset asymmetrical seizures (seizures that affect one body side more than the other) can indicate structural brain lesion contralateral to the more affected body side (e.g. facial twitches on the left side indicate a right forebrain lesion).

Dogs and cats with seizures secondary to extra-cranial causes can have similar neurological deficits, but they are usually symmetrical in presentation. The clinical signs might be waxing and waning.

The inter-ictal neurological examination can be normal for extra-cranial and functional intra-cranial causes, as seizures can be the only clinical sign of forebrain dysfunction. Post-ictal cerebral dysfunction can cause neurological deficits for hours to days. The clinician should therefore repeat the neurological examination, if neurological deficits are found in close proximity to the last seizure event.

Define the lesion

An easy way to refine your lesion is to use what we have called a 'five-finger' (Figure 8.2) rule:

1. Onset
2. Clinical course
3. Lateralisation (asymmetrical neurological deficits)
4. Pain
5. Neuroanatomical localisation.

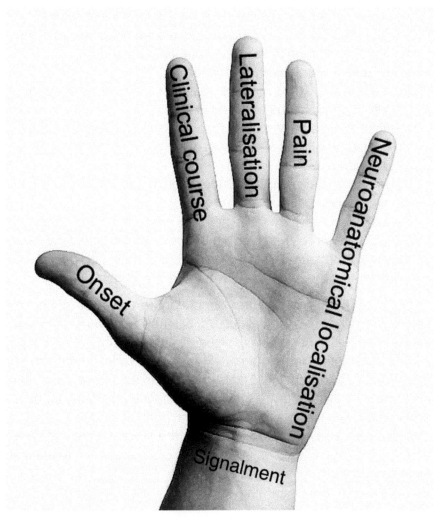

Figure 8.2 The five-finger rule.

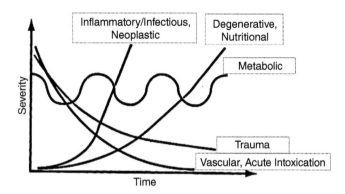

Figure 8.3 The onset and clinical course of a disease can narrow down aetiologies to be considered to unravel the riddle of a case presentation.

Signalment should be considered last to reduce the impact of breed and age-specific biases in clinical decision-making.

Think pathophysiologically – the onset and clinical course of a disease is relative specific to certain aetiologies (Figure 8.3), as is lateralization or asymmetry of neurological deficits, which are more commonly seen with diseases affecting CNS structure, and pain, which is more commonly seen with inflammatory/infectious or neoplastic causes.

Vestibular attacks

The diagnostic work-up may vary greatly between central (brainstem/cerebellum) vs. peripheral disease. Depending on the onset and clinical course, diseases can be grouped into acute onset, non-progressive or progressive and chronic progressive (Figure 8.3, Tables 8.2 and 8.3). Furthermore, thinking pathophysiologically, diseases that can be associated with pain are inflammatory, infectious or neoplastic conditions. Apart from checking for neck pain and palpating the skull and ear area, you can also check if the animal has pain opening its mouth.

The use of the five-finger rule (Figure 8.2) can help you reduce your differential list. For example, an animal with a chronic, progressive, painful, left-sided peripheral vestibular disease most likely has an inflammatory, infectious or neoplastic middle/inner ear condition.

Table 8.2 Potential differential diagnoses for central vestibular disease. Lesions that can be associated with pain are shown in italics.

Category	Acute non-progressive	Acute progressive	Chronic progressive
Anomalous degenerative			(*Hydrocephalus*) Neurodegenerative diseases Storage diseases
Metabolic		Hypothyroidism	Hypothyroidism
Neoplastic		*Metastatic*	Primary: *choroid plexus tumour*, glioma, meningioma, *lymphoma*
Nutritional		Thiamine deficiency (usually bilateral)	
Inflammatory/ infectious		*MUA*	*MUA*
		FIP, canine distemper Protozoal, fungal	*FIP, canine distemper Protozoal, fungal*
Toxic		Lead Hexachlorophene Metronidazole (usually bilateral)	Lead Hexachlorophene
Traumatic vascular	Fracture/bleed Infarction Haemorrhage		

FIP, feline infectious peritonitis; MUA, meningoencephalomyelitis of unknown aetiology.

Table 8.3 Potential differential diagnoses for 'peripheral' vestibular disease. Lesions that can be associated with pain are shown in italics.

Category	Acute non-progressive	Acute progressive	Chronic progressive
Degenerative			Congenital vestibular syndrome (often also deaf)
Metabolic		Hypothyroidism (diabetes mellitus; indirect)	Hypothyroidism

Table 8.3   (Continued)

Category	Acute non-progressive	Acute progressive	Chronic progressive
Neoplastic		Metastatic	Soft-tissue tumours
			Nerve-sheath tumour
Inflammatory/ infectious		*Otitis media/interna (bacterial/fungal)*	*Otitis media/interna (bacterial/fungal)*
		Protozoal	Protozoal
Idiopathic	Idiopathic	Sterile otitis media with effusion	Sterile otitis media with effusion
Traumatic	*Fracture*		
Toxic		Streptomycin	Streptomycin
		Gentamycin	Gentamycin
Vascular	Infarction		
	Haemorrhage		

Narcolepsy

Narcolepsy can usually be identified by characterising the episode. If you are uncertain, you can trigger an episode by food and/or excitement or pharmacologically (e.g. physostigmine).

Paroxysmal behaviour changes

It can be difficult sometimes to differentiate paroxysmal behavioural changes from seizures that mainly affect the behaviour of an animal. If you are uncertain whether the episode could be a seizure or find inter-episodic neurological deficits, then follow the work-up scheme presented as follows for seizure disorders.

Paroxysmal movement disorders

Currently, we have only very limited availability to characterise these *paroxysmal movement disorders*. Genetics has improved our understanding of these disorders and will continue to do so. It is therefore recommended to search the internet when you suspect an episode to be a movement disorder; for example, a gene defect in *BCAN* has been *identified for* episodic falling in Cavalier King Charles Spaniels, and a gene test is available.

Syncope

The differential diagnoses for syncope are presented in Table 8.4.

Table 8.4 Potential differential diagnoses for syncope.

Category	Differentials	Diagnostics
Cardiovascular	Left-sided heart failure	Thoracic radiographs, echocardiography
	Paroxysmal arrhythmias	Electrocardiography, echocardiography
	Heartworm disease	Thoracic radiographs, antigen detection, microfilaria detection
	Severe anaemia	Haematology (and see Chapter 10)
	Hyperviscosity syndromes	Haematology, serum biochemistry, protein electrophoresis
Respiratory	Severe upper airways disease	Endoscopy, radiographs/computed tomography (CT)
Metabolic	Hypoglycaemia	(Fasted) blood glucose

Epileptic seizures

Extra-cranial vs. intra-cranial

Epileptic seizures are caused by either extra-cranial or intra-cranial diseases, which alter cerebral function (Figures 8.4–8.6).

Intra-cranial causes

Intra-cranial causes can be further subdivided into the following:
- Functional diseases
  - Idiopathic epilepsy (a genetic component is suspected)
    - No visible structural changes of the brain on magnetic resonance imaging (MRI) or gross pathological examination
    - Unremarkable inter-ictal neurological examination
- Structural diseases
  - Structural epilepsy
    - Presence of gross structural changes of the brain causing asymmetrical neurological deficits or asymmetrical seizures, for example, neoplasms, inflammatory/infectious causes, vascular accidents or cerebral anomalies.

Please be aware that intra-cranial disease cannot be ruled out completely if the animal is completely normal between seizures.
- This is especially so when dogs are younger than 6 months or older than 6 years of age and cats are older than 7 years of age. Usually, these animals will not respond adequately to anti-seizure treatment.
- Structural lesions that are too small to cause neurological dysfunction other than seizures or are in a relatively 'silent' area of the forebrain may not manifest in any way other than seizures.

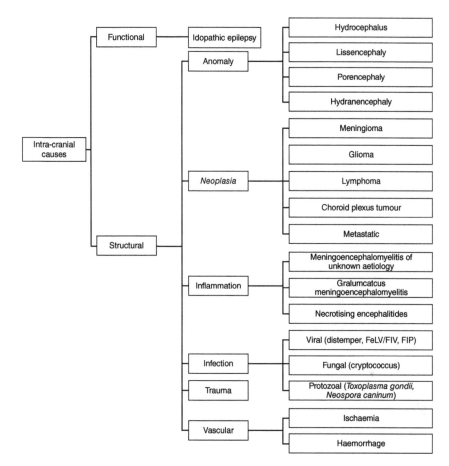

Figure 8.4 Intra-cranial causes for epileptic seizures.

We have shown that finding asymmetrical neurological deficits on the inter-ictal neurological examination increases significantly (by 25 times) the likelihood of finding intra-cranial structural brain disease. Finding symmetrical deficits, cluster seizures and focal-onset (usually asymmetrical) seizures also significantly increases the chance of finding intra-cranial pathology. If you then take age and breed into account, you can refine your differential list substantially. The neurological examination is a powerful tool! Some animals might have other neurological deficits unrelated to the seizure disorder (e.g. chronic disc disease), so always make sure you take a holistic view on the case.

Generalised onset (symmetrical) seizures are more common with idiopathic epilepsy, metabolic, toxic and degenerative causes and

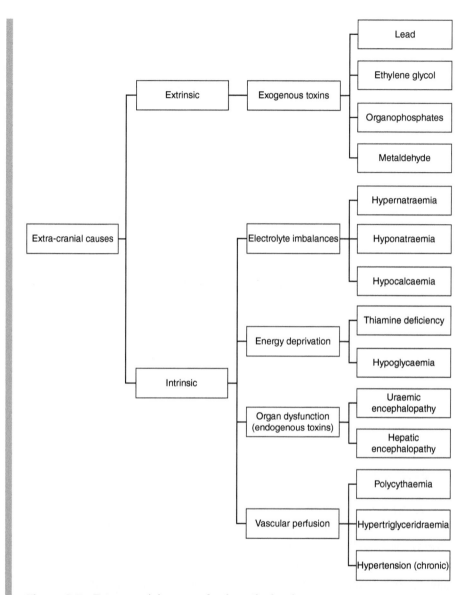

Figure 8.5 Extra-cranial causes for (reactive) seizure.

with hydrocephalus. Since metabolic and toxic disease tends to have diffuse, symmetrical effects on the brain, seizures tend to be generalized and symmetrical in onset. The lack of inter-ictal neurological deficits and clinical examination findings are the most important predictors for the diagnosis of idiopathic epilepsy. If you also

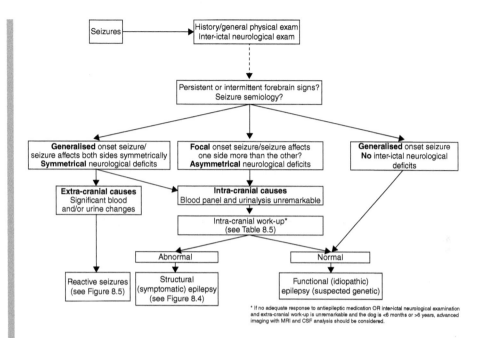

Figure 8.6 Flowchart to help define the lesion.

consider breed (especially familial history of seizures) and the age of onset (6 months–6 years), you have more than a 95% chance that idiopathic epilepsy is the cause of the seizure disorder.

Many breeds are predisposed to have epilepsy. A hereditary and familial basis for idiopathic epilepsy has been proposed in a number of breeds, including the golden retriever; Labrador retriever; Australian, German and Belgian shepherd (Tervuren); Bernese mountain dog; beagle; Irish wolfhound; English springer spaniel; keeshond; Hungarian vizsla; standard poodle; border collie and Lagotto Romagnolo. There is currently only a gene test for the Lagotto Romagnolo and Belgian Tervuren for idiopathic (genetic) epilepsy.

Extra-cranial causes

Extra-cranial causes can impair the function of the CNS and cause reactive seizures. Seizures will stop when the metabolic or toxic cause is rectified. For example:

- Reduced delivery of nutrients and/or oxygen to the brain
  - Glucose and thiamine
  - Impairment of vascular function

o Hyperviscosity syndrome (hypertriglyceridaemia and polycythaemia) and hypertension
• Changes in the internal milieu of neurons that alter their function
  o Calcium and sodium imbalances
• Exposure to extrinsic or intrinsic toxins
  o For example, metaldehyde and portosystemic shunt.

The lesion can be further defined by considering the history and
clinical examination findings. Observations more commonly reported
in seizures caused by extra-cranial metabolic disease include the
following:
• Waxing and waning clinical signs (often involving the level of
mentation)
• Chronological association of clinical signs to feeding
• Gastrointestinal disturbances
• Increased or decreased appetite
• Pica
• Hypersalivation.

Extra-cranial disease may or may not cause clinical signs in addition to seizures. Metabolic disturbances such as hyperkalaemia due
to hypoadrenocorticism and hypocalcaemia most commonly will
also cause signs of malaise, such as gastrointestinal dysfunction,
but there are occasional reports of dogs with these disorders where
seizures were the only presenting sign. Hypoglycaemia will frequently cause seizures with no other clinical signs. Confirmation of
hypoglycaemia may be problematical, as homeostatic mechanisms
(adrenaline and cortisol release) will come into play when the blood
glucose falls to a critical level and increase the blood glucose tem-
porarily. It is important to obtain a fasting blood glucose sample
when investigating metabolic causes of seizures.

The clinician should also always ensure asking the owners if
exposure to a toxin is possible. Only a few toxins can be easily identified on blood work analysis, and there are few laboratories available that can analyse samples for toxins and provide guidance for
companion animals. Good history taking is therefore essential. The
most commonly reported toxins causing seizures are lead, ethylene
glycol, organophosphates and metaldehyde.

Diagnostic approach to the patient presenting with fits or strange episodes

Your diagnostic approach will be determined by the aforementioned problem-solving path. Most of the diagnostics for diseases that present as paroxysms can be performed in general practice.

Vestibular attacks

Apart from intoxication, metabolic and nutritional causes, the differentiation of the various central vestibular diseases will usually require advanced imaging (Table 8.2). This is the most important reason for vestibular disorders to localise the lesion correctly, as it will change the work-up of the case. It is generally believed that lesion localisation has to do with determining the prognosis. However, the prognosis is determined by the diagnosed disease process, *not* by the location of the lesion.

Animals have been diagnosed with soft-tissue sarcomas invading the middle ear (poor prognosis), and conversely, dogs have been diagnosed with cerebellar infarcts causing paradoxical vestibular disease (good prognosis). Structural lesions affecting the brain parenchyma will not be seen with conventional radiography. These lesions may be mass lesions, infarcts or just areas of inflammation that will enhance on MRI with contrast. For the definitive diagnosis of inflammatory/infectious central vestibular disease, cerebrospinal fluid (CSF) evaluation is required.

Given a peripheral vestibular location, radiography of the skull with oblique views and open mouth can be considered (especially in cats), but the main investigation will be an otoscopic examination of the external ear canal and the tympanic membrane (Figure 8.7). If the potential for otitis media exists, then myringotomy is a diagnostic option, although it does require general anaesthesia. Cultures (fungal and bacterial) and cytology should be obtained from within the bullae. Cytology, in particular, will allow differentiation of active infection from normal middle ear flora, bearing in mind that the middle ear communicates with the oral cavity via the eustachian tube. Take note that the tympanic bullae of the dog are anatomically different from those of the cat. The tympanic bulla of both species contains two compartments. In the cat, there is a near-closed membrane

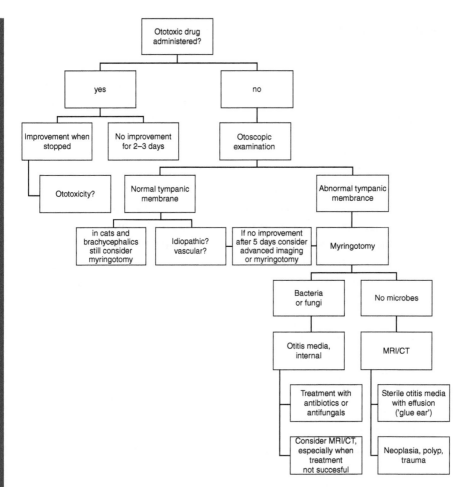

Figure 8.7 Algorithm for peripheral vestibular work-up.

between the two, whereas in the dog, both compartments communicate with each other.

Myringotomy should be performed in the ventrocaudal quadrant of the tympanic membrane where the resultant puncture in the membrane is quick to heal. Wound healing can be prolonged in patients treated with, for example, systemic glucocorticoids, or systemic disease, such as diabetes mellitus.

The vestibular attack, which can be challenging to diagnose and can be confused with seizure secondary to idiopathic epilepsy, might be a transient ischaemic vestibular attack. No pathology can be identified, and the only way to differentiate these episodes from seizures is by the presence of cardinal signs of vestibular dysfunction.

Syncope

Your physical examination findings will guide your work-up. Depending on the clinical signs and the system you have identified, following differentials and work-up need to be considered (Table 8.4).

Narcolepsy

Familial (e.g. Labrador retriever and Doberman pinscher) and sporadic forms have been described. Make sure that you ask if other animals in the litter or the breeding line have been affected. A gene test is available for the familial form, which is caused by a defect in the hypocretin receptor 2 gene. To identify the sporadic form, an intra-cranial work-up (MRI and CSF analysis) is required. Special laboratories can measure CSF hypocretin levels, which might be reduced in the sporadic form. An extra-cranial work-up needs to be considered (see the following section) if you are not completely confident that the 'strange' episode(s) observed can be explained by narcolepsy.

Paroxysmal behaviour changes and paroxysmal movement disorders

Follow the work-up scheme presented as follows for seizure disorders, especially when a trigger was not identified, there are interepisodic neurological deficits, they do not respond to medication or no genetic cause was identified.

Seizures

Most of the diagnostics for extra-cranial causes of seizures (metabolic or toxic) can be performed in first-opinion practice (detailed history, blood and urine tests, blood pressure measurements, examination of the retina [convoluted and/or dilated blood vessels, bleeding] for signs of hypertension and imaging modalities accessible in first-opinion practice such as ultrasonography; Table 8.5).

Table 8.5 Diagnostic tests to consider for dogs and cats presenting with seizures.

Extra-cranial	Intra-cranial

• Haematology
• Serum biochemical profile
• Pre- and post-prandial bile acids
• Ammonium biurate crystals (urine)/ammonia (blood)
• Urinalysis
• Blood pressure/fundus examination
• Serology/PCR, for example, *Toxoplasma gondii*, *Neospora caninum*, canine distemper, feline leukaemia virus (FeLV)/feline immunodeficiency virus (FIV), FIP, *Cryptococcus*
• Genetic characterization, for example, *Epm2b*, *LGI2,* L2-hydroxyglutaric aciduria, neuronal ceroid lipofuscinosis
• Serum lead concentration
	• Advanced imaging
	  ○ MRI
	  ○ CT
	• CSF analysis
	  ○ Cytology
	  ○ Protein
	  ○ PCR (*Toxoplasma gondii, Neospora caninum*, canine distemper virus, feline enteric coronavirus [FeCoV])
	• Electroencephalogram

The suspicion of an intra-cranial lesion usually requires advanced imaging techniques (CT or ideally MRI) and CSF analysis to help differentiate the various aetiologies. Hydrocephalus can often be diagnosed with a brain ultrasound through an open fontanelle (common in animals affected with a congenital hydrocephalus). Most infectious diseases can be tested for by serology or PCR.

Some breeds have a predisposition, genetic susceptibility or causative mutation for diseases that are or can be associated with seizures. Examples include:

- Mutation in Epm2b causing Lafora body storage disease and progressive myoclonic epilepsy described in wire-haired dachshunds, beagles and basset hounds
- L2-hydroxyglutaric aciduria in Staffordshire bull terriers
- Neuronal ceroid lipofuscinosis in border collies, English setters, Australian shepherds, American bulldogs, dachshunds, American Staffordshire and Tibetan terriers
- Gliomas in boxers
- Meningoencephalomyelitis of unknown aetiology in certain terrier breeds.

In conclusion

Syncope, narcolepsy/cataplexy, pain, compulsive behaviour disorders, vestibular attacks, certain movement disorders, neuromuscular weakness and seizures are paroxysmal events that share some commonalities in clinical presentation, but using a stepwise approach, you will not only be able to differentiate these episodes but also be able to determine the most likely diagnosis.

Key points

As a result of reading this chapter you should be able to:
- Recognise the importance of clearly defining the problem by taking a detailed history and conducting a thorough clinical examination to differentiate paroxysmal episodes
- Recognise that 'thinking pathophysiologically' is essential to rank in appropriate order the body systems under consideration
- Recognise that 'thinking pathophysiologically' and using the five-finger rule can help you narrow down your differential list
- Recognise that by following this approach, many diseases can be diagnosed in first-opinion practice.

Questions for review

- How can the owner's description of pre-, inter- and post-episodic time period help me in differentiating the various paroxysmal episodes?
- How can my understanding of the five-finger rule help me differentiate pathologies?

Case example

- 'Poppy' is a 3-year-old female neutered Labrador retriever. Poppy had a history of having three fits over the previous week. Fits were described as rhythmic movements of all limbs accompanied by hypersalivation. She was on her side during the episode, fits lasted around a minute or 2 and she appeared dazed for up to an hour afterwards. No triggers or changes were noted prior to the episode. She was unable to look the owner in the eye during the episode, and she did not come to the owners when called. The most recent fit occurred 12 hours ago.

- During the consult "Poppy" started to have left facial twitching.
- Poppy has been up to date with vaccination and worming. She has not had any other problems in the past.
- Her appetite has been slightly reduced, no vomiting or diarrhoea has been noted and her water intake is unchanged.

Define the problem

- Poppy's problem is defined as epileptic seizures and can further be defined as subacute, episodic, lateralising, recurrent focal seizure disorder with secondary generalisation.
- Epileptic seizures are most likely, as she showed rhythmic movement during the episode, episodes last 1-2 minutes, consciousness is impaired and autonomic signs and a post-ictal period are present.

Define the system

- Epileptic seizures always have their origin in the CNS, specifically in the forebrain. The forebrain can be affected primarily or secondarily. As the dog had a witnessed asymmetrical/lateralized epileptic seizure affecting the left side of its face, there is a high chance of the dog having a right forebrain lesion and therefore structural epilepsy.
- A neurological examination remains important to help re-assess the system +/- location +/- differentiate focal from multifocal disease processes.
- Neurological examination findings:
- Mentation: unremarkable quality and level
- Posture/gait: unremarkable
- Postural reactions: unremarkable
- Cranial nerves: reduced menace response on the left side
- Good facial sensation
- Spinal reflexes: intact
- Palpation: unremarkable.
- Nociception: not tested as appears to have good sensation.

Define the location

The neurological examination confirms that the lesion affects mainly the right forebrain.

Define the lesion

We can summarise our findings with the five-finger rule as subacute, episodic, non-painful, asymmetrical forebrain disorder. The differential diagnoses list can be narrowed down to:

1. Anomaly (porencephaly, cortical dysplasia,. . .)

    Advanced imaging would be needed unless the animal has an open fontanelle, then you can use an ultrasound probe.

2. Inflammatory/infectious
    - CSF tap.
    - Use CSF and/or blood for PCR for *Toxoplasma gondii*, *Neospora caninum* and canine distemper virus or you can do a Toxoplasma IgG/M, neospora titre or/and an LCAT for *Cryptoccocus* (depending where you live).
    - Otherwise, advanced imaging – ideally MRI.

3. Neoplasia
    - Check for generalised lymphoma.
    - Check for other tumours such as haemangiosarcoma.
    - Otherwise, advanced imaging – best, MRI.

4. Vascular – a possibility but less likely.

    Listen to the heart to make sure there is no heart murmur – might indicate vegetation.

    Check for coagulopathies and potential lung-worm infection.

    Otherwise, advanced imaging – ideally MRI.

Case outcome

To evaluate general health status, haematology and biochemistry were run, which were unremarkable.

CSF tap revealed a pleocytosis of 20 cells/ μL (normal <5 cells/ μL), which was mainly mononuclear. Protein levels were also elevated 0.5 g/l (normal <0.25 g/l). An MRI was not performed due to client cost constraints.

Tests for infectious agents were unremarkable, and an inflammatory brain disease was suspected. Poppy was treated with immunomodulatory drugs and anti-seizure medication, which she responded well to.

CHAPTER 9

Sneezing, coughing and dyspnoea

David B. Church

Department of Clinical Science and Services, The Royal Veterinary College, London, UK

The why

- Certain clinical signs commonly observed in veterinary practice can be considered characteristic or typical of compromised respiratory function.
- These include sneezing and nasal discharge, coughing and dyspnoea/tachypnoea.
- Respiratory signs can be due to primary disorders of the respiratory tract or disorders outside of the respiratory tract that compromise respiratory function.
- A logical approach that defines the problem and the location within the respiratory tract is essential to help determine whether the problem is a result of primary respiratory pathology or secondary to malfunctioning of another body system.
- Of particular relevance in small animal practice is the relationship between the cardiovascular and respiratory systems because of the relatively common occurrence of cardiac disease, which may or may not be compromising respiratory function.

Introduction

Diseases that alter respiratory function can be classified as primary or secondary respiratory problems. Primary problems of the respiratory system (e.g. neoplasia, bronchiectasis, laryngeal collapse, etc.) usually result in structural changes to a specific part of the respira-

Clinical Reasoning in Veterinary Practice: Problem Solved!, Second Edition.
Edited by Jill E. Maddison, Holger A. Volk and David B. Church.
© 2022 John Wiley & Sons Ltd. Published 2022 by John Wiley & Sons Ltd.

tory tract. Often the clinical signs can provide clues as to which part of the respiratory tract is compromised.

A traditional approach to determining what part of the respiratory tract is involved has been based on 'upper' or 'lower' respiratory problems. Unfortunately, there is no clear agreement as to where this division exists. The author believes a more helpful delineation is based on compartmentalising the respiratory system into five broad areas:

1 Nasal cavity, cranial sinuses and the cranial oropharynx
2 Caudal oropharynx and larynx
3 Trachea and larger airways
4 Smaller airways and alveoli
5 The pleural space.

Respiratory function can also be affected by secondary respiratory disorders, in other words, dysfunction of the respiratory system caused by malfunction of another body system. This situation may result in altered structure of the respiratory tract (e.g. pulmonary oedema due to left-sided heart failure) or may simply produce derangements that alter respiratory function without directly affecting the respiratory system's structures at all (e.g. tachypnoea or dyspnoea in a severely anaemic animal).

Similar to the logical approach to diarrhoea, where definition of location in the GI tract can assist in defining the system, definition of the problem and location for patients who are sneezing, coughing or dyspnoeic can help resolve the essential generic question, *What system is involved and how is it involved?*

To aid in determining what part or parts of the respiratory tract are involved, it can be helpful to think of the problems as:

• Sneezing and nasal discharge
• Coughing with minimal dyspnoea
• Dyspnoea with minimal coughing
• Coughing with dyspnoea.

As mentioned, it is important to differentiate primary from secondary causes of respiratory dysfunction as well as to recognise respiratory dysfunction may be part of a broader, multisystem disorder such as a viral or fungal infection or multisystem neoplasia.

Sneezing and Nasal Discharge

 Define the location

Sneezing and nasal discharge are typically signs of disease affecting the nasal cavity, the nasal sinuses, the cranial oropharynx and the dental arcade. On rare occasions when a disorder is both erosive and sufficiently well established, lesions of the hard palate may also result in nasal discharge and sneezing.

 Define and refine the problem

The clinical signs of nasal disease are principally excessive snorting or sneezing with nasal discharge that may have varying consistencies, contain various amounts of blood (epistaxis) and be either unilateral or bilateral. Ulceration or excoriation of the nares, discharging sinuses from the maxillary bones forming the lateral walls of the nasal cavity or irritation of parts of the nasal cavity are uncommon findings but generally significant when present. Less commonly, distortions of the bones surrounding or adjacent to the nasal cavity may be detected as well as increased prominence of one or both ocular globes.

It is important to note the character of the nasal discharge if present, as this may assist in determining the diagnostic approach and potential differentials. Nasal discharge may be serous, bloody (epistaxis) or mucopurulent or may be a combination of these.

Patients with primary nasal disease generally do not cough or wheeze. Dogs will also not have significant dyspnoea unless forced to breathe through their nose as occurs when they sleep in positions that result in their mouth being closed. While their nasal cavity may be totally occluded with no air movement evident at the external nares, this will not result in dyspnoea unless their mouth is forced closed, as they will accommodate readily by breathing through their open mouth.

Cats seem to be far less comfortable in breathing through their mouth, hence nasal cavity obstruction in the cat may also result in degrees of dyspnoea, although when the nasal disease is this severe, the clinical picture is generally dominated by the discharge and sneezing, which focuses attention on the nasal cavity as the part of the respiratory tract primarily affected.

Define and refine the system

Sneezing is a coordinated protective respiratory reflex that arises due to stimulation of the upper respiratory tract, particularly the nasal cavity. The cause may be local disease or systemic disease causing nasal irritation and inflammation, for example, respiratory viruses, allergic rhinitis.

Sneezing may be associated with a nasal discharge or a nasal discharge may present without sneezing. Broadly speaking, a serous nasal discharge is most consistent with a systemic cause such as viral disease or allergy; a mucopurulent disease indicates bacterial infection (almost always secondary in the dog and cat) that may be due to local or systemic disease; epistaxis may be due to local disease or systemic disease (discussed further in Chapter 12).

Whether the discharge is unilateral or bilateral may assist in determining if the pathology is local and confined to the nasal cavity or systemic. Unilateral mucopurulent or haemorrhagic nasal discharge supports the presence of local nasal disease, although a systemic cause of epistaxis (e.g. coagulopathy) cannot be ruled out.

Other evidence that supports local nasal pathology is signs of facial/nasal distortion (neoplasia) and ulceration of the nares (fungal).

Define the lesion

Inflammatory nasal disease may occur as part of a systemic infection, for example, calicivirus or herpes infection in cats or a systemic allergic reaction. Or it may occur due to a local pathology.

With local nasal problems, it is important to ascertain if the problem is acute or chronic, as many acute problems such as inhalation of irritants like dust and sand resolve with minimal, if any, therapy.

Chronic nasal discharge +/– sneezing may be due to

- A nasal foreign body
- Fungal disease, for example:
  - Aspergillosis (dog)
    - Due to the fungi's tendency to cause vasculitis and secondary ischaemic necrosis, infection tends to result in turbinate destruction and loss of intra-nasal structures.

- The most common clinical signs are chronic, profuse, san-guinopurulent nasal discharge with sneezing and epistaxis.
- The severity of the nasal discharge helps to differentiate this condition from nasal neoplasia, where the discharge tends to be less voluminous and often not quite as haemorrhagic or have had a longer period of prior non-haemorrhagic nasal discharge.
- Discomfort around the nostrils, mouth or bridge of the nose and face is commonly encountered, as are excoriations of the external nares. These superficial abnormalities are uncommon in nasal neoplasia.
  - Cryptococcosis (cat)
    - Infection usually involves the nasal cavity.
    - Skin, subcutis and the central nervous system have been implicated as additional common sites for infection.
    - However, the vast majority of animals with cryptococcosis have nasal disease as the predominant clinical feature.
- A tooth root abscess that has become continuous with the maxillary sinus and thus indirectly the nasal cavity or the nasal cavity itself
- Neoplasia within the nasal cavity, the mouth or the cranial oropharynx
  - Nasal neoplasms commonly include squamous cell carcinoma, fibrosarcoma, lymphoma and various adenocarcinomas.
  - Most nasal tumours in dogs and cats are malignant, and prognosis is poor (except perhaps nasal lymphoma in cats).
- Non-infectious inflammatory disease – lymphocytic/plasmacytic rhinitis or allergic rhinitis
- Nasopharyngeal polyps
  - These are benign growths that have been mainly reported in kittens and young adult cats.
  - The clinical signs are usually referable to upper airway obstruction, noisy breathing and serous to mucopurulent nasal discharge.

Diagnostic approach

Patients with structural nasal discharge are likely to require the following diagnostic procedures:

- Imaging of the nasal cavity, sinuses and oropharynx

- o Diagnostic precision is substantially enhanced if computed tomography (CT) imaging can be used, although if not available, standard radiological views may be helpful in a proportion of cases.
- Rhinoscopy – both antegrade and retrograde views are essential
- Nasal biopsies
- Serology and/or culture for specific pathogens such as *Cryptococcus* (LCAT rather than lateral flow testing). Remember *Aspergillus* is a commensal of the nasal cavity of dogs so its presence on a nasal culture cannot be considered significant.

In general, the use of nasal washings and standard bacterial cultures is of little, if any, value, as primary bacterial inflammation of the nasal cavity is almost never encountered.

In view of the invasive nature of these procedures and/or the need for significant immobilisation, it is most practical to perform all of the procedures at one time, avoiding multiple anaesthetics. Unsurprisingly, imaging should be performed before any interventions are undertaken.

COUGHING

 ## Define the problem

The act of coughing is a forced expiratory effort against an initially closed glottis that then opens, resulting in the explosive release of air from the lungs through the larynx and mouth. There is generally an initial increased inspiration before the cough allowing the respiratory muscles to work to greater mechanical advantage.

Coughing is usually easily recognised by owners and unlikely to be confused with another clinical sign. However, as mentioned in Chapter 3, gagging after vomiting or regurgitation may be interpreted by owners as coughing, so this is an occasional source of confusion. Conversely, animals may retch after coughing, and the owner may therefore think the problem is vomiting.

At this stage let's review our understanding of why animals cough. The cough reflex is initiated by irritant and mechanical receptors located predominantly in the trachea and major bronchi. There are fewer cough receptors in the smaller bronchi, and they are absent beyond the bronchioles. The receptors can be activated by irritation from mucus, dust, foreign material or chemical irritation, as well as sudden or marked changes in airway lumen diameter resulting in accelerated airflow. Coughing is therefore likely to be associated with respiratory pathology of the trachea and airways but not when there is pathology of other parts of the respiratory tract without involvement of the airways (e.g. laryngeal disease or the early stages of progressive pulmonary fibrosis).

Refining the problem

Coughing may or may not be associated with dyspnoea. This is an important clinical distinction as the location of the pathology within the respiratory tract in a patient that is coughing with no or minimal dyspnoea is often different from the location of the pathology in a patient that is coughing *and* dyspnoeic.

Haemoptysis

Haemoptysis refers to the expectoration of bloody material – that is, coughing up blood. It confirms the presence of significant structural bronchoalveolar disease and is most commonly associated with severe inflammatory disease secondary to such parasitic infestations as Dirofilariasis or Angiostrongylosis, neoplasia and coagulopathies, for example, due to rat bait toxicity.

Coughing with minimal dyspnoea

 Define the location (and system)

Coughing with minimal dyspnoea is generally associated with tracheal or large airway disease. The system involved is always primary respiratory. Disorders of these structures often produce coughing that has a harsh 'hacking' sound, will frequently occur in paroxysms and may be followed by retching.

Many of the disorders that affect the trachea and large airways will not be associated with dyspnoea as it is difficult to significantly occlude the lumen of these relatively wide airways. There is one notable exception however – tracheal hypoplasia. This is a congenital malformation of the trachea that results in a significant narrowing of the trachea generally starting at the thoracic inlet and mainly affecting varying amounts of the cranial intra-thoracic trachea. The reduction in luminal diameter can be dramatic and result in varying degrees of dyspnoea. Tracheal hypoplasia can be one component of the so-called BOAS complex (brachycephalic obstructive airway syndrome) and as such has been reported to be overrepresented in a number of brachycephalic breeds as well as Rhodesian ridgebacks.

Additionally, while disorders that affect the bronchi may be associated with coughing and minimal dyspnoea, certain bronchial disorders may be more likely to produce coughing *and* dyspnoea or, when active bronchoconstriction is present (cats but rarely dogs), dyspnoea with minimal coughing.

In other words, depending on the type of lesion, bronchial disease may present with predominantly coughing, predominantly dyspnoea or both.

In cats in particular, inflammation of the airways due to various hypersensitivities produces inflammation and varying degrees of bronchospasm. The latter results in dyspnoea that is usually expiratory.

 Define the lesion

As previously mentioned, disorders of the trachea and large bronchi usually result in coughing with minimal dyspnoea. While coughing with minimal dyspnoea suggests tracheal involvement and possibly bronchial disorders with no or minimal luminal narrowing, various disorders of the smaller bronchi may also cause a significant amount of dyspnoea. As thoracic respiratory sounds are predominantly generated by airflow in the airways, whenever bronchial disease is present thoracic auscultation invariably results in increased levels of audible wheezes and crackles.

The most common types of pathology affecting the trachea and bronchi include:

- Inflammation
  - In the dog inflammatory disorders rarely produce bronchoconstriction and may or may not be particularly exudative. Causes include:

- Infectious causes – the most common is infectious tracheobronchitis or 'kennel cough', a result of a mixture of viral and bacterial agents that albeit clinically dramatic tends to be self-limiting.
  - Non-infectious causes such as immune-mediated disease.
  o In the cat inflammatory disorders are most commonly immune-mediated with possibly secondary infectious agents further compromising function.
    - Because of the release of specific cytokines, inflammatory bronchial disorders can result in varying degrees of bronchoconstriction and/or exudative inflammation.
    - Cats with bronchial disease can subsequently present with predominantly coughing, predominantly dyspnoea or both.
- Degenerative disorders
  o Most commonly seen in toy and small breed dogs where variably progressive chondromalacia results in tracheal and/or bronchial collapse.
  o This will be characterised by persistent coughing and, at least initially, minimal dyspnoea.
  o The coughing is caused by altered airflow and increased turbulence because of the deformity of the airway lumen as well as the increased compliance, meaning on inspiration and expiration luminal narrowing results in opposing airway surfaces touching and activating cough receptors.
- Neoplasia
  o Neoplasia of the airways is generally carcinoma and tends to produce coughing with minimal dyspnoea – at least initially.
- Malformations
  o These include, for example, tracheal hypoplasia, bronchiectasis and ciliary dyskinesia.

Diagnostic approach

Confirming a number of these disorders will require cytology obtained either from a transtracheal aspirate, bronchial wash or bronchoalveolar lavage. Thoracic radiology may be of limited value. While there may be indications of increased radiodensity of the airways (a so-called 'bronchial pattern'), this may not always be apparent. In many cases of symptomatic allergic bronchospasm, the airways will be difficult to find due to general pulmonary over-inflation. Also, in many cases of 'dynamic airway disease' (or so-called 'collapsing trachea'), diagnosis requires either flouroscopy or endoscopy (although rarely both) as airway collapse can usually only be demonstrated when the patient coughs – an action not conducive to obtaining a good radiograph.

DYSPNOEA

 Define the problem

Increased respiratory effort (dyspnoea and/or tachypnoea) indicates impaired oxygen exchange due to either reduced delivery of air to the alveoli (pathology affecting the respiratory tract) or impaired delivery of appropriately unoxygenated haemoglobin to the alveoli. This impaired delivery of unoxygenated haemoglobin can be a result of either *reduced* pulmonary arterial *perfusion* of *normal* levels of *unoxygenated* haemoglobin or *normal perfusion* of *reduced* levels of *unoxygenated* haemoglobin.

Dyspnoea can be characterised as being expiratory dyspnoea (the effort in breathing occurs with exhalation) or inspiratory dyspnoea (the effort of breathing occurs with inspiration). This classification can assist in localising the lesion – expiratory dyspnoea occurs with intra-thoracic disease; inspiratory dyspnoea occurs with laryngeal disease and occasional large airway pathology such as tracheal hypoplasia.

The problem of dyspnoea can also be further refined by determining whether it is associated with significant coughing or associated with no or minimal/inconsequential coughing.

Coughing *and* dyspnoea

 Define the location

Coughing accompanied by dyspnoea is most often a reflection of certain forms of bronchial disease with varying degrees of alveolar disease. In contrast to laryngeal disease, where the dyspnoea tends to be more inspiratory, the dyspnoea associated with bronchopulmonary disease tends to be most notable on expiration or throughout inspiration and expiration.

Bronchoalveolar problems that produce coughing and dyspnoea may also result in excessive amounts of fluid (mucus, exudate, oedema fluid or blood) within the alveoli and airways. The fluid means the coughing tends to have a moist sound and results in the fluid from the airways being delivered to the oral cavity. Usually, the animals demonstrably swallow the material. Rarely, expectoration occurs and can be confused with vomiting.

The presence of this material lining airways will reduce airway diameter and increase turbulent airflow in the airways (which may be exacerbated by increased respiratory effort). This increased turbulence results in increased thoracic respiratory sounds. Almost all dyspnoeic animals with bronchoalveolar disease will have abnormalities on thoracic auscultation heard most prominently over the affected area(s) of the thorax.

Normal lung sounds

Normally thoracic auscultation reveals bronchial and vesicular sounds.
- Bronchial sounds are tubular sounds similar to those heard over the trachea and are more prominent in the hilar areas.
- Vesicular sounds are likened to 'wind through the trees', are softer and are heard more peripherally.

Abnormal lung sounds

Abnormal lungs sounds are described as crackles or wheezes.

- *Crackles* are non-musical, discontinuous noises similar to cellophane being 'crumpled' or bubble-wrap 'popping'.
  - Crackles are usually associated with alveolar abnormalities with secondary exudate/oedema within airways.
- *Wheezes* are more musical, continuous high-pitched whistling sounds.
  - Wheezes suggest narrowing of airway diameters through the presence of excessive amounts of material such as exudate, thickening of the airway walls, active bronchoconstriction or increased compliance of the airways resulting in their collapse whenever there is a significant increase in intra-thoracic pressure (e.g. with expiration) or various combinations of all of the above.

Define the system – coughing –/– dyspnoea

Coughing and dyspnoea can be due to primary respiratory pathology or secondary pathology e.g. pathology outside of the respiratory system that has caused changes within it. The main example of this is congestive heart failure causing pulmonary oedema.

Define the lesion – coughing +/– dyspnoea

The disorders of the airways that can cause coughing as well as dyspnoea are bronchoconstrictive disorders and bronchoalveolar disease. Bronchoconstrictive disorders may also present as dyspnoea *without* coughing, and these are discussed in more detail in the next section.

Bronchoalveolar disease
Most patient with bronchoalveolar disease have coughing accompanied by dyspnoea (either during expiration or throughout the respiratory cycle).
   Causes of bronchoalveolar disease include:

- Inflammation (infectious)
  - Infectious causes include bacterial and in certain geographic areas fungal aetiologies.
  - As a general rule, bacterial inflammatory bronchoalveolar disease is likely to be secondary to a significant inciting event, such as an inhaled foreign body or aspiration secondary to oesophageal dysfunction.
- Inflammation (non-infectious)
  - Non-infectious immune-mediated inflammation may have an allergic aetiology, although the underlying cause is often ill-defined.
- Parasitic
  - *Dirofilaria immitis*.
  - *Angiostrongylus vasorum* (dogs).
  - *Aelurostrongylus abstrusus* and *Eucoleus aerophilus* (cats).
- Congestion and oedema
  - This is most commonly a result of left atrial hypertension and resultant pulmonary venous hypertension.
  - The most common causes in small animal practice are the acquired cardiac disorders myxomatous degenerative mitral valve disease, dilated cardiomyopathy and hypertrophic cardiomyopathy.
  - Pulmonary oedema may also occur with high-output cardiac disease (as seen in various congenital abnormalities) and with

increased pulmonary vascular permeability as is seen with adult respiratory distress syndrome where abnormalities in permeability occur as a result of damage to alveolar epithelial and microvascular barriers.

- Neoplasia
  - Primary pulmonary tumours, metastatic neoplasia and multicentric neoplasia can all involve pulmonary parenchyma.
  - Most primary pulmonary tumours that are malignant metastases are not common in the early phases of the disease; consequently, complete surgical removal provides an opportunity for a significant postoperative period of remission.
  - Clinical signs are usually chronic and slowly progressive, although peracute manifestations may occur with complications such as pneumothorax or thromboembolism.
- Emphysema.

Diagnostic procedures

Patients with coughing accompanied by dyspnoea usually require some combination of the following diagnostic procedures for further elucidation of their bronchopulmonary disease:

- Thoracic radiography
  - Inflammatory pulmonary parenchymal disease generally results in exudative inflammation. The exudate fills the alveoli with fluid, resulting in increased radio-opacity of the pulmonary parenchyma. As the small airways located adjacent to these fluid-filled alveoli still contain air, the characteristic appearance is of fluffy white areas with black lines running through these white areas – a so-called 'alveolar pattern' of increased pulmonary radio-opacity. In more severe cases there may also be areas of consolidation, which is frequently more severe in the dependent regions.
  - In patients with pulmonary neoplasia, thoracic radiography frequently reveals focal areas of increased radiodensity with obliteration of all underlying structures. Margins are often distinct, and cavitation may be present. Metastatic or multicentric disease tends to result in a diffuse interstitial pattern with or without nodular changes.
- CT
- Transtracheal washings

- o In a proportion of cases, transtracheal aspirate provides a definitive diagnosis. Its advantages are that it can be performed with the animal awake (although usually sedated) and produces an uncontaminated sample. The disadvantage of this procedure is that the yield can be disappointing and thus non-diagnostic.
- Bronchial washings or bronchoalveolar lavage
  - o This process generally provides the most information about the process and its underlying aetiology; however, it requires general anaesthesia, which of course is not necessarily an attractive option in a patient with significant thoracic disease.
- Haematology and C-reactive protein
  - o A peripheral leukogram may reflect an inflammatory, allergic or parasitic process although a normal leukogram does not preclude a significant inflammatory disease. In dogs, a reliable indication of the latter can frequently be gained by determining the patient's serum C-reactive protein concentration.
- Transthoracic pulmonary aspirates
- 'Systemic' tests for both primary and secondary causes of structural bronchopulmonary disease
  - o These might include sampling for various primary causes for structural disease such as serology for *Dirofilaria immitis* or faecal examination for *Angiostrongylus* larvae or for a secondary cause of structural bronchopulmonary disease such as cardiac disease resulting in heart failure and pulmonary congestion and oedema (estimating N-terminal pro-B type natriuretic peptide: NT-pro-BNP).
- Arterial blood gas analysis
- Thoracoscopy and/or open-chest lung biopsy.

Dyspnoea with minimal coughing

Define the system

Dyspnoea with minimal coughing can be due to primary respiratory disorders affecting the larynx and intra-thoracic structures (resulting in reduced delivery of oxygen to the alveoli) or primary or secondary disorders resulting in impaired delivery of unoxygenated haemoglobin to normally aerated alveoli.

Define the location

Patients with dyspnoea and/or tachypnoea and minimal coughing will have impaired oxygen exchange in their alveoli in the absence of significant airway disease. Only rarely do animals with predominantly tracheobronchial disease present with dyspnoea as a major problem, and almost all of these patients will have coughing as a prominent concurrent sign.

The parts of the respiratory tract likely to be involved in primary respiratory disease causing impaired alveolar ventilation and not involving the airways (thus causing dyspnoea with minimal coughing) are going to fall into two fairly broad categories:

- Those with dyspnoea and minimal coughing produced by laryngeal dysfunction
- Those with dyspnoea and minimal coughing produced by various intra-thoracic abnormalities
  - Space-occupying disorders of the pleural cavity
  - Constrictive bronchial inflammation
  - Primary alveolar disorders.

Initial differentiation of these two broad regions of the respiratory tract is essential if the most effective diagnostic aids are to be used. This differentiation is best achieved, at least initially, through auscultation.

By localising the area where the respiratory sounds are most audible, it is often possible to differentiate laryngeal from intra-thoracic causes of dyspnoea. Furthermore, laryngeal dysfunction may produce a stridor (high-pitched sound heard during inspiration) as well as dysphonia and occasionally deglutition problems.

More severe cases with laryngeal dysfunction may develop cyanosis and respiratory distress. The respiratory distress is a result of upper airway obstruction. Typically, it occurs during inspiration as negative intra-airway pressures tend to suck surrounding tissues into the airway lumen. Expiration is often rapid and effortless.

Key points
- Dyspnoea with minimal coughing suggests laryngeal or various forms of intra-thoracic disease.

- Patients with *laryngeal* dysfunction have predominantly *inspiratory* dyspnoea and *rarely cough unless there is secondary tracheal irritation*.
- Patients with various forms of *intra-thoracic* disease are more likely to have *expiratory* dyspnoea.

Dyspnoea without coughing can also be due to secondary disorders where the cause of the dysfunction lies outside the respiratory system. Examples of secondary disorders include cardiac disease and pulmonary thromboembolism.

 ## Define the lesion – laryngeal disorders

Laryngeal disorders commonly encountered in companion animal practice can be broadly classified as:
- Inflammatory
  - Most commonly associated with feline viral infections
- Malformations
  - Such as seen with the BOAS complex of abnormalities in brachycephalic dogs
- Degenerative
  - Most commonly seen in severe cases of chondromalacia and hence accompanying so-called 'collapsing trachea'
- Neoplastic
  - Most commonly lymphoid malignancies in cats and adenocarcinomas in cats and dogs
- Paresis
  - May be affecting laryngeal innervation only as seen on older large breed dogs or be part of a more generalised neuropathy.

Diagnostic procedures

Cases with suspected primary laryngeal disease require thorough inspection of the caudal pharynx and larynx (laryngoscopy). Laryngoscopy allows visualisation of the larynx and pharynx for assessment of structural and functional abnormalities of the arytenoid cartilages and vocal cords. As functional problems need to be considered, *restraint without pharmacological modification of laryngeal function is imperative*.

Appropriate sedation

Generally, a light dose (2-4 mg/kg) of propofol given to effect is a reliable means of avoiding anaesthetic-induced 'excitement' and examining the area thoroughly in a suitably tractable patient. Both a laryngoscope and a small rigid endoscope help in illuminating the region and enhancing visualisation. The animal should be in sternal recumbency to minimise any asymmetry due to positioning.

Once laryngeal function has been assessed, anaesthesia should be deepened and the caudal pharynx and larynx examined for structural abnormalities, foreign bodies or tumours and, where appropriate, samples obtained for histopathology.

It should be remembered that prolonged upper airway obstruction results in the soft tissues being 'pulled' into the lumen by increased negative pressure. Eversion of the laryngeal saccules, thickening and elongation of the soft palate and inflammation with thickening of the pharyngeal and laryngeal mucosa can occur. The laryngeal cartilages can become soft and deformed, and in severe cases they will collapse medially, virtually occluding airflow.

Define the lesion – space-occupying disorders of the pleural cavity

When there are clinically significant amounts of material in the pleural space, although there is increased movement of the chest wall, the lungs are frequently not expanding normally, reducing the velocity of airflow and the volume of air and oxygen delivered to the alveoli and available for exchange.

While the patient will have dyspnoea, the reduced airflow (remember thoracic respiratory sounds are produced by the airflow in the small and large airways) together with the greater distance between the airways and the chest wall combine to produce reduced thoracic respiratory sounds for the degree of thoracic excursion, sometimes described as 'muffled' respiratory sounds.

Space-occupying disorders of the pleural cavity can be attributed to the presence of significant amounts of air, fluid (blood, chyle, transudates and exudates - see Chapter 6 for more information about transudates and exudates) as well as ectopic normal abdominal organs (because of disruption of the diaphragm) or neoplasms.

Common causes of pleural effusion include:

- Pyothorax
- Chylothorax
- Heart failure (right sided in dogs, left or right sided in cats)
- Neoplasia
- Diaphragmatic hernia.

Pleural fluid characterisation can be clarifying in determining possible causes.

- An inflammatory exudate suggests a primary inflammatory process.
- Transudates are usually a result of either increased systemic venous pressure or decreased oncotic pressure, although the latter is usually associated with generalised oedema.
  - As a result, they generally indicate respiratory dysfunction secondary to a problem in another body system.
  - In dogs increased systemic venous pressures tend to suggest some form of right atrial hypertension and right-sided heart failure.
  - However, in cats thoracic transudates and chylous effusions can also occur as a result of increased left atrial pressure, presumably because a number of the pleural veins drain into the left atrium rather than the right.
- Chylous effusions can also develop as a result of increased systemic venous pressure or lack of integrity of some part of the thoracic lymphatic system.

Diagnostic approach

In patients with suspected pleural disorders, thoracic imaging can help clarify whether the problem is air, fluid or tissue.

While cytology and general fluid analysis can be helpful in determining possible causes for the thoracic effusion, ultrasonography is likely to be the most rewarding diagnostic aid in clarifying potentially displaced normal or simply abnormal structures present in the thoracic cavity. This is particularly true if there is some pleural effusion to increase the acoustic window. The detection of abnormal structures within the pleural cavity should be further evaluated by fine-needle aspirates whenever possible.

Thoracocentesis is another valuable aid in determining the nature and possible aetiology of the pleural fluid. However, it should always be remembered that any pleural effusion is likely to produce bizarre reactive mesothelial cells that may be mistaken for poorly differentiated neoplastic cells.

Should I remove the fluid?

As a broad guide, compromised respiratory function is only going to be seen once the volume of pleural fluid exceeds 30–50 ml/kg. In some severely affected individuals, removal of pleural fluid may significantly improve the respiratory reserve, and this should be considered once thoracic ultrasonography has been performed. Fluid removal may also provide improved radiological definition of the pleural structures. Significant amounts of pleural fluid are most conveniently and thoroughly removed using surgically implanted chest drains.

 Define the lesion – constrictive bronchial inflammation

As stated above, while many bronchial disorders will result in coughing, few are likely to result in dyspnoea with minimal coughing.

The one notable exception to this generalisation is those disorders of the smaller bronchii characterised by marked bronchoconstriction. Because the overall diameter of the bronchial system will be reduced and decrease oxygen delivery to the alveoli, these animals will have dyspnoea as a marked clinical characteristic, and if the cause for the bronchoconstriction does not illicit an exudative response, cough receptor activation can be marginal and there will be minimal coughing. However, if there is an exudative response, these patients will also cough. Due to the turbulence in airflow created by the luminal narrowing, patients will have dramatically increased airway sounds and hence increased thoracic respiratory sounds, which are frequently generalised.

By far the most common type of pathology resulting in generalised narrowing of the diameter of the bronchial tree is the constrictive inflammation seen as a result of the release of various inflammatory cytokines, which stimulate bronchoconstriction.

Interestingly, this is almost never seen in dogs, as they generally do not release 'bronchonconstricting cytokines' in response to airway inflammation. Hence, most dogs with bronchial inflammation will not be characterised by bronchoconstriction and present with coughing as their major clinical sign. In contrast, cats with bronchial disease may have coughing with minimal dyspnoea or dyspnoea with minimal coughing or, of course, both coughing and dyspnoea.

Diagnostic approach

Diagnostic procedures that may be helpful include:
- Thoracic imaging - thoracic radiology or CT
  - However, as dyspnoea with minimal coughing due to bronchial disease is likely to be predominantly constrictive inflammation with minimal exudate present, the chest is likely to appear normal regardless of the imaging modality.
  - Indeed, with standard thoracic radiography, the airways may be difficult to find due to general pulmonary over-inflation.
  - However, the presence of a normal thoracic radiograph in a dyspnoeic cat with minimal coughing, normal laryngeal and cardiac auscultation and generalised, increased thoracic respiratory sounds is strongly suggestive of constrictive bronchial inflammation.
- Transtracheal aspirate
- Bronchial wash/bronchoalveolar lavage
- Haematology looking for a degree of eosinophilia.

 ## Define the lesion – primary alveolar disease

Patients with degenerative disorders of the respiratory tract that primarily affect the alveoli and spare the bronchi will also present with dyspnoea and minimal coughing, as they will have reduced surface areas for oxygen exchange but no significant damage to their airways.

Pathology primarily affecting the alveoli is uncommon but includes degenerative pulmonary fibrosis.

Define the lesion – secondary disorders

When compromised alveolar oxygen exchange is due to impaired delivery of appropriately unoxygenated haemoglobin to the alveoli, this can be a result of either *reduced delivery of normal haemoglobin* or *normal delivery of abnormal haemoglobin*. In either case the patient is likely to be dyspnoeic with minimal coughing, as oxygen exchange is compromised in a patient with normal airways.

Reduced delivery of normal haemoglobin

The secondary disorders that can result in reduced delivery of normal haemoglobin include:
- Any cardiac disorder that results in clinically significant impaired cardiac output
  - This is the reason why one of the markers of adequate control of patients with congestive heart failure is a resting respiratory rate of less than 30 breaths per minute.
- Pulmonary thromboembolic disease
- Pulmonary oedema.

Pulmonary thromboembolism

Thromboemboli generally form as a result of disease in organs other than the lungs. Circulating emboli such as bacteria, fat, air, parasites and circulating parts of thrombi from elsewhere in the body can be trapped in the pulmonary vascular system.

Thrombi can develop within vessels as a result of:
- Venous stasis
- Turbulent blood flow
- Endothelial damage
- Systemic hypercoagulability.

The most common conditions associated with clinically significant thromboembolism include:
- Dirofilariasis (in regions where this disease is endemic)
- Glomerulopathies with urinary protein loss and hence loss of antithrombin 3
- Immune-mediated haemolytic anaemia
- Cushing's syndrome.

Clinical signs

The sudden onset of hypoxia produces peracute dyspnoea and tachypnoea. Occasionally coughing or abnormal lung sounds are present. In cases with recurrent disease there may be right cardiomegaly or split-second heart sounds; evidence for pulmonary hypertension.

Diagnosis

Diagnosis is based on thoracic radiography, angiography and nuclear scintigraphy. In many cases of pulmonary thromboembolism thoracic radiographs are normal despite severe respiratory signs and blood gas evidence for marked ventilation-perfusion abnormalities. Such inconsistency is highly suspicious for pulmonary vascular disease.

More frequently definitive diagnosis requires angiographic demonstration of truncation and/or intra-vascular filling defects using contrast-enhanced thoracic CT.

Pulmonary oedema

Aetiology

Causes of pulmonary oedema:
- Pulmonary venous hypertension
- Increased pulmonary vascular permeability
- Reduced plasma oncotic pressure.

Pathophysiology

Whatever the cause, fluid initially accumulates in the interstitium, then rapidly spreads to alveolar spaces and, in severe cases, the airways. Respiratory function is adversely affected as alveolar compression and reduced surfactant create atelectasis and decreased pulmonary compliance.

Clinical signs

Animals with pulmonary oedema present with dyspnoea with or without coughing. The cough is usually soft. When the airways are involved. the patient may cough, but if the fluid is only in the alveolar they will not. The onset may be peracute or more gradual.

Causes of pulmonary oedema

Cardiac disease

The most common cause of pulmonary oedema in dogs and cats is left atrial hypertension and consequently pulmonary venous hypertension. Any cardiac disease that results in left atrial hypertension may produce pulmonary oedema.

By far the most common causes in small animal practice are the acquired cardiac disorders myxomatous degenerative mitral valve disease (MMVD), dilated cardiomyopathy and hypertrophic cardiomyopathy.

Additionally, pulmonary oedema may also occur with high-output cardiac disease with no left atrial hypertension. The marked increase in pulmonary blood flow results in extravasation of fluid at a rate that exceeds pulmonary lymphatic capacitance. This form of high-output pulmonary oedema may occur in some congenital cardiac anomalies such as patent ductus arteriosis or ventricular septal defect.

When pulmonary oedema is due to cardiac failure, cardiac abnormalities will also be detectable. These may include:

- Absence of a normal sinus rhythm (always)
- Alterations in palpable or audible cardiac impulse
- Reduced pulse amplitude
- Tachyarrhythmias
- Murmurs consistent with mitral insufficiency, aortic stenosis or murmurs suggesting left to right shunting.

The detection of MMVD in a coughing dog makes the assumption that the coughing is due to cardiac disease appealing. However, it should be remembered that many dogs with MMVD have no clinical signs for long periods after the valve dysfunction is detected through an audible murmur. Thus, while explaining two abnormal findings with one disease is attractive, in this case it will not always be appropriate, and it is essential that all aspects of the history and physical examination be used to make this assessment.

For MMVD to cause clinical signs, including exercise intolerance, coughing or dyspnoea, there needs to be some degree of heart failure and hence recruitment of various compensatory mechanisms that should also be detectable. The absence of any evidence to suggest recruitment of compensatory process such as tachycardia should alert the clinician to the possibility that the coughing may *not* be a consequence of the MMVD.

Neurogenic oedema
- Neurogenic pulmonary oedema results from massive sympathetic stimulation. The sympathetic discharge raises peripheral resistance and systemic blood pressure, resulting in a massive shift in blood volume from the systemic to pulmonary circulation.
- Pulmonary venous pressure rises dramatically and fluid is extravasated. Both central venous and pulmonary venous pressures usually return to normal within 30 minutes, avoiding acute heart failure.
- However, the hypertension and hypervolaemia damages the capillary endothelium, causing increased permeability and persistence of pulmonary oedema.

Adult respiratory distress syndrome
- In adult respiratory distress syndrome pulmonary oedema occurs due to increased pulmonary capillary permeability without an increase in pulmonary venous pressure.
- It is a common response of the lung to many forms of injury.
- The abnormalities in permeability that occur are the result of damage to alveolar epithelial and microvascular barriers.
- Multiple mediators are likely to be involved in causing increased permeability and include:
  - Endotoxins (directly toxic to vascular endothelium)
  - Inflammatory cells
  - Various inflammatory mediators (cytokines, eicosanoids)
  - Platelets
  - Platelet activating factor
  - Complement.
- These mechanisms can be activated by many conditions including inhaled toxins, sepsis, pancreatitis, aspirating gastric contents and various drugs.

Reduced oncotic pressure due to hypoproteinaemia
When reduced oncotic pressure is the inciting agent, pulmonary oedema is likely to be just one manifestation of generalised subcutaneous oedema.

Normal delivery of abnormal haemoglobin
Causes include animals with significant disorders of the haematopoietic system such as patients with marked anaemia or with dysfunctional haemoglobin such as methaemoglobinaemia.

Key points

As a result of reading this chapter you should be able to:
- Develop a rational approach to the diagnosis of patients manifesting any of the following clinical signs: sneezing, nasal discharge, cough or dyspnoea
- Recognise that respiratory dysfunction can be due to primary respiratory disease or secondary respiratory disease
- Recognise that patients with primary nasal disease invariably do not cough, wheeze or have significant dyspnoea unless forced to breathe through their nose
- Recognise that patients with laryngeal disease present with dyspnoea and minimal coughing and that focused auscultation can help alert the clinician to the likely presence of laryngeal dysfunction
- Understand the relevance of the location of the lesion in the context of patients that cough with minimal dyspnoea vs. those that have cough and dyspnoea vs. those with dyspnoea with minimal coughing
- Recognise the importance of ascertaining whether inspiratory or expiratory dyspnoea is present
- Recognise that patients presenting with dyspnoea without coughing fall into two groups: those with laryngeal dysfunction and those with intra-thoracic disease
- Understand that the characteristics of a cough can be valuable in localising the anatomic site of a respiratory lesion.

Questions for review

- What clues might help you assess whether a patient with a nasal discharge has local or systemic disease?
- What are some causes of local nasal disease?
- Where are the cough receptors located in the respiratory tract?

- What is the likely location of the pathology in a patient with inspiratory dyspnoea?
- What is the likely location of the pathology in a patient with expiratory dyspnoea?
- What are some primary respiratory causes of:
  - Coughing without dyspnoea
  - Coughing with dyspnoea
  - Dyspnoea with minimal coughing?
- What is a difference between canine and feline bronchial disease?
- What clinical signs in a coughing dog with a murmur would alert you to the fact that the cough was *unlikely* to be due to primary cardiac disease?
- What are some examples of secondary respiratory pathology that can cause dyspnoea without coughing?

Case example

'George' is an 11-year-old male Shih Tzu who presented with a 12-month history of progressive coughing and exercise intolerance. His coughing was harsh and dry and worsened with exercise and excitement. Approximately 2 months ago he started to develop wheezing and progressive dyspnoea.

On physical examination he was found to be bright and alert and a little overweight (BCS 6/9). He had a normal rectal temperature, heart rate of 120 bpm, respiratory rate of 48 bpm. Mucous membrane colour was pink with a CRT of <2 sec.

He had a grade IV/VI systolic murmur audible over the left cardiac apex region. A sinus arrhythmia was present with a heart rate of 100 and normal pulse quality. There was a generalised and substantial increase in thoracic respiratory sounds with increased expiratory effort. A harsh paroxysmal cough occurred spontaneously and following tracheal palpation.

Define the problem

George has two major respiratory signs with differing chronology. He had a harsh cough without evidence of dyspnoea for 10 months, then developed signs of wheezing and dyspnoea more recently.

Define the location

Where is the problem in the respiratory system?

The initial harsh cough without dyspnoea indicates large airway disease – trachea or large bronchi. The reaction to a tracheal pinch and the paroxysmal nature of the cough indicate tracheal disease.

The more recent respiratory signs of wheezing and dyspnoea suggest the smaller airways are affected – small bronchi.

The development of the dyspnoea might be due to a progressive respiratory problem, that is, something that has progressed from tracheal disease to tracheobronchial disease, or the dyspnoea might indicate a new problem has developed that might be a primary or secondary respiratory problem.

Define the system

Does George have primary or seconary respiratory disease?

George definitely has a mitral valve murmur, but there are few clinical signs suggesting impaired cardiac function or indeed any recruitment of compensatory processes. He is not tachycardic; he has a sinus arrhythmia that is a normal finding (and is usually absent once compensatory mechanisms are recruited as the heart fails), and there is no mention in the history of a soft cough, poor perfusion or weak pulses that may indicate congestive heart failure.

Thus, it is likely that George has primary respiratory disease involving initially the large airways and now both large and smaller airways.

Define the lesion

Differentials for the harsh cough include:
- Degenerative airway disease, for example, tracheal collapse, chronic bronchitis.

Differentials for the wheezing and dyspnoea include:
- Bronchoconstriction
- Bronchial thickening
- Exudate or fluid within the bronchial lumen
- Masses within airways.

Case outcome

The diagnostics planned to assess the differentials were:

- Thoracic radiographs, which showed a distinct bronchial pattern
- A transtracheal aspirate showed an increased numbers of inflammatory cells – mostly non-degenerate neutrophils and occasional eosinophils
- Bacterial culture and PCR for mycoplasma was negative
- George was referred for fluoroscopic examination, which confirmed tracheal collapse.

George's final diagnosis was tracheal collapse and chronic bronchitis of unknown aetiology. He was moderately well managed with glucocorticoids and antitussive treatment.

CHAPTER 10

Anaemia

Jill E. Maddison[1] and Lucy McMahon[2]

[1]Department of Clinical Science and Services, The Royal Veterinary College, London, UK

[2]Anderson Moores Veterinary Specialists, Winchester, UK

The why/what

- Anaemia is characterised by a significant decrease of red blood cells (RBCs), haematocrit/packed cell volume (HCT/PCV) and/or haemoglobin. Its clinical importance can vary from being the patient's primary life-threatening problem to being relatively clinically inconsequential.
- Anaemia is a common clinical problem with a multitude of causes. A structured approach to investigation leads to faster diagnosis and treatment. This chapter will describe a logical approach to the diagnosis of anaemia in small animals.
- Becoming familiar with interpretation of the haemogram and blood film evaluation are useful ways to further characterise anaemia as these give clues to the underlying pathological process.
- It is important to note the severity of anaemia and whether it is responsible for an animal's clinical signs. Mild anaemia may not require direct investigation or treatment but is often a flag for underlying disease that should be investigated. Moderate to severe anaemia requires prompt investigation and treatment.

Clinical Reasoning in Veterinary Practice: Problem Solved!, Second Edition.
Edited by Jill E. Maddison, Holger A. Volk and David B. Church.
© 2022 John Wiley & Sons Ltd. Published 2022 by John Wiley & Sons Ltd.

Define the problem

Animals with anaemia present with pale mucous membranes. The first step is, therefore, to define the problem and system involved – that is to differentiate those animals with pale mucous membranes due to poor peripheral perfusion (e.g. due to hypovolaemia, cardiogenic shock) from those that have anaemia. Animals with pale mucous membranes due to poor peripheral perfusion will typically have prolonged capillary refill time and/or weak femoral pulses.

PCV or HCT are used to measure red cell mass and represent the percentage of blood that is composed of red blood cells. The terms are interchangeable but PCV is determined by centrifugation and HCT is calculated by automated haematology analysers from the RBC count and MCV (mean corpuscular volume).

Anaemia can easily be confirmed by measurement of the PCV/HCT. It is possible to have anaemia *and* poor peripheral perfusion; this is most commonly seen following acute blood loss. Note that splenic relaxation following sedation or anaesthesia leads to RBC sequestration in the spleen and can result in a significant drop in PCV/HCT, and animals may appear falsely anaemic if samples are taken at that time. Also note that severe dehydration may lead to a false increase in the PCV/HCT and may mask mild anaemia until an animal is rehydrated. It is normal for puppies and kittens to have a lower PCV/HCT than adult animals until approximately 4 months of age.

Once it has been confirmed that 'true' anaemia is the cause of the animal's pale mucous membranes, it is important to assess whether the anaemia is the primary disease process or secondary, that is, whether it is causing the animal's presenting clinical signs or whether it is secondary to a more significant underlying disorder. Often, the clinical significance of mild to moderate anaemia is overestimated. The most common cause of mild anaemia is anaemia of inflammatory disease, which is a feature of many infectious, inflammatory or neoplastic disorders (discussed later in the chapter).

The assessment of clinical disease onset and progression is important to help differentiate possible causes. The rapidity with which anaemia develops will also influence its clinical effect. For example, a dog with a PCV of 20% may show only mild clinical signs if the anaemia has developed slowly but will be more severely affected if the PCV has decreased suddenly.

Define the system

The system involved in the problem of anaemia is the haemopoietic system. The system may be further refined by determining how the haemopoietic system is affected, that is, by destruction or loss of RBCs (usually, though not always, causing regenerative anaemia) or by a failure to effectively produce RBCs (causing non-regenerative anaemia).

Non-regenerative anaemia can be refined further to consider whether the problem is a structural problem of the bone marrow or whether the problem is functional (i.e. local vs. systemic bone marrow disease).

Assessment of anaemia – refine the system

It is imperative to ascertain whether the anaemia is regenerative or non-regenerative. An important caveat to note is that peracute anaemia may be pre-regenerative, that is, it may initially appear to be non-regenerative because it takes 2–5 days for the bone marrow to fully respond to the loss of red cell mass. However, usually after 48 hours of blood loss or haemolysis, there will be some evidence of a regenerative response even if it is not complete.

The diagnostic approach and possible aetiologies for regenerative and non-regenerative anaemia are by and large different (although there is some overlap), and full evaluation of the haemogram for clues relating to regeneration is essential.

Regenerative anaemia

There are many clues within the haemogram that can be used to determine whether anaemia is regenerative or non-regenerative, although the reticulocyte count is the most reliable way to confirm this. RBC parameters such as size as well as morphology should be evaluated. Evidence for regeneration includes the following:
- Presence of increased numbers of reticulocytes (Figure 10.1). In the dog an absolute reticulocyte count of >95,000/μl and in cats an absolute aggregate reticulocyte count of >60,000/μl is compatible with adequate regeneration.
- Increased RBC size – macrocytosis (increased MCV) – note that macrocytosis can also be seen due to other causes.
- Variation in RBC staining and size (polychromasia and anisocytosis; Figure 10.2).
- Presence of nucleated RBCs (although these can also occur with lead toxicity and splenic pathology; Figure 10.2).

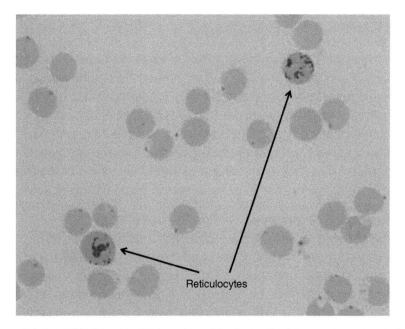

Figure 10.1   Blood smear from a dog showing reticulocytes. New methylene blue stain. (Courtesy of Dr Balazs Szladovits.)

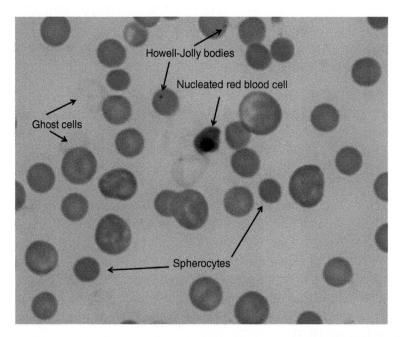

Figure 10.2   A blood smear from a dog with immune-mediated haemolytic anaemia with strong evidence of regeneration, including anisocytosis and poly-chromasia (variations in size and staining of red blood cells), nucleated red blood cells, Howell-Jolly bodies and also shows numerous spherocytes and ghost cells (indicating extravascular and intravascular haemolysis, respectively). Wright's stain. (Courtesy of Dr Balazs Szladovits.)

Define the location

Acute pre-regenerative or regenerative anaemia can occur in only one of two ways – as a result of haemorrhage, haemolysis or occasionally both. Superficially, it might appear simple to differentiate haemorrhage from haemolysis as the cause of the anaemia, but sometimes, differentiation poses a significant diagnostic dilemma.

Haemorrhage vs. haemolysis

Clues that can assist in deciding whether haemorrhage or haemolysis is present include the following:
- Clinical signs/physical examination/imaging
  - Evidence for external haemorrhage?
  - Evidence for internal haemorrhage?
- Plasma protein concentration – typically reduced in acute haemorrhage and chronic external haemorrhage. Normal to increased in haemolysis
- Presence of autoagglutination – in the blood tube or during saline agglutination test?
- Presence of prominent spherocytosis (see below)
- Plasma appearance
  - Haemolysis?
  - Icterus?
- Urine
  - Haemoglobinuria?
  - Bilirubinuria?

Haemorrhage

The key question when haemorrhage is detected is whether it is due to local disease (e.g. trauma, bleeding tumour) or systemic disease (e.g. coagulopathy). This then permits the possible lesions to be defined. Coagulopathy is discussed in detail in Chapter 12.

If haemorrhage is acute, there may initially be no change in the PCV, as both plasma and RBCs have been lost. However, after a few hours, the plasma will equilibrate, and the reduced PCV will become apparent.

Acute haemorrhage is often associated with decreased plasma protein concentrations, especially if the haemorrhage is external. If a patient has developed acute regenerative anaemia and the plasma protein is high normal or above normal, then haemolysis is more likely than external haemorrhage. If there is evidence for external haemorrhage but the plasma protein is in the upper reference range or above, then consider that haemolysis may also be contributing to the anaemia or that the animal may have hyperglobulinaemia.

Chronic external haemorrhage (e.g. gastroduodenal ulceration, bleeding gastrointestinal tumour, intestinal parasites such as hookworms and severe flea infestation) will eventually cause iron deficiency, although the anaemia often remains moderately regenerative initially. Anaemia due to chronic gastrointestinal haemorrhage may be associated with mild hypoproteinaemia. The platelet count is often normal or elevated in chronic blood loss (unless thrombocytopenia is the reason for the bleeding).

Internal haemorrhage into a body cavity may be difficult to detect, particularly intra-abdominal or retroperitoneal haemorrhage. With internal haemorrhage, the protein usually is less reduced than with external haemorrhage, because the protein is not 'lost' and plasma concentrations will increase more quickly after the bleed.

Intra-thoracic haemorrhage will usually cause acute, specific signs of compromised respiratory function unless the bleed is very small. In contrast, intra-abdominal haemorrhage may be more difficult to identify. In particular, intra-abdominal haemorrhage is rapidly resorbed into the circulation (the peritoneum is a very large and efficient absorption surface), and thus, an acute splenic bleed of small volume, for example, in a dog with haemangiosarcoma, may not be detectable by abdominocentesis within a few hours of the bleed.

Haemolysis
Anaemia resulting from haemolysis or internal haemorrhage tends to be more regenerative than that due to external blood loss, as all the iron is preserved and can be re-used. Haemolysis may occur extravascularly (RBCs are broken down in the reticuloendothelial system – the spleen predominantly, but also the liver and bone marrow) or intravascularly (RBCs are broken down within the bloodstream, releasing haemoglobin). Increased serum bilirubin and bilirubinuria are observed in the majority (but not all) cases of extravascular haemolysis, although overt jaundice may be less common than with intravascular haemolysis. The diagnosis of haemolysis (e.g. caused by immune-mediated

haemolytic anaemia) should, therefore, never be excluded due to the absence of jaundice.

Intravascular haemolysis can be easily demonstrated, as the plasma of a centrifuged sample will be red if the intravascular hae-molysis is moderate to severe (not to be confused with artefactual haemolysis, which happens during sampling). Haemoglobinuria is usually present in cases of intravascular haemolysis, and jaundice is common. Haemoglobinuria should be differentiated from haematu-ria by centrifuging urine and observing the supernatant – it will be clear if haematuria is present, as the RBCs settle to the bottom of the tube but will remain red if haemoglobinuria is present.

Clues to the presence of IMHA include prominent spherocytosis (Figure 10.2). Spherocytes are common in IMHA and large numbers are pathognomic for IMHA, but small numbers can be hereditary (rare) or occur in animals with oxidative RBC damage, microangio-pathic anaemia, hypersplenism (e.g. splenic lymphoma, haeman-giosarcoma or haemophagocytic variant of histiocytoma) and envenomation. Evaluation for spherocytes should be done in the monolayer of the blood smear to avoid artefactual RBC change. They cannot be reliably identified in cats, as their RBCs normally lack central pallor. Spherocytes are commonly present in transfused patients, thus they cannot be used as an indicator of IMHA following blood transfusion.

The direct Coombs test can be used to identify anti-RBC antibodies if autoagglutination is not present after RBC washing. This test cannot differentiate between associative and non-associative IMHA, however. False-positive and false-negative results can also sometimes occur.

 Define the lesion

Causes of haemolytic anaemia
Immune-mediated haemolytic anaemia (IMHA)
IMHA can be defined as associative or non-associative. Associative IMHA is when a concurrent disease process has been identified and may be the cause of the IMHA (*secondary IMHA*). Or the disorders may be concurrent but unrelated to the IMHA. Potential secondary causes of IMHA include infection, drugs and neoplasia.

Non-associative IMHA is the most common form in dogs and can also affect cats, although this species appears to present more commonly with non-regenerative IMHA. Non-associative IMHA includes *primary* (idiopathic) IMHA or cryptogenic (obscure or unknown) causes of IMHA.

In both species, it is important to investigate for concurrent disease before treatment if budget allows, particularly in cats or dogs where history taking or physical examination has revealed increased risk (e.g. a cat or dog living in, or having travelled from, an area endemic for common infectious causes of IMHA; unexpected physical examination findings).

Infectious haemolytic anaemia

Mycoplasmosis or haemoplasmosis (infection usually with *Mycoplasma haemofelis*) is a potential cause of haemolytic anaemia in the cat. It should be noted that if a cat is positive for *M. haemofelis* but does not have a regenerative anaemia, other underlying disease should be sought. Older male non-pedigree cats are believed to be at increased risk for *M. haemofelis* infection, although younger cats may be more likely to show signs of disease. The significance of infection is difficult to assess, as asymptomatic carrier cats exist. Diagnosis should be made on the basis of PCR results (not blood smear alone) and should be interpreted in light of other clinical information. Anaemia due to *M. haemofelis* infection may be more likely in immunocompromised cats.

Babesiosis can cause haemolytic anaemia, which can mimic idiopathic IMHA. In endemic areas, it is often the most common cause of haemolytic anaemia. In non-endemic areas, the key question is travel history – if a dog has travelled outside a country such as the United Kingdom, then PCR testing for *Babesia* spp. is often appropriate. Rarely, *Babesia* infection can be found in untravelled dogs in non-endemic areas.

Drug/toxins

Drugs such as sulphonamides, penicillins, cephalosporins and methimazole have been associated with haemolytic anaemia, usually immune mediated. Causes of direct haemolysis include zinc toxicosis, snake envenomation and severe hypophosphataemia in both cats and dogs.

Ingestion of oxidants including onions or onion products, garlic, paracetamol in cats, propylene glycol, vitamin K, benzocaine, methylene blue and naphthalene (mothballs) has also been reported to cause haemolysis. Heinz bodies are commonly seen in anaemia due to oxidation injury, although low numbers can be normal in cats. Methaemoglobinaemia can also develop following some forms of oxidation injury and can be detected clinically as brown discolouration of mucous membranes and plasma. History, serum biochemistry and plain radiography (zinc foreign bodies) can aid in ruling out these causes of haemolytic anaemia.

Hereditary haemolytic anaemia
Haemolytic anaemia may occur in certain dog and cat breeds with congenital defects of RBC metabolism, for example, pyruvate kinase deficiency (basenji, West Highland white terrier, Abyssinian, Somali), phosphofructokinase deficiency (English springer spaniel), osmotic fragility (Abyssinian, Somali) and porphyria (cat).

Hereditary anaemias can occur in some breeds not listed here and occasionally occur in unexpected breeds. Affected animals may present young but in some disorders can present when mature. Haemolytic crises can occur with some disorders.

Microangiopathic anaemia
Microangiopathic anaemia is a variant of haemolysis where the RBCs are physically damaged. Examples are numerous and include:
• Mechanical injury
  o Disseminated intravascular coagulation
  o Caval syndrome
  o Glomerulonephritis
  o Valvular stenosis
• Damage due to abnormal endothelium
  o Haemangiosarcoma
  o Vasculitis
  o Splenic torsion
  o Hepatic disease
  o Cutaneous renal and glomerular vasculopathy (CRGV or Alabama rot)

- Thermal injury
  - Heatstroke
  - Severe burns
- Osmotic injury
  - Freshwater near-drowning.

In microangiopathic anaemia abnormal RBC morphology may be seen including schistocytes, acanthocytes and keratocytes (see Figure 10.3). Acanthocytes are spiculated RBCs that can be seen in microangiopathic anaemia and also in disorders where there is altered lipid composition of the RBC membrane (e.g. liver disease).

Microangiopathic anaemia can be non-regenerative, as the underlying disorder can be associated with cytokines that suppress RBC production in the bone marrow.

Causes of haemorrhage
These will be discussed in Chapter 12.

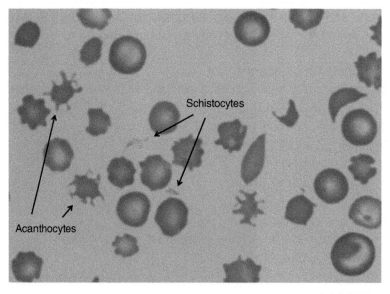

Figure 10.3 Blood smear from a dog with schistocytes and acanthocytes indicating shear damage to the erythrocytes. Wright's stain. (With permission of Dr Balazs Szladovits.)

Define the location

Non-regenerative anaemia

Non-regenerative anaemia is typically associated with RBCs that are of normal size and colour (normocytic normochromic anaemia), although macrocytic and microcytic non-regenerative anaemia is sometimes seen due to specific causes. Non-regenerative anaemia is caused by decreased or ineffective RBC production. Decreased or ineffective RBC production can be caused by numerous mechanisms, and often these mechanisms overlap.

Non-regenerative anaemia must be differentiated from pre-regenerative anaemia, which can be present within the first few days following haemolysis or haemorrhage.

 ## Define the lesion

Causes of non-regenerative anaemia

Anaemia of inflammatory disease

Anaemia of inflammatory disease is the most common cause of non-regenerative anaemia. It is usually clinically innocuous and does not require specific treatment. However, it is an indication that there is an underlying disease present and warrants a vigorous search for its cause.

Anaemia of inflammatory disease can occur with infectious, inflammatory or neoplastic diseases and is so named because the anaemia is caused by inflammatory cytokines that lead to suppression of RBC production as well as decreased RBC lifespan. It is almost always normocytic, normochromic although depending on the underlying disease abnormal RBC morphology may be present (e.g. RBC fragments may be seen if disseminated intravascular coagulation [DIC] is present) and is usually mild (PCV 25–36% in dogs and 18–26% in cats). It should resolve if the underlying systemic disease is treated successfully.

Chronic kidney disease

Anaemia is more likely with advanced stages of chronic kidney disease (CKD) (IRIS stages 3 and 4). It is simple to rule out by checking urea, creatinine and urine specific gravity. CKD causes anaemia via multiple mechanisms including decreased erythropoietin production, suppression of RBC production due to uraemic toxins and inflammatory cytokines, chronic blood loss in the gastrointestinal tract and lack of essential minerals due to malnutrition.

Bone marrow disorders

Clues to bone marrow disease as the cause of non-regenerative anaemia include the following:

- RBCs are usually normocytic and normochromic but are occasionally macrocytic.
- Anaemia is often severe (PCV <15%) and clinical signs may be minimal despite the low PCV as the anaemia has usually developed slowly.
- The haemogram often contains major clues such as other cytopenias.
  - Thrombocytopenia and neutropenia are most common along with anaemia in bone marrow disease.
  - Other leukocytes are relatively long lived and are less likely to be affected in bone marrow disease.
  - Note that lymphopenia is relatively common and usually seen as part of a stress leukogram rather than as an indicator of bone marrow disease.
- If the animal has leukaemia or myelodysplasia, abnormal circulating cells may be seen on blood smear, which may elevate the overall white blood cell (WBC) count.
  The bone marrow may be affected by the following disorders:
- Infection
  - Parvovirus/panleukopenia
  - Feline leukaemia virus (FeLV)
  - Ehrlichiosis
- Toxins/drugs
  - Oestrogen
  - Chemotherapeutic/cytotoxic agents
  - Hydroxyurea
- Immune-mediated disease
  - Precursor-directed immune-mediated anaemia (PIMA)
  - Pure red cell aplasia

- o Immune response to administration of erythropoietin
- Neoplasia
  - o Primary haemopoietic neoplasia, for example,
    - Lymphoma
    - Multiple myeloma
    - Leukaemia
  - o Infiltrative neoplasia
    - Neoplastic cells compete for space and nutrients and release inhibitory factors; this is known as myelophthisis
- Myelodysplasia
  - o Abnormal maturation or production of cells in the bone marrow
- Myelofibrosis
  - o Normal haemopoietic tissue is replaced by fibrous tissue
    - The cause of this is not always known, and it may occur secondary to some immune-mediated anaemias.

Iron deficiency

Iron deficiency is a relatively uncommon cause of anaemia in small animals, but it can be overlooked because it doesn't tend to fit into the neat classification of regenerative or non-regenerative anaemia. It can be moderately regenerative to non-regenerative in nature. Fortunately, once established, iron-deficiency anaemia is easy to identify as it is fairly characteristic usually resulting in:
- Microcytosis (low MCV)
- Hypochromasia (low mean corpuscular haemoglobin concentration [MCHC])
- Poikilocytosis – specifically acanthocytes, schistocytes, keratocytes
- Thrombocytosis if due to chronic haemorrhage.

Iron deficiency in cats (rare) and early iron deficiency in dogs may be normocytic and normochromic. The most common cause of iron deficiency in adult small animals is chronic external blood loss (e.g. from the gastrointestinal or urinary tract). Internal blood loss does not cause iron deficiency, as the iron is absorbed across the peritoneum and recycled. Puppies and kittens have low iron stores and are more prone to development of iron deficiency if they are fed an iron-deficient diet or have heavy parasite burdens (fleas or hookworms).

Key points

As a result of reading this chapter you should be able to:

- Define the problem – the first step in an animal with pallor is to *define the problem* – to differentiate between anaemia and poor peripheral perfusion using clinical examination and measurement of the PCV. Some animals have both, for example, in acute blood loss.
- Define and refine the system – once anaemia is defined, the haemopoietic system is known to be affected (*define the system*) but this can be further refined as whether there is RBC loss or destruction (usually, but not always, *regenerative anaemia*) or inadequate RBC production (*non-regenerative anaemia*).
- Define the location – we can then *define the location* by considering if regenerative anaemia is caused by blood loss or haemolysis (or sometimes both). Blood film examination, total protein measurement, haemolysis clues and clinical examination can help to differentiate between these two causes. Non-regenerative anaemia can be mild (e.g. in anaemia of inflammatory disease) or severe (e.g. in bone marrow disease). Diagnostic testing must be tailored to the likely underlying cause. Mild, non-regenerative anaemia often requires investigation to identify the underlying disease. Severe non-regenerative anaemia often requires prompt patient support with blood transfusion and bone marrow examination to diagnose the underlying cause.
- Define the lesion – once the location is defined – haemolysis, haemorrhage or bone marrow dysfunction – the cause can be sought, that is, *define the lesion*.
- Remember that the numbers in a haemogram may not give you the whole picture. It is vitally important to assess RBC morphology and indices to progress your understanding of the type of anaemia present and its possible causes. Always perform a smear and submit this to an external laboratory if you or your team does not have the confidence to adequately assess it in your practice. Advice of a clinical pathologist is recommended in all cases, but in-house examination can result in prompt diagnosis and treatment out of hours.

Questions for review

- What are the key methods used to differentiate between regenerative and non-regenerative anaemia? Why is this important?
- How can diagnostic testing help to distinguish between blood loss anaemia and haemolytic anaemia? Is specialised equipment necessary to do this?
- What is the most common reason for mild, non-regenerative anaemia? How should this finding be approached clinically?

Case example

'Edith' is a 5-year-old female neutered cocker spaniel. She presents for lethargy, reduced appetite and exercise intolerance of 1 week duration. She 'flopped down' on a walk on the day of presentation and had to be carried back to the car. Edith has not travelled outside the UK, and toxin exposure is very unlikely. Routine parasite treatment and vaccinations are up to date.

Edith's mucous membranes are pale on examination, and capillary refill time is not easy to assess as a result. Her heart rate is 140 bpm and her femoral pulses feel 'bounding' and are synchronous with the heartbeat. Skin turgor is normal and examination is otherwise unremarkable.

Define the problem

Edith has multiple problems including mucous membrane pallor, tachycardia, exercise intolerance, reduced appetite and lethargy. Pallor is the most specific problem and may be caused by poor peripheral perfusion or anaemia. Poor perfusion typically results in reduced pulse quality, which is not present in this case. Anaemia tends to be associated with strong or bounding pulses unless poor perfusion is also present concurrently. Thus, Edith is likely to be anaemic – this can be easily confirmed by measurement of packed cell volume or haematocrit. Manual PCV is performed and the result is 22% (reference interval 37–55%). Edith is confirmed as anaemic.

Define the system

The haemopoietic system is affected in anaemia. This can be refined further by looking at how the system is affected: is there increased destruction or loss of RBCs or is there reduced or ineffective production of RBCs? This question can be answered by determining whether the anaemia is *regenerative or non-regenerative*. The most straightforward and useful way to differentiate between regenerative and non-regenerative anaemia is to look at the absolute reticulocyte count. Edith has an absolute reticulocyte count of 180,000/μl, which is compatible with *regenerative* anaemia.

Define the location

We know that regenerative anaemia is caused by either blood loss or haemolysis. There is no physical or historical evidence of blood loss in this case but loss into body cavities cannot be ruled out.

Assessment of total protein and blood smear evaluation can add to the library of information that we compile when assessing an animal with anaemia. Edith's total protein is within normal range (60g/l, reference range 50-75) which is more typical for haemolytic anaemia than blood loss anaemia.

Blood smear evaluation shows moderate anisocytosis, polychromasia, increased numbers of nRBCs and marked spherocytosis. These findings are typical findings in IMHA although there are other less common causes of spherocytosis.

A Direct Coombs' test was positive adding strength to the diagnosis of IMHA.

Define the lesion

Edith has findings compatible with a diagnosis of IMHA. In the majority of dogs this is an idiopathic condition (non-associative) although history taking (e.g. drug and travel history) and further diagnostics (infectious disease testing, imaging, organ sampling) can be done to look for concurrent disease (associative IMHA).

Case outcome

Edith also had serum biochemistry performed, which showed mild hyperbilirubinaemia (22 μmol/l, reference range 4–12). Hyperbilirubinaemia is common in haemolytic anaemia and frequently leads to clinically detectable jaundice (once the serum level exceeds about 45 μmol/l) and bilirubinuria. History and further diagnostic testing did not identify a trigger for IMHA. She was successfully treated with immunosuppressive drugs – prednisolone and mycophenolate.

CHAPTER 11

Jaundice

Jill E. Maddison[1] and Lucy McMahon[2]

[1]*Department of Clinical Science and Services, The Royal Veterinary College, London, UK*

[2]*Anderson Moores Veterinary Specialists, Winchester, UK*

The why/what

- Jaundice or icterus is a relatively common clinical sign.
- It is not necessarily noted by owners and is usually detected by the veterinarian during the clinical examination of an unwell patient.
- It may also be observed in serum or identified in biochemistry results.
- The diagnostic approach to jaundice is straightforward, although confirming the final cause can be challenging.

 ## Define the problem

Jaundice or icterus is a yellow discolouration of body tissues caused by increased serum concentrations of bilirubin. The normal liver has a large capacity to take up and excrete bilirubin. Therefore, jaundice will be observed clinically only when there is a large, persistent increase in bilirubin production or a major impairment in bilirubin excretion.

The issue of defining the problem in relation to jaundice is not that it can be confused with another clinical sign but that it may be missed if the clinical examination is not sufficiently rigorous. Jaundice is most easily seen on sclerae, mucous membranes and non-pigmented skin. Specific examination of the sclerae during the clinical examination is important, concentrations as they are not always obvious when observing an animal's face. Increased serum of bilirubin can be defined as a problem even if the animal isn't overtly jaundiced.

Clinical Reasoning in Veterinary Practice: Problem Solved!, Second Edition.
Edited by Jill E. Maddison, Holger A. Volk and David B. Church.
© 2022 John Wiley & Sons Ltd. Published 2022 by John Wiley & Sons Ltd.

Physiology

Bilirubin is primarily formed from the breakdown of haemoglobin from aged red blood cells in the reticuloendothelial (RE) system of the spleen, liver, bone marrow and lymph nodes. A small amount is derived from myoglobin and haem-containing liver enzymes. Haemoglobin is split to release a protein molecule and haem (iron-containing porphyrin). The iron is released and stored in RE cells or re-used for haem synthesis. The remainder of haem is converted to biliverdin and then to bilirubin.

Bilirubin is transported to the liver in blood tightly bound to albumin – unconjugated bilirubin. Unconjugated bilirubin is not water soluble and is not filtered by the renal glomeruli or excreted by renal tubules.

Dogs (males more often than females) have a low resorptive threshold for bilirubin. They also have renal enzyme systems that produce and conjugate bilirubin to a limited extent. Therefore, mild bilirubinuria (up to 2+) can occur in normal dog urine with a specific gravity greater than 1.025. Bilirubinuria will develop before overt jaundice in dogs due to the low renal threshold.

In contrast, cat kidneys cannot conjugate bilirubin, and their renal threshold is nine times higher than in dogs; therefore, bilirubinuria in a cat is always pathological.

In the liver, bilirubin is conjugated in hepatocytes and excreted into bile canaliculi and thence transported to the bile ducts and intestine.

Conjugated bilirubin is water soluble, dialysable and filtered by the kidneys – therefore, it can appear in urine. Conjugated bilirubin excreted through the bile duct into the small intestine is converted by colonic bacteria to urobilinogen (colourless), which is oxidised to urobilin (orange).

Some urobilinogen is reabsorbed by the intestine, enters the enterohepatic circulation and is re-excreted into the bile. A small amount is also excreted into urine (about 5%). Urobilinogen remaining in the intestinal tract is converted to stercobilinogen that is oxidised to stercobilin, which imparts normal faecal colour.

The hepatic excretion of conjugated bilirubin into bile is the rate-limiting step in bilirubin metabolism, and this phase will be over-loaded first if there is excessive production of bilirubin.

The metabolic pathway for bilirubin is illustrated in Figure 11.1.

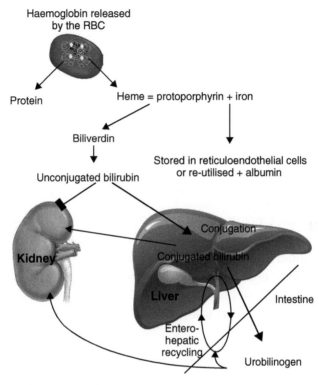

Figure 11.1   Bilirubin metabolism.

Define the system *and* location

The strict 'define the system then location approach' to problem-solving theoretically is applicable to jaundice as a problem, but in practice, we tend to assess the system and location together. The system question relates to consideration of haematopoietic causes i.e. haemolytic causes of jaundice vs. hepatobiliary causes, and this is the first key question. The combined system/location question relates to, *Is the jaundice due to pre-hepatic, hepatic or post-hepatic mechanisms?* It is relatively easy to differentiate haemolytic from hepatobiliary causes but more challenging to differentiate hepatic from post-hepatic causes of jaundice.

Pre-hepatic jaundice
Pre-hepatic jaundice occurs when there is significant *red blood cell (RBC) haemolysis*, which results in the bilirubin conjugation process in the liver being overwhelmed.

Animals with RBC haemolysis that is severe enough to result in jaundice will *always have a significant anaemia*, which is usually regenerative assuming (i) that the bone marrow has had time to respond and (ii) that the patient doesn't have immune-mediated haemolytic anaemia (IMHA) with antibodies directed against RBC precursors as well as mature RBCs.

Rarely, jaundice may occur when there is significant tissue haemorrhage when the subsequent breakdown of RBCs may overwhelm the capacity of the liver to take up, conjugate or secrete bilirubin.

Hepatic jaundice

Hepatic jaundice occurs with *hepatocellular disease*, which results in both conjugated (as the excretory capacity of liver is impaired) and unconjugated bilirubinaemia. There must be significant hepatocellular disease present before jaundice occurs. Jaundice is more likely to occur with hepatic disorders that involve primarily the periportal hepatocytes rather than centrilobular hepatocytes.

Post-hepatic jaundice

Post-hepatic jaundice occurs with obstruction, inflammation or rupture of the biliary tract. It may result in primarily conjugated bilirubinaemia.

Other causes of jaundice

Animals with sepsis, systemic inflammation and cats with hyperthyroidism may develop mild hyperbilirubinaemia, although overt jaundice is very unusual.

 Define the lesion

Pre-hepatic jaundice

Causes of haemolytic anaemia are discussed in detail in Chapter 10 and include the following:
- IMHA
- Infectious anaemia (e.g. haemoparasites)
- Drugs/toxins
- Hereditary disorders
- Microangiopathic anaemia.

Hepatic jaundice

Hepatic disorders causing jaundice in *dogs* include:

- Chronic hepatitis
- Copper-associated liver disease
- Cirrhosis/end-stage liver disease
- Neoplasia (usually diffuse or extensive, e.g. hepatic lymphoma)
- Infectious hepatitis (e.g. viral, bacterial, protozoal, fungal, parasitic – causes variable depending on geographic location)
- Toxin ingestion (e.g. Amanita fungi, aflatoxin, blue-green algae, xylitol, Sago palm)
- Drug related – dose-dependent toxicity or idiosyncratic reactions.

Hepatic disorders causing jaundice in *cats* include:

- Cholangitis
  - Most cases of cholangitis involve the biliary ductules within the liver. The previous terminology was cholangiohepatitis (which will still be found referred to in various sources), but the name was changed because the hepatic parenchyma cells themselves are not inflamed (the meaning of hepatitis)
  - The type of inflammatory infiltrate as well as chronology of clinical signs determines the classification and management of these disorders. They are:
    - Acute neutrophilic cholangitis (previously termed suppurative)
    - Chronic neutrophilic cholangitis
    - Lymphocytic cholangitis
    - Cholangitis due to liver flukes (in endemic areas)
- Feline infectious peritonitis
- Diffuse hepatic neoplasia
- Hepatic lipidosis
- Toxoplasmosis
- Toxin ingestion – in general cats are less likely to ingest toxins than dogs
- Drug related as above.

A liver biopsy is usually required to identify the type of pathology involved, although some disorders where cells exfoliate easily such as lymphoma, mast cell tumours or hepatic lipidosis can be diagnosed by fine-needle aspirate (FNA). Liver biopsy is not always indicated, particularly in acute, fulminant hepatic failure when identification of the tissue pathology may not assist in determining the aetiology and there is a particular risk of a coagulopathy.

Post-hepatic jaundice

Post-hepatic jaundice in cats and dogs occurs when there is pathology affecting the common bile duct, cystic duct and/or the gall bladder. The pathology may cause extra-hepatic bile duct obstruction (EHBDO), which can be partial or complete.

Causes of post-hepatic jaundice include:
- Intra-luminal pathology, for example,
  - Mucocoele
  - Cholecystitis
  - Cholelithiasis
  - Inspissated bile
- Intra-mural pathology, for example,
  - Stricture
  - Neoplasia, for example, biliary carcinoma
  - Choledochitis/cholangitis
    - Classified as post-hepatic if only the common bile duct is inflamed. However, in most cases, it is the biliary ductules within the liver that are affected, thus cholangitis is primarily defined as causing hepatic jaundice
- Extra-luminal pathology
  - Pancreatitis (including abscesses, pseudocysts)
  - Neoplasia (e.g. pancreatic, biliary, duodenal)
  - Duodenal foreign body (at the opening of the bile duct)
  - Fibrosis secondary to peritonitis
  - Diaphragmatic hernia (rare)
- Rupture of the biliary tract (trauma, inflammation, iatrogenic damage, mucocoele).

Other causes of jaundice

Increased bilirubin levels may occur in patients with sepsis or severe inflammatory disease. Bacterial products and inflammatory mediators impair biliary excretion by downregulating bile transporters. In addition, inflammatory cytokines cause upregulation of nitric oxide, which inhibits secretion of bile by biliary ductules. However, overt jaundice is rarely evident.

Mild hyperbilirubinaemia (but not overt jaundice) may occur in a proportion of hyperthyroid cats; this may be due to increased degradation of hepatic haem proteins.

Differentiating causes of jaundice

Pre-hepatic

Pre-hepatic jaundice is generally easy to differentiate from hepatic and post-hepatic causes of jaundice, as in pre-hepatic jaundice the animal will have a significant and usually regenerative anaemia (see also comment above the about the pre-regenerative state).

Animals with pre-hepatic jaundice may also have mild to moderately increased liver enzymes (due to hypoxic hepatopathy and systemic inflammation), but the predominant feature is regenerative anaemia without blood loss (the total protein is usually normal or increased).

Take care if there are signs of intestinal haemorrhage with jaundice, as this could be caused by either:

- Pre-hepatic jaundice such as IMHA in combination with immune-mediated platelet destruction and resulting blood loss due to mucosal bleeding
- Severe hepatocellular disease and associated gastrointestinal (GI) ulceration and/or coagulopathy caused by hepatic disease, disseminated intravascular coagulation (DIC) or severe cholestasis.

The key test to further assess for haemolysis is blood smear evaluation (See Chapter 10).

Hepatic vs. post-hepatic

Hepatic and post-hepatic causes of jaundice are more difficult to distinguish and usually require imaging to differentiate with confidence. However, there may be clues in other clinical information, although these clues are not a substitute for a correct diagnosis.

While an animal with only conjugated bilirubinaemia would most likely have post-hepatic jaundice and an animal with predominantly unconjugated bilirubinaemia will have haemolysis, the majority of animals with pre-hepatic, hepatic or post-hepatic jaundice will have increased levels of both unconjugated and conjugated bilirubinaemia, and the relative increase of one vs. the other is unpredictable.

Haemolysis causes cholestasis, postulated to be as a result of hypoxia and increased production of bilirubin. Post-hepatic obstruction will cause secondary hepatocellular damage due to the toxic effect of accumulated bile salts on hepatocytes or cholestasis-induced decreases in the hepatic transporters that take up unconju-gated bilirubin from blood. As previously mentioned, bilirubin excretion is the first process to become disordered in primary hepatocellular disease. Therefore, in most cases measurement of conjugated vs. unconjugated bilirubin in small animals is usually not useful in determining the underlying cause of jaundice and is no longer included on many biochemical panels.

Signalment and history

History may reveal information regarding vaccination status, parasite exposure, drug history and potential toxin ingestion. Certain dog breeds are known to be predisposed to particular disorders such as chronic hepatitis, gall bladder mucocoele and pancreatitis.

Clinical signs and physical examination

It can be difficult to reliably use clinical signs and physical examination to differentiate between hepatic and post-hepatic jaundice, as either can present with abdominal effusion, abdominal pain, anorexia, vomiting and dehydration. Animals can appear to be relatively well with chronic clinical signs or more acutely and severely unwell with both hepatic and pre-hepatic jaundice.

Clinical pathology

Liver enzyme activities may give clues but cannot be relied upon for diagnosis of hepatic vs. post-hepatic jaundice. Traditionally we think of either 'cholestatic' patterns or 'hepatocellular' patterns in liver enzymology. Cholestatic patterns may occur in post-hepatic jaundice and typically lead to significant increases in ALP, GGT and cholesterol along with mild to moderate increases in ALT and AST. Hepatocellular patterns may occur in hepatic jaundice and typically lead to moderate to severe increases in ALT, AST and ALP and sometimes reduction in BUN/urea, albumin, cholesterol and occasionally glucose.

These patterns are not always reliable to differentiate hepatic and post-hepatic causes of jaundice. In some instances, the magnitude of increase in liver enzymes will not always fit the expected 'pattern' of the underlying disease. For example, ALP is elevated by both intra- and extra-hepatic cholestasis and thus is increased in hepatic and post-hepatic disease.

The relative degree of increase of each enzyme is also not helpful – in fact, if ALP is substantially increased and ALT normal or only slightly increased, non-hepatic disease such as hyperadrenocorticism or exogenous corticosteroid administration is more likely to be present, though of course these patients will not be jaundiced.

Cholesterol is more likely to be elevated in post-hepatic jaundice and more likely to be reduced in hepatic jaundice. However, cholesterol may be elevated in endocrine conditions such as hyperadrenocorticism and hypothyroidism, which often result in abnormal ALT and ALP activities but should not cause jaundice. Other conditions that may coexist with hepatobiliary disease and that may lead to increased serum cholesterol include nephrotic syndrome, obesity and familial hyperlipidaemias.

Measurement of serum bile acids is not useful in differentiating between hepatic and post-hepatic jaundice, and it is not useful or cost effective to perform this test in jaundiced animals.

Diagnostic imaging
Ultrasound is arguably the most useful imaging modality available to most veterinary surgeons for the investigation of hepatobiliary disease, as it can give valuable information about the echogenicity of hepatic parenchyma, appearance of hepatic contours, gall bladder content and wall thickness, biliary tree, vascular structures, pancreas and local lymph nodes. Hepatic size can also be subjectively assessed, although this may be less reliable than with some other imaging techniques.

As with all specialised techniques, its usefulness is determined partly by operator training and experience and partly by the quality of the equipment used. Patient factors also contribute to image quality. It is important to bear in mind that great care should be taken to not over-interpret ultrasonographic lesions, particularly without biopsy or without careful consideration of other clinical information. For example, a liver with benign nodular hyperplasia might appear sonographically similar to a liver with multiple nodules due to neoplasia. In some situations, ultrasound can also be relatively insensitive, and some diseased livers will appear ultrasonographically normal.

Ultrasound is very useful for diagnosis of hepatic or biliary tract masses and biliary disease in general and is valuable for obtaining percutaneous ultrasound-guided liver biopsies. In a jaundiced animal, ultrasound is usually the next diagnostic step once pre-hepatic jaundice has been ruled out. As ultrasound is sensitive for post-hepatic disorders, it can be used to differentiate between these and hepatic causes of jaundice. If the gall bladder, bile ducts and pancreas appear normal during ultrasound examination, the jaundice is very likely to be hepatic in origin, providing pre-hepatic jaundice has been ruled out. However, the converse is not always true because the appearance of the liver itself can sometimes be an unreliable indicator – some diseased livers can appear relatively normal in contour and echogenicity, whereas some functionally healthy livers may have abnormal echogenicity.

Cytology, culture and histopathology

Liver biopsy is usually needed to diagnose the underlying pathology in primary hepatic jaundice, although it is not necessary in all cases such as acute toxic or infectious liver diseases and acute liver disease that appears to be resolving. However, biopsy is very useful to guide optimal treatment in chronic conditions such as copper-associated hepatitis, chronic idiopathic hepatitis and feline cholangitis/cholangiohepatitis.

FNA is sometimes useful for diagnosis of liver diseases that exfoliate well and can be easily recognised cytologically, such as round cell neoplasia e.g. lymphoma affecting the liver. However, cytologic evaluation of the liver has been shown to frequently disagree with histopathology, so FNA cytology results should be interpreted with caution and in light of other clinical information. Bile cytology and culture are sometimes performed to guide antibiotic treatment in neutrophilic cholangitis and septic cholecystitis.

Liver biopsy carries risk of complications including haemorrhage. This risk can be increased in dogs and cats with coagulopathy related to hepatobiliary disease. Prior to liver biopsy, clinicians should be aware of how to assess for and minimise these risks. Some dogs and cats will be poor candidates for anaesthesia and biopsy and may even acutely decompensate following the procedure.

Why bother to differentiate?

The reason that it is important to determine whether an animal has hepatic or post-hepatic jaundice is that treatment may be quite different including mandatory surgery for some post-hepatic causes (bile peritonitis, progressive or severe biliary obstruction). In contrast, surgery is usually only indicated in primary hepatocellular disease to obtain biopsies, and hepatic biopsies may be obtainable by other, less invasive, means (such as ultrasound-guided percutaneous biopsy).

Most jaundiced animals are poor anaesthetic and surgical candidates and so the decision to operate should be made carefully, particularly as many underlying causes resolve with medical therapy alone. If biliary surgery is performed, it is essential to have excellent knowledge of the relevant anatomy and the ability to perform biliary diversion techniques if required (magnification is very useful). Perioperative care should be intensive and of a high standard. If specialist referral is not an option, it is often useful to discuss these cases with a specialist in medicine or soft-tissue surgery prior to operating.

Treatment of jaundice is aimed at the treatment of the underlying disease. For example, immunosuppression in idiopathic or non-associative IMHA, antibiotic treatment in canine leptospirosis and feline neutrophilic cholangitis, and corticosteroids in feline lymphocytic cholangitis. Supportive care is often required and should be tailored to the individual patient. Fluid therapy, analgesia, anti-emetics, antacids, hepatoprotective and cholerectic medications, appetite stimulants and feeding tubes may be indicated depending on the underlying disorder.

Summary

Jaundice is a clinical problem that may be detected on clinical examination or by laboratory testing. It almost always indicates serious pathology, the location of which can be the haematopoietic system (haemolysis), liver, the biliary tract or peri-hepatobiliary structures such as the pancreas. Mild hyperbilirubinaemia can also be caused by severe inflammation and sepsis. A rational approach involves appreciation of the relevant pathophysiology, as well as recognition that differentiating hepatic from post-hepatic causes can be challenging and often requires a multi-modal diagnostic approach.

Key points

As a result of reading this chapter you should be able to:
- Understand how bilirubin is metabolised and how dysfunction at different levels may cause jaundice
- Appreciate that bilirubinuria can have a different pathophysiological significance in dogs and cats
- Appreciate the importance of determining whether jaundice is pre-hepatic, hepatic or post-hepatic in origin
- Appreciate the limitations of clinical pathology tests in the differentiation of hepatic and post-hepatic jaundice
- Appreciate the importance of differentiating hepatic from post-hepatic jaundice.

Questions for review

- List four (4) causes of hepatocellular jaundice in dogs and four in cats.
- List four (4) causes of post-hepatic jaundice (dogs or cats).
- What is the value in attempting to differentiate non-invasively hepatic and post hepatic causes of jaundice? What diagnostic tool/s are most helpful to do this?

Case example

'Dusty' is a 12-year-old male neutered border collie. He presents with a 6-day history of lethargy, vomiting, reduced appetite and weight loss. He has no prior medical history of note and is not receiving any medication. He is a keen swimmer, and his owner reported that rats were known to live around the lake where he swims. He has been regularly vaccinated against core and non-core vaccines appropriate for his geographic area including leptospirosis.

Dusty is bright on examination. His sclerae and oral mucous membranes are icteric. Cardiac and thoracic auscultation are unremarkable. Heart rate, pulse quality and capillary refill time are within normal limits. Abdominal palpation appears to cause discomfort cranially, but no other abnormalities are identified. Peripheral lymph nodes are normal on palpation. Rectal temperature is normal.

Define the problem

Dusty has multiple problems including jaundice, suspected abdominal pain, vomiting, reduced appetite, weight loss and lethargy. Jaundice is the most specific problem and is not easily confused with other problems. Abdominal pain is a relatively specific problem. As many of the causes of jaundice may also cause abdominal pain, the two problems will be considered together.

Define the system

Jaundice may be caused by pre-hepatic, hepatic or post-hepatic disorders. Occasionally jaundice can be caused by other disorders such as sepsis, but this is relatively rare and unlikely in a dog that presents bright and cardiovascularly stable.

Pre-hepatic jaundice can be relatively easily differentiated from hepatobiliary causes of jaundice by measurement of packed cell volume. Dusty's packed cell volume was 39% (reference range 37–55%) with normal total protein (76 g/l) so pre-hepatic jaundice was ruled out. Thus, the jaundice was either primary hepatic or post-hepatic in origin.

Define the location

Dusty's serum biochemistry confirmed the presence of hyperbilirubinaemia (bilirubin 119 µmol/l, reference range 0–15). Liver enzyme activities were elevated (ALT 8 × upper limit of the reference range; ALP 9 × upper limit of the reference range). Hypercholesterolaemia (12.6 mmol/l, range 2.84–8.26) and mild hypertriglyceridaemia were also present. Globulins were mildly raised. Haematology showed changes compatible with an inflammatory leukogram but was otherwise unremarkable.

The biochemical findings showed some indications of cholestasis, but the marked increase in ALT activity meant that primary hepatic disease was also possible. Aside from raised bilirubin there were no other possible indicators of decreased hepatic function (albumin, urea and glucose were normal). Imaging was required to further differentiate between hepatic and post-hepatic jaundice.

A patient-side ELISA test for Leptospira serovars was negative. Coagulation was assessed by measurement of prothrombin time and activated partial thromboplastin time (PT and APTT). Both parameters were within normal limits. A sample was submitted to an external laboratory for measurement of Spec cPL® – this is a relatively sensitive test for pancreatitis, although results should always be interpreted in light of other clinical information as false-negative and false-positive results can occur - the test in isolation can neither definitely rule in or rule out the diagnosis of pancreatitis.

Define the lesion

Abdominal ultrasound was performed following administration of analgesia and sedation to facilitate relaxation of the abdominal wall. This showed subjective, mild hepatomegaly with hyperechoic hepatic parenchyma in comparison with the spleen; the pancreas was enlarged and irregular with diffusely hypoechoic parenchyma; the peripancreatic mesentery was hyperechoic; the pancreatic duct was mildly dilated; the common bile duct and intra-hepatic bile ducts were mildly distended; the gall bladder wall appeared mildly thickened/oedematous and contained normal, anechoic bile.

The changes seen on ultrasound were compatible with acute pancreatitis and suspected partial bile duct obstruction/inflammation. Primary hepatic disease could not be ruled out even with only mild ultrasound changes.

In view of the hepatic changes seen during ultrasound examination, percutaneous fine-needle aspirates were taken from the liver using ultrasound guidance and bile was collected via transhepatic cholecystocentesis. Platelet count had been previously confirmed as normal on haematology. Liver cytology was compatible with cholestasis and mild vacuolar hepatopathy. There was no evidence of inflammation or neoplasia. These changes were most likely secondary to acute pancreatitis and extra-hepatic cholestasis leading to a reactive hepatopathy. Bile cytology was unremarkable and bile culture was negative.

The Spec cPL result was 467 µg/l (reference interval <200), which was consistent with a diagnosis of acute pancreatitis.

Case outcome

Acute pancreatitis could explain Dusty's clinical signs and was considered to be the most likely cause of his jaundice. Pancreatitis can cause jaundice due to inflammation and physical compression of the bile duct leading to post-hepatic jaundice. This in turn can lead to a secondary, reactive hepatopathy.

Dusty was hospitalised and treated with supportive care including analgesia, anti-emetics, appetite stimulants, intravenous fluid therapy and initially a low-fat, highly digestible diet. Hepatoprotective and choleretic medications were also given (SAMe and ursodeoxycholic acid [UDCA]). He didn't vomit again, and his appetite and abdominal comfort improved within a few days. Dusty was discharged with oral medication after 4 days of hospitalisation.

One week later Dusty was rechecked. He seemed back to normal in his owner's opinion. His sclerae were mildly jaundiced but subjectively this was reduced compared to his original presentation. He was eating well and had gained weight but was not yet at his normal body weight. Repeat blood testing showed significant improvement of all liver enzyme abnormalities and reduction in hyperbilirubinaemia. Oral medication was discontinued apart from SAMe and UDCA.

One month after presentation, Dusty had returned to normal but remained in lean body condition. Repeat blood testing showed complete resolution of all of the previous abnormalities. Oral medications were stopped, and Dusty was gradually transitioned to a moderate-fat content, highly digestible diet. His owners were advised to avoid high-fat treats, and ongoing monitoring of his weight was recommended.

Pancreatitis is a common disease and can sometimes lead to jaundice. The majority of dogs and cats with jaundice due to pancreatitis recover with supportive care only – surgical intervention is not usually necessary.

CHAPTER 12

Bleeding

Jill E. Maddison

*Department of Clinical Science and Services, The Royal Veterinary College,
London, UK*

The why

- Bleeding is a potentially life-threatening clinical sign, which often requires prompt assessment and management.
- As with all clinical signs, a structured approach is the key to ensuring that important differentials are not overlooked.
- Understanding the pathophysiology of bleeding is also important, particularly in relation to interpreting relevant clinical pathology.
- Three major bleeding sites are discussed in this chapter, but the principles of the approach apply to any site of bleeding; most importantly – is this animal bleeding because of local disease or systemic disease?

Diagnostic approach to the bleeding patient

Define the problem

The potential for confusing bleeding as a clinical sign with another clinical sign is variable dependent on the site of bleeding.

Epistaxis
Epistaxis is defined as bleeding from the nose. It is unlikely that identification of the problem will pose any difficulties, although confirming the blood is coming from within the nasal cavity as opposed to perinasal skin is important (the latter almost always due to local trauma or skin pathology).

Melaena

Melaena is the presence of digested blood in the faeces and is manifested as black tarry faeces. It can also be detected using tests for occult faecal blood.

Before assuming melaena indicates bleeding in the gastrointestinal (GI) tract, it is important to determine whether the melaena is due only to the animal having eaten a meal very high in raw red meat (therefore, obtaining a dietary history is important. A high red meat meal is unlikely to cause true melaena but can cause the faeces to be very dark) or has swallowed blood – that is, is bleeding in the mouth or nasal cavity, coughing up blood then swallowing it or licking a bleeding wound (thus the physical examination is crucial).

Red urine

Red urine may be due to haematuria, haemoglobinuria, myoglobinuria or even ingestion of beetroot (beeturia). Hence, for the animal presenting with what the owner describes as 'blood in the urine', an important first step is to confirm that the urine discolouration is in fact due to the presence of red blood cells.

Clinical signs may assist (see the following sections), or a simple method is to centrifuge a sample of urine and examine the sediment and supernatant. In cases of 'pseudohaematuria', the supernatant will remain discoloured.

Note that urine dipsticks cannot differentiate between lysed blood cells, 'pure' haemoglobin and myoglobin.

Other clinical signs of bleeding

Bleeding disorders may manifest as a variety of other clinical signs including bruising, petechiation, haemoptysis, haematemesis, haematochezia, abdominal, pleural and pericardial haemorrhage or prolonged bleeding from a wound.

Define and refine the system

Is it local or systemic?

Bleeding may be due to local disorders or systemic disorders – this is the key question to answer, which has a profound impact on the diagnostic pathway and potential differentials.

Systemic disorders include bleeding disorders (coagulopathy), hypertension, polycythaemia, hyperviscosity and systemic vasculitis.

Local disorders causing bleeding

Define the lesion: local causes of epistaxis

Local disorders that can cause epistaxis include the following:
- Neoplasia
- Inflammatory/infectious
  - Immune-mediated or allergic rhinitis
  - Fungal infection
  - Local vasculitis
- Severe dental disease, for example, tooth root abscess
- Trauma
- Foreign bodies.

Clues
The diagnostic approach to local disorders or systemic disorders is obviously very different; thus, the initial goal should be to try to identify clues from the physical examination and history that suggest whether local or systemic disease is present.

Site of bleeding
Careful examination for any signs of bleeding at other sites (mucous membranes, skin, haematuria, melaena and retina) is essential. Whether the epistaxis is unilateral or bilateral may also be helpful – a bleeding disorder is less likely to cause a unilateral discharge, although this is by no means an absolute finding.

Character of the nasal discharge
Neoplasia, fungal infections and foreign bodies will often cause a mucopurulent as well as haemorrhagic nasal discharge. The animal may have a history of sneezing (more likely with local nasal lesions than bleeding disorders, but sneezing can still occur with systemic causes).

Nasal examination
Local disorders causing epistaxis may be associated with swelling or deformity along the nasal cavity, ulceration of the nares (fungal disease) and/or evidence of disruption/displacement of the nasal septum on radiographs.

If the animal has only epistaxis with no mucopurulent component, no signs of swelling or pain and no history of sneezing, a bleeding disorder should be considered even if there is no other site of haemorrhage detected (unusual).

Local disorders causing epistaxis – diagnostic approach

If a local disorder is suspected (other than trauma), a systemic disorder such as a coagulopathy has been ruled out from either the physical examination and diagnostic testing *and* the patient cannot be referred for computed tomography (CT) (see the following sections and Chapter 9), the diagnostic approach should involve nasal biopsies via aggressive intra-nasal aspiration and washings, radiography (maxillary views – 'radiographic plate in the mouth' technique) and/or rhinoscopy if the equipment is available.

Note that haemorrhagic/mucopurulent nasal discharge may occur with severe dental disease, so this should obviously be excluded as a cause before embarking on intra-nasal investigations.

Exploratory surgery of the nasal cavity is a messy and invasive procedure, and it is prudent to avoid it if possible. The following guidelines pertinent to local nasal disorders apply:

- Fungal and neoplastic causes of epistaxis are relatively common.
  - o Aspergillosis is the most common fungal disease observed in various countries.
  - o Neoplasia includes adenocarcinoma, squamous cell carcinoma, lymphosarcoma, fibrosarcoma, chrondosarcoma, haemangiosarcoma and osteosarcoma.
- Nasal biopsy/washings are best performed with some type of relatively rigid catheter, which is forcefully inserted into the nasal cavity as far as possible.
  - o Measure externally the length from the nares to the frontal sinus – cut a large stiff urinary catheter to this length (or mark it) and insert.
  - o Forceful aspiration is mandatory – gentle nasal washings with saline are usually unrewarding.

- Radiology is often of value if you can obtain radiographs of the maxilla only – that is, an intra-oral radiograph or ventrodorsal open mouth views.
  - o Both neoplasia and fungal disease will cause turbinate and septum destruction, but septal deviation is usually only caused by neoplasia.
- CT scanning is an extremely useful diagnostic tool in the diagnostic work-up of the patient with epistaxis due to local disease and should be considered as a diagnostic option if at all possible ahead of the previously mentioned procedures.

Define the lesion: melaena due to GI ulceration

Melaena can occur due to GI ulceration or due to bleeding disorders. In the latter case, there is no overt ulceration, and the use of anti-ulcer drugs in the management of these cases is not indicated.

Melaena due to GI ulceration may occur due to:

- *Primary GI* disease
  - o Neoplasia
  - o Parasites (e.g. *Ancylostoma caninum, Ancylostoma braziliense, Uncinaria stenocephala*)
  - o Foreign bodies
  - o Severe inflammatory disease

OR

- *Secondary GI* diseases that cause ulceration, for example,
  - o Hepatic disease
  - o Mast cell tumours (at any site)
  - o Gastrinoma
  - o Non-steroidal anti-inflammatory drug (NSAID) toxicity
  - o Hypoadrenocorticism.

Local disorders causing melaena – diagnostic approach

It is clear from reviewing the local and systemic causes of melaena that it is important you do not immediately assume that the presence of melaena indicates primary GI disease, even if vomiting is also present. Many of the secondary GI causes of ulceration will also cause vomiting (see Chapter 3). Failure to recognise this may result in *very* inappropriate diagnostic procedures (e.g. endoscopy) being performed on a patient with a coagulopathy or systemic disease causing ulceration.

The diagnostic approach to the patient with melaena will vary depending on the patient's signalment and concurrent clinical signs. Systemic causes are investigated (after ensuring a complete history, including drug access, is taken and a thorough physical examination performed) through haematology, biochemistry, abdominal imaging and/or endocrine testing.

Primary GI disease is investigated by faecal testing for parasites, abdominal imaging, endoscopy and/or exploratory surgery.

Define the lesion: Local causes of haematuria

Haematuria is most commonly due to local disease but, similarly to other sites of bleeding, can occur as a consequence of systemic disease.

The causes of haematuria due to local disease include the following:
- Urinary calculi
- Neoplasia
  - o Bladder neoplasia (most commonly transitional cell carcinoma)
  - o Neoplasia of the renal pelvis
  - o Polyps
- Inflammatory/infectious causes
  - o Bacterial cystitis
  - o Prostatitis
  - o Interstitial cystitis (cats)
- Idiopathic
  - o Idiopathic renal haemorrhage
- Vascular anomalies
- Trauma, for example, road traffic accident.

Clues
- Inflammatory lower urinary tract disease is usually associated with dysuria and/or pollakiuria.

- If the animal has haematuria without signs of pollakiuria or dysuria, then renal or ureteral haemorrhage (from any cause), cystic neoplasia, polyps or a systemic bleeding disorder should be considered.

 ### Define the location

The location of the bleeding in relation to the process of micturition may give some clues.
- If bleeding occurs at the beginning of urination, disorders of the lower urogenital tract – bladder neck, urethra, prostate, vagina, vulva, penis or prepuce – should be considered.
- Dogs with prostatitis will often drip blood unrelated to urination.
- Blood occurring at the end of urination or throughout urination is usually due to upper urinary tract disorders – bladder, ureters or kidneys.

Local disorders causing haematuria – diagnostic approach

- Identification of the cause of haematuria due to local disorders usually requires urinalysis +/– culture and sensitivity +/– diagnostic imaging.
- If a lesion has not been identified by these methods and a bleeding disorder has been ruled out (see the following sections), exploratory surgery may be required.

Systemic bleeding disorders

Physiology

Diagnosis and understanding of systemic bleeding disorders require an understanding of the normal process of coagulation.

When a vessel wall is damaged, a number of processes come into play to attempt to heal the vascular damage. The factors involved in forming a haemostatic plug are interdependent, and a defect at any level can result in a bleeding disorder.

Classically, three systems (the vascular wall, the primary haemo-static system and the secondary haemostatic system) are considered to be responsible for healing vascular damage. This classical approach to the coagulation system forms a basis for understanding many of the commonly used clinical coagulation tests. However, the classical approach does not explain all of the clinically observed findings relating to coagulation abnormalities. These include:

- The observation that Factor XII deficiency is not clinically significant, whereas Factor VII deficiency results in a severe coagulopathy.
- The fact that fibrinolysis is part of healthy healing, and this is clinically relevant with hyperfibrinolysis in *Angiostrongylus*, disseminated intravascular coagulation (DIC) and (to a much lesser degree – as in not very frequently an issue) greyhounds with bleeding post-surgery.

This has resulted in the development of an alternative or 'cell-based' model of coagulation. The reader is referred to other texts if they wish to delve more deeply into this area of physiology and pathophysiology.

As Figure 12.1 demonstrates (in a *very* simplified manner) vessel wall function, platelet function and the coagulation cascade are all involved in the formation of a clot after vascular damage has occurred.

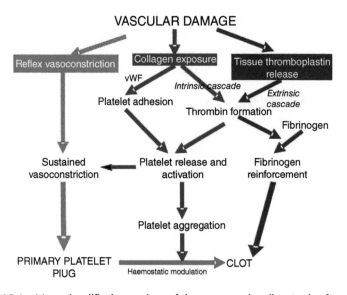

Figure 12.1 *Very* simplified overview of the process leading to the formation of a clot after vascular damage. vWF, von Willebrand factor.

Diagnosis of bleeding disorders

There are a range of tests that can be used to assess the coagulation system. The changes in coagulation tests that occur with different bleeding disorders are summarized in Table 12.1.

Table 12.1   Changes in coagulation tests associated with bleeding disorders.

Bleeding disorder	Coagulation tests results
Disorders of the intrinsic coagulation pathway, for example, • Haemophilia A *(Factor VIII deficiency)* • Haemophilia B *(Factor IX deficiency)*	• Prolonged activated clotting time (ACT) • Prolonged whole blood clotting time (WBCT) • Prolonged activated partial thromboplastin time (APTT) • Normal prothrombin time (PT)
Disorders of the extrinsic coagulation pathway • *Factor VII deficiency*	• Prolonged PT • Normal APTT
Disorders of the common pathway or multifactor disorders • Hereditary common pathway defects *(Factor II or X deficiency)*	• Prolonged PT, PTT, WBCT and ACT
• Acquired multiple factor deficiencies *(DIC, liver disease)* • Vitamin K disorders *(warfarin toxicity, malabsorption of vitamin K, liver disease, Devon Rex coagulopathy)*	• Thrombin time (TT) will also be abnormal in DIC, and FDPs will be increased • PT is prolonged before PTT in Vitamin K disorders due to the short half-life of Factor VII
von Willebrand's disease	• WBCT, ACT, PT, APTT and TT will usually be normal • PTT can be prolonged though not to a great degree – von Willebrand factor (vWF) binds with Factor VIII and increases its half-life • Buccal mucosal bleeding time and clot retraction will be prolonged
Acquired or congenital platelet dysfuction	• Buccal mucosal bleeding time and clot retraction will be prolonged

In general, prolongation of clotting times is regarded as significant if the patient time is more than 33% greater than the control sample. When using reference ranges, remember that 5% of the normal population will fall outside of the reference range (as the range is mean ±2 SD), so interpret with great care results that are only a few seconds outside the reference range. Decreased clotting times *may* be indicative of a hypercoagulable state.

Clinical signs
- Reduced platelet numbers or impaired platelet function usually manifests as bleeding from mucosal surfaces, for example, petechiation.
- In contrast, clotting factor deficiencies (from any cause) usually manifest as deeper tissue (ecchymosis) and body cavity haemorrhages.
- Petechiation and ecchymosis can also occur with vasculitis and local trauma.

Platelet count
- Ensure that you specifically request a manual platelet count from your laboratory if you are investigating a bleeding disorder, as many laboratories assess platelet numbers only qualitatively unless specifically requested.
- Although in-house haematology machines may be useful, they may also be inaccurate, and clinicians should be familiar with the assessment of platelet counts on a fresh blood smear.
  - Generally 8–15 platelets per high-power field (×100) would be considered normal.
  - Clinical bleeding is unlikely unless the platelet count drops below 50×10^9/L (usually $<30 \times 10^9$/L), which is approximately 3–4 platelets per high-power field.
  - The presence of multiple platelet clumps in the feathered edge is likely to represent numbers adequate for haemostasis.

Activated clotting time (ACT)
- An abnormal ACT indicates a defect in the coagulation cascade, specifically the intrinsic (Factors VIII, IX, XI and XII) and common (Factors V and X) pathways.

- The ACT does not assess platelet number or function. However, as platelets are essential for activation of the clotting cascade, the ACT may be prolonged in the presence of severe thrombocytopenia ($<10 \times 10^9$/L).
- A prolonged ACT suggests the presence of a severe coagulopathy.
- As the ACT is a relatively insensitive screening test, it may miss patients with mildly defective secondary haemostasis.
- The activated partial thromboplastin time (APTT) (see the following section) evaluates the same clotting pathways as the ACT but is more sensitive. Therefore, it is possible for a patient to have a normal ACT but a prolonged APTT.

Activated partial thromboplastin time (APTT)
- APTT assesses the *intrinsic* coagulation and common pathways (see above).
- In factor-deficient states, there must be at least a 30% deficiency of a factor before the APTT is increased.

Prothrombin time (PT)
- Measurement of PT assesses the *extrinsic* coagulation pathway (Factor VII).
- The PT is very sensitive to warfarin toxicity or vitamin K deficiency due to the short half-life of factor VII.

Thrombin time (TT)
- The TT measures the reactivity of fibrinogen to exogenous thrombin.
- It is independent of the intrinsic and extrinsic coagulation pathways.
- TT is prolonged in conditions causing hypofibrinogenaemia (DIC, liver disease) or dysfibrinogenaemia (liver disease).
- The TT may also be prolonged by thrombin inhibitors such as fibrin degradation products (FDPs) and heparin.

Thromboelastometry/theromboelastography
- These tests are currently mostly run in specialist hospitals but will probably become more available in practice in the future. They assess hypo- and hyperfunctional stages of the clotting process.

Platelet function

Platelet function can be assessed in-house by various crude methods including buccal mucosal bleeding time (most commonly) or clot retraction.

Buccal mucosal bleeding time

- The buccal mucosal bleeding time is a crude screening test for platelet function.
- A platelet count must be performed first – the test should only be used to assess thrombocytopathia, not thrombocytopenia.
- In animals with platelet dysfunction (e.g. von Willebrand disease), it will often be the only readily available test that can confirm that a tendency to bleed is present.
- Buccal mucosal bleeding time can be measured easily but does require a standard cut being made in the buccal mucosa and strict attention to detail when timing the formation of a clot. The test is quite subjective, and intra- and inter-observer variability is high.
- It is usually performed using a commercial device such as the Surgicutt® on the buccal mucosa. Two to four minutes is considered normal.

Clot retraction

This is performed as follows:

- Place a sample of blood into a glass test tube and leave it to stand for 4–6 hours.
- Clot retraction can be calculated by measuring the height of the clot compared to the height of the total sample in the tube.
- In a normal animal, the clot should separate from the serum and contract to approximately 50% of the original volume by 4–6 hours.

Clot retraction will be reduced if there is platelet dysfunction or if there is a significant thrombocytopenia. Hence, like buccal mucosal bleeding time, the test is mainly useful once thrombocytopenia has been ruled out as a cause of the coagulopathy.

In addition, disorders such as hypertension and hyperviscosity will increase the tendency for exudation to occur and will perturb platelet function.

Define the lesion: bleeding disorders

Bleeding may occur if there is:
- An abnormality of the *vessel wall*
  - Trauma (local)
  - Vasculitis
    - Local or systemic
- Reduced platelet numbers
  - Thrombocytopenia
- Platelet dysfunction (thrombocytopathia)
  - Lack of or decreased vWF
  - Defect in platelet activation and aggregation
- A defect in the extrinsic or intrinsic coagulation cascade
  - Haemophilia A and B
  - Vitamin K deficiency disorders, for example,
    - Rodenticide toxicity
    - Fat malabsorption
    - Devon Rex coagulopathy
- DIC
- Hyperfibrinolysis
  - Congenital
  - Acquired, for example, liver disease.

With particular reference to systemic bleeding disorder, the most common causes of impaired coagulation are:
- Immune-mediated thrombocytopenia (ITP or IMT)
- von Willebrand disease
- Drug-induced platelet dysfunction
- Rodenticide poisoning
- DIC
- *Angiostrongylus vasorum* infection (in endemic areas).
  Other less common causes include the following:
- Inherited platelet dysfunction
- Inherited coagulation factor deficiencies
- Malabsorption of vitamin K
- Acquired disorders of platelet function.

Define the lesion: thrombocytopenia

Thrombocytopenia may occur due to:
- Inadequate *production* of platelets
- Excessive *consumption* of platelets
- Excessive *destruction* of platelets
- *Infectious* causes (often a combination of mechanisms).

Unless there is a concurrent platelet function defect, haemorrhage due to thrombocytopenia will usually not occur until the platelet count is well below normal, usually at or below 30×10^9 cells/L (normal range $200–400 \times 10^9$ cells/L).

As acute haemorrhage can cause moderate to marked thrombocytopenia, moderately sub-normal platelet counts should not be over-interpreted, as they may be a consequence rather than a cause of haemorrhage. Platelet numbers are rarely reduced below 50×10^9 cells/L as a result of haemorrhage alone.

Inadequate production
Inadequate production of platelets by the bone marrow is associated with:
- *Primary bone marrow disorders* such as myelophthisis (replacement of blood-forming cells by neoplastic or inflammatory tissue).
- *Drugs* such as oestrogen and cytotoxic agents, which may suppress platelet production.
  - Various other drugs such as phenobarbitone and methimazole can also cause thrombocytopenia – many also cause anaemia and/or neutropenia.
  - In general, thrombocytopenia due to bone marrow failure will be associated with depression of other blood-forming cells.
  - An exception is the haemogram seen in the early stages of oestrogen toxicity when a neutrophilia is usually observed (neutropenia develops later).
  - Endogenous oestrogen toxicity due to testicular or ovarian tumours causing thrombocytopenia has been reported but is rare.
- *Retroviral infections* (feline leukaemia virus [FeLV], feline immunodeficiency virus [FIV]) in cats, which can cause thrombocytopenia and should be considered in a thrombocytopenic cat with no history of previous medication.

Excessive destruction

- Excessive destruction of platelets is usually a result of immune-mediated processes. ITP is the most common cause of thrombocytopenia in dogs but is rare in cats.
  o ITP can be a primary autoimmune disorder, induced by live vaccines or drugs or secondary to underlying pathology such as neoplasia and infection.
- Sepsis can also cause excessive destruction of platelets.

A definitive diagnosis of ITP can be difficult and requires measurement of anti-platelet antibodies (not widely available) and/or a bone marrow examination (reveals 'maturation arrest' of megakaryocytes).

However, at least in dogs, a diagnosis of ITP can usually be made from the haemogram alone if:

- Oestrogen toxicity can be ruled out from the history.
- There is no prior history of drug administration or vaccination that could cause thrombocytopenia.
- There is no evidence of underlying disease that might cause DIC (or it is ruled out by normal coagulation tests).
- Infectious causes are ruled out due to geography or lack of a travel history.
- The platelet count is sufficiently low to cause haemorrhage ($<30 \times 10^9$).

In cats, FeLV and FIV infection and other causes of decreased platelet production should be thoroughly investigated, as immune-mediated platelet destruction is a rare cause of thrombocytopenia.

Excessive consumption

Excessive consumption of platelets occurs in DIC. DIC occurs as a result of intravascular activation of coagulation together with fibrinolysis. As a result, thrombosis occurs in multiple organs, platelets and coagulation factors are consumed and become depleted and FDPs interfere with platelet function.

Excessive consumption or sequestration can also occur in micro-angiopathy (this can also be associated with intravascular haemolytic anaemia).

Infectious causes

- Tick-borne disease such as canine erlichiosis, Rocky Mountain spotted fever, cyclic thrombocytopenia, anaplasmosis and babesiosis can all cause thrombocytopenia and should be considered if these diseases are endemic to the area or the patient has travelled to endemic areas. Rarely, *Babesia* infection can be found in untravelled dogs in non-endemic areas.
- Leptospirosis may cause thrombocytopenia.
- The bleeding diathesis that can occur in a proportion of dogs with *Angiostrongylus vasorum* infection can be associated with a variety of coagulation abnormalities including thrombocytopenia.
  - The mechanism of coagulopathy has not been definitely established, but it is believed to be a hyperfibrinolytic disorder with thrombocytopenia due to the bleeding.

Miscellaneous causes

Rare causes of clinically significant thrombocytopenia due to consumption and/or sequestration and/or destruction of platelets include:
- Haemolytic uraemic syndrome
- Thrombotic thrombocytopenia purpura
- Sepsis
- Vasculitis
- Splenomegaly
- Splenic torsion
- Acute hepatic necrosis.

Define the lesion: platelet function defects (thrombocytopathia)

Inherited disorders of platelet function
Von Willebrand disease

- The most common hereditary platelet function defect is von Willebrand disease (vWD).
- vWD is due to a deficiency in von Willebrand factor (vWF, previously termed Factor VIII-related antigen).
  - vWF is associated with primary haemostasis and mediates the adhesion of platelets to exposed endothelial surfaces in sites of fast blood flow (i.e. not capillaries).

- vWD has a higher incidence in breeds such as Dobermans and German shepherds but has been reported in at least 54 different breeds.

Other inherited disorders
- There are a variety of inherited disorders of platelet function, but they are rare.
- Dysfunction of various components of platelet release or aggregation functions have been described, and the reader is referred elsewhere to more details about these disorders.
  - Breeds where inherited disorders have been reported include basset hounds, otter hounds, German shepherds, cocker spaniels and Persian cats.

Acquired disorders of platelet function
Platelet function (adhesion, release of vasoactive substances and/or aggregation) is impaired in a relatively large number of clinical disorders that may have clinical relevance to the patient. Disorders where platelet function may be impaired include:
- Uraemia
- Liver disease
- Pancreatitis
- Hypothyroidism
- Dysproteinaemia (e.g. multiple myeloma)
- Myeloproliferative disorders
- Drug-induced platelet dysfunction
  - Aspirin and other NSAIDs inhibit cyclo-oxygenase I and thus the synthesis of thromboxane by platelets.
    - As thromboxane is the most important factor in stimulating platelet aggregation, deficiency of thromboxane can severely impair platelet function.
  - The enzyme inhibition is irreversible with aspirin and phenylbutazone (i.e. persists for the life of the platelet), but with other NSAIDs the effect only appears to last while the drug is in circulation.
  - Clopidogrel is used therapeutically to decrease platelet activation and function, for example, in cats with hypertrophic cardiomyopathy or dogs with immune-mediated haemolytic anaemia.

In conclusion

As with many other clinical signs, the assessment of the bleeding patient requires a structured approach. This must be underpinned by appreciation of pathophysiology so that the results of diagnostic tests can be appropriately assessed.

The very first step when faced with a bleeding patient is to define the system – is the bleeding due to local or systemic disease? The answer can be obvious or require investigation, but the aim is to avoid a serious clinical error by neglecting to ensure that coagulation is normal before proceeding with invasive diagnostic tests to assess local disease, such as biopsy.

Key points

As a result of reading this chapter you should be able to:
- Recognise the importance of identifying whether bleeding from any site is due to local disease or a systemic bleeding disorder
- Recognise that diagnosis and understanding systemic bleeding disorders requires an understanding of the normal process of coagulation
- Develop a basic understanding of the process of coagulation
- Recognise the interaction that occurs between platelet function, the coagulation cascade and fibrinolysis
- Understand the basis of the clinical pathology tests used to diagnose bleeding disorders
- Understand how to interpret tests of coagulation
- Develop a rational approach to the diagnosis of bleeding disorders.

Questions for review

- List five broad mechanisms by which bleeding may occur.
- Identify the coagulation factors involved in each of the intrinsic, extrinsic and common coagulation pathways.

- What coagulation tests will be abnormal if there is a defect in each of the intrinsic, extrinsic and common coagulation pathways?
- What role do platelets play in the clotting process?
- List the mechanisms by which thrombocytopenia can occur.

Case example

'James' is a 2-year-old male neutered Pomeranian. He presented to the veterinarian because the owner was concerned he was passing black tarry diarrhoea and had had reduced appetite for 1 week.

On physical examination he was extremely nervous. His mucous membranes appeared pale. His heart rate was 160 bpm, pulses were synchronous and strong. His capillary refill time was <2 seconds. The rest of the physical exam and other vital signs were unremarkable other than obvious melaenic faeces on the rectal thermometer. There was no evidence of bleeding from any other location, no petechiation or echymoses.

He was fed a standard commercial diet with the occasional table scrap. He was fully vaccinated and up to date with appropriate parasite control. He lived in the UK and did not have a travel history.

The problem list

1. Melaena
2. Pale mucous membranes
3. Tachycardia.

Define the problems

Melaena
Due to a raw meat diet, swallowed blood or GI bleeding? *In this case, the melaena appears to be due to GI bleeding*.

Pale mucous membranes
Due to decreased peripheral perfusion or anaemia or both? *He is tachycardic, but there is no evidence of decreased perfusion so it is likely that he is anaemic. A packed cell volume (PCV) will help confirm this*.

Tachycardia
A heart rate of 160 is probably increased (reference range for small dogs = 80–140 bpm, though some references cite up to 160).

Define the system

Melaena
Is this due to:
- Primary GI disease?
- Secondary GI disease causing GI ulceration?
- A coagulopathy?

Pale mucous membranes
Blood work will be required to assess whether the anaemia is regenerative or not.

Tachycardia
- This could be physiological (he is very nervous) +/- pathological.
- If pathological the key question is whether it is due to primary cardiac pathology or extra-cardiac pathology, for example, anaemia, fever, pain. In this case anaemia is likely contributing.

Diagnostic results

- PCV = 18% (35–55)
- MCV (mean corpuscular volume) = 78 (60–74)
- Reticulocyte count (corrected) = 4.4%
- Platelet count = 100 x 10^9 (200–500)
- Total protein = 50 g/L (55–75)
- All biochemistry normal
- Faecal flotation negative
- Plain abdominal radiographs unremarkable
- Urinalysis unremarkable.

Revised problem list

1. Melaena
2. Pale mucous membranes due to significant regenerative anaemia
3. Tachycardia
4. Thrombocytopenia
5. Hypoproteinaemia.

Define the lesion

Is the *melaena* due to primary GI disease, secondary GI disease or a coagulopathy?

- No evidence for swallowed blood.
- Not sufficiently thrombocytopenic to result in spontaneous haemorrhage unless platelet dysfunction is present.
- Need to fully assess coagulation now to rule out a coagulopathy.
- If a coagulopathy is ruled out, then there is primary GI lesion that may be inflammatory, parasitic, due to a partial foreign body or neoplasia.

Is the *anaemia* due to haemorrhage or haemolysis?

- Hypoproteinaemia suggests that GI loss is likely in the absence of any other evidence for protein loss (renal loss or hepatic failure).

Further diagnostics and case outcome

- The coagulation profile was normal.
- Blood film review: *platelets are clumped and decreased; mild anisocytosis, mild polychromasia, mild hypochromasia, mild macrocytosis = consistent with regenerative anaemia; there are occasional mast cells present.*
- Ultrasound examination indicated thickened bowel loops.
- Post-mortem and histopathology confirmed infiltrative GI mast cell neoplasia.

CHAPTER 13

Polyuria/polydipsia and urinary incontinence

Jill E. Maddison and David B. Church

Department of Clinical Science and Services, The Royal Veterinary College, London, UK

The why

- Polyuria/polydipsia (PU/PD) is a relatively frequent presenting complaint in small animal practice.
- A wide range of disorders ranging from clinically inconsequential to life threatening may cause polydipsia and/or polyuria, and an ordered, rational diagnostic approach to the problem, as well as an understanding of the underlying pathophysiological processes, is invaluable in the successful investigation and management of these cases.
- When impaired urinary concentrating ability is identified during case assessment, this may lead to recognition of a range of potential causes of renal dysfunction.
- Urinary incontinence is also a relatively common problem in small animal practice – it may or may not be related to or associated with PU/PD.

Polyuria/polydipsia

Define the problem

The initial step in assessing the patient presenting with polydipsia is to ensure true polydipsia is present, that is, that increased drinking is not an appropriate physiological response. For example, animals with profuse watery diarrhoea will often drink more water than usual

---

Clinical Reasoning in Veterinary Practice: Problem Solved!, Second Edition.
Edited by Jill E. Maddison, Holger A. Volk and David B. Church.
© 2022 John Wiley & Sons Ltd. Published 2022 by John Wiley & Sons Ltd.

to maintain their hydration status. In addition, animals with gastritis will often drink large amounts of water but will vomit immediately and are not truly polydipsic. Increased levels of exercise and/or high ambient temperatures may also induce an animal to drink more than usual – another appropriate physiological response.

Those animals that drink excessively and subsequently urinate excessively (or vice versa) require investigation to determine the cause of their disordered water intake. These animals are defined as having polyuria/polydipsia (PU/PD).

It is important to be aware that a polyuric animal may present for urinary incontinence, and the owner may not be aware, or may not volunteer, that the animal is drinking more than usual. Owners may confuse pollakiuria (increased frequency of urinating small amounts) with polyuria. A logical approach to investigating urinary incontinence is discussed later in the chapter.

Confirmation of polydipsia
Polydipsia is usually defined in dogs as water intake that is twice maintenance requirements - approximately 100 mL/kg day. In cats, ingestion of greater than 50 mL/kg day is probably excessive and indicative of polydipsia. It may be necessary to measure the animal's water intake to ensure that it is polydipsic. However, particularly in the stressful hospital environment, a polydipsic animal may reduce its water intake for a period of time, and it is therefore desirable, if possible, to ask the owner to measure the intake at home.

Measurement at home, of course, may be very difficult or impossible if the owner has multiple animals and/or the pet drinks from uncontrolled sources such as a swimming pool, ponds, rain puddles or toilets. If the owner has noticed the dog or cat is drinking substantially more often (especially cats), they may be able to estimate roughly what the patient is drinking (e.g. 'I normally only have to fill the water bowl once per day but now I have to fill it three times per day').

Determine urine specific gravity (SG)
Having confirmed that an animal is truly polydipsic or polyuric, usually the initial and most important diagnostic step is to determine the urine SG – without this information, appropriate interpretation of other pathology results can be difficult.

However, it is also important to consider the other clinical signs the patient may have, as this will have an important influence on consideration of realistic differentials. For example, if the patient also has polyphagia and weight loss, the limited number of explanations (e.g. diabetes mellitus, hyperthyroidism) allows the clinician to make a rational assessment of the likely diagnostic possibilities even before a urine sample is obtained.

- Urine with an *SG of less than 1.008* (1.006 in cats) has been actively diluted (hyposthenuria).
- Urine with an *SG of 1.008–1.012* has neither been diluted nor concentrated (isosthenuria).
- Urine with an *SG of greater than 1.012* has been concentrated to some degree (hypersthenuria). However, whether the degree of concentration for the patient is *appropriate* must now be determined.

Normal animals may have a urine SG of any value depending on the physiological circumstances. It is therefore essential to always interpret urine SG *in relation to the hydration status of the patient*. Although urine with an SG greater than 1.012 has been partially concentrated, the degree of concentration may not be appropriate if there is any reason to suspect the patient has a diminished glomerular filtration rate (GFR) – in other words, *if it is dehydrated, or azotaemic or both*. On the other hand, a urine SG of 1.012 in an animal that is not polydipsic, dehydrated or azotaemic may be perfectly normal for that animal at that time on that day.

Before progressing, we should discuss relevant pathophysiological principles as they underpin our understanding of how to interpret urine SG as well as azotaemia.

Pathophysiology

Classifying the mechanisms of polyuria/polydipsia

Polydipsia and polyuria can only occur for two reasons – either the animal is drinking too much water and thus has polyuria as a normal consequence of increased water intake, or it has impaired renal concentrating capacity resulting in increased urine volume and thus must increase water intake to maintain neutral water balance.

When the cause is increased water intake with adequate urinary concentrating ability, the problem can be categorised as *primary polydipsia*. If the polydipsia occurs to compensate for impaired renal concentrating ability, the problem is categorised as *primary polyuria*. The concentrating ability of the kidney is dependent on a number of factors; impairment of any can result in primary polyuria and consequently polydipsia.

Primary polydipsia

Effectively, primary polydipsia is a behavioural abnormality or a form of cerebrocortical dysfunction and can be thought of as either a primary (intra-cranial) or a secondary (extra-cranial) abnormality (see Chapter 8). A number of well-defined endocrine disorders can result in a range of clinical signs that includes primary polydipsia. However, many patients with primary polydipsia are otherwise clinically unremarkable.

Primary polyuria

The reader is referred elsewhere to refresh his/her knowledge and understanding of renal physiology. There are several mechanisms by which the ability to modify urine concentration is compromised to a degree where primary polyuria occurs.

Reduced nephron number and/or function

Creation of a highly concentrated renal interstitium with a gradient of increasing concentration from renal cortex to renal medulla is essential for the formation of concentrated urine. The creation and maintenance of this gradient is dependent upon *normal numbers* of *normally functioning nephrons*. Consequently, reduced nephron numbers and/or reduced nephron function results in a diminished concentration gradient within the renal interstitium and impaired capacity to modify tubular filtrate and hence urine concentration.

Disorders that result in markedly reduced numbers of nephrons, or where nephron numbers are normal but their function is impaired, will result in increased urine volume and compensatory polydipsia.

Absent, deficient or impaired anti-diuretic hormone function

The second mechanism resulting in an impaired ability to concentrate urine occurs when the part of the nephron responsible for water moving from the tubular filtrate down its concentration gradient to the concentrated interstitium (the collecting tubule) remains impermeable to water.

The permeability of the collecting tubule to water and urea is a direct result of anti-diuretic hormone (ADH) binding to its receptors on the collecting tubules. A primary ADH deficiency or systemic factors interfering with ADH's binding to, or activation of, its receptors will impair this process.

Altered osmolarity of the glomerular filtrate

The third means by which urine-concentrating mechanisms can be impaired occurs when the tubular filtrate itself contains greater than normal numbers of osmotically active particles. When this occurs, the osmotic gradient between the tubular filtrate and the renal interstitium is reduced, and less water can be withdrawn from the tubular filtrate, even though both the renal interstitial osmotic gradient and the permeability of the collecting tubule are completely normal.

Summary

PU/PD can be due to:

1. *Primary polydipsia*

   Some of the disorders that can produce PU/PD through this mechanism include the following:

   - Psychogenic causes
   - Hyperadrenocorticism (part of the explanation – may also cause impaired urine concentration through the effect of cortisol on ADH function +/- concurrent urinary tract infection)
   - Hepatic encephalopathy (part of the explanation – may also cause impaired urine concentration, though the mechanism is uncertain)
   - Hyperthyroidism
   - Hypothalamic lesion affecting thirst receptors (rare)
   - Drug effect on thirst centre (e.g. phenobarbitone).

2. *Primary polyuria* due to:

   a. *Structural renal tubule damage (>75% loss of nephrons) resulting in reduced medullary hypertonicity*

   The disorders most likely to result in PU/PD through this mechanism include the following:

   - Chronic kidney disease (CKD)
   - Pyelonephritis

- Nephrocalcinosis
- Bilateral renal neoplasia

b. *Impaired nephron function resulting in reduced medullary hypertonicity*

The disorders most likely to result in PU/PD through this mechanism include the following:

- Hyponatraemia, for example, caused by
  - Hypoadrenocorticism
  - Profound gut sodium loss
  - And other disorders including urological and cardiac disorders, sepsis
- Decreased urea concentration in medullary interstitium
  - ADH deficiency/dysfunction (see point c)
- Liver disease causing decreased urea? (not resolved)
- Endotoxemia including pyometra and pyelonephritis – disrupts the medullary osmotic gradient
- Hypokalaemia – disrupts the Na-K pump in the ascending loop of Henle resulting in increased sodium loss
- Hypercalcaemia – disrupts the Na-K pump in the ascending loop of Henle resulting in increased sodium loss

c. *Absence of, or interference with, ADH function*

The disorders that can produce PU/PD through this mechanism include the following:

  - Diabetes insipidus
  - Hyperadrenocorticism
  - Hypercalcaemia
  - Hypokalaemia
  - Pyometra
  - Pyelonephritis especially if due to *E. coli*

d *Osmotic diuresis*

The disorders that can produce PU/PD through this mechanism include the following:

  - Glucosuria
    - Diabetes mellitus
    - Renal tubular defect.

Table 13.1 details the pathophysiological mechanisms causing PU/PD in various disorders.

Table 13.1   Pathophysiology of PU/PD.

Disorder	Pathophysiology
	PRIMARY POLYDIPSIA
Psychogenic polydipsia	• Psychogenic polydipsia is a behavioural disorder causing primary polydipsia, which causes compensatory (and appropriate) polyuria. • The cause is unknown, but it is speculated that anxiety may be a cause in some animals.
Hyperadrenocorticism	• Dogs with hyperadrenocorticism can usually reduce their water intake and urine output when initially hospitalized, confirming that they have primary polydipsia. • PU/PD does not occur in humans with hyperadrenocorticism or in humans on corticosteroid medication, which is a fascinating species difference. • Clinical impressions are that cats become polydipsic after corticosteroid treatment much less frequently than dogs, which also suggests an interesting species difference.
Hepatic disease	• The mechanism by which hepatic disease, especially portosystemic encephalopathy, causes polyuria remains controversial. • Various theories have been proposed – decreased urea concentration in the medullary interstitium may be a factor suggesting a primary polyuria. • However, dogs with portosystemic shunts can generally concentrate their urine when challenged by a water deprivation test, suggesting primary polydipsia may be the more likely explanation. • It is possible that this maybe a neurobehavioral consequence of encephalopathy.
Hyperthyroidism	• The mechanism by which hyperthyroidism causes PU/PD is multifactorial. • Thyroxine increases effective renal blood flow due to dilation of the pre-glomerular arterial vessel, which causes increased GFR and hyperfiltration. ○ It has been suggested that increased renal blood flow may also impair urine-concentrating ability by causing medullary solute washout, but this has never been confirmed. • It is also possible that thyrotoxicosis produces a primary, compulsive polydipsia due to disturbance of hypothalamic function. ○ People with hyperthyroidism have their osmoreceptors reset and therefore feel thirstier than they should on the basis of their plasma osmolarity. ○ It is thought that this may also be an important factor in causing polydipsia in cats.

(Continued)

Table 13.1   (Continued)

Disorder	Pathophysiology
PRIMARY POLYURIA – EXTRA-RENAL CAUSES	
Diabetes insipidus	• Central diabetes insipidus is due to the absence of ADH, which results in impaired water and urea reabsorption from the distal collecting duct. • This causes water loss as well as reduced osmolarity of the medullary interstitium due to reduced resorption of urea, which further reduces water reabsorption from the thin loop of Henle. • Diabetes insipidus may be congenital or acquired (e.g. due to neoplasia, trauma or idiopathic). • Nephrogenic diabetes insipidus is defined as lack of response to ADH. The most common cause is acquired impaired renal response to ADH, as noted in Table 13.2. ○ Congenital nephrogenic insipidus is very rare.

Hypercalcaemia	• Hypercalcaemia impairs the action of ADH on the collecting duct, although the exact mechanism has not been identified.
	• A protein, apical extracellular calcium-sensing receptor (CaSR), is believed to be involved.
	  ○ When luminal calcium increases, CaSR decreases ADH-induced permeability of the collecting duct.
	• In addition, there may be downregulation of the formation of water channels (aquaporin 2) in the collecting duct.
	  ○ The effect may be partial or total.
	• Other mechanisms proposed include:
	  ○ Impaired NaCl transport in the loop of Henle.
	• Hypercalcaemia will also decrease the GFR by causing vasoconstriction of afferent arterioles, which results initially in reversible azotaemia.
	  ○ Eventually, tubular function may become permanently impaired, causing azotaemia due to nephrocalcinosis (if the calcium × phosphate product is high), though this is not inevitable.

Hypokalaemia	• Hypokalaemia results in mild to moderate impairment of urinary concentrating ability through ADH resistance. ○ Aquaporin 2 is downregulated, resulting in decreased permeability of the collecting duct to water.
Pyometra	• Bacterial infection *(E. coli)* in pyometra causes decreased responsiveness to ADH, although urine dilution is still possible.

Table 13.1   (Continued)

Disorder	Pathophysiology
Hypoadrenocorticism	• Hyponatraemia due to any cause will impair urine concentration, although PU/PD may not be an overt clinical sign. • The cause is related to decreased medullary osmolarity as a result of sodium loss. • Low sodium also impairs the natural osmotic stimuli for ADH secretion (low serum osmolality) and so promotes formation of dilute urine despite dehydration.
Diabetes mellitus	• Primary polyuria in diabetes mellitus is due to the osmotic effect of glucose in the urine.

PRIMARY POLYURIA – RENAL CAUSES

Chronic kidney disease	• Both urine concentration *and* dilution are impaired in CKD. • As the number of functioning nephrons decreases, primary polyuria occurs partially due to osmotic diuresis as the remaining nephrons adapt and increase the fractional excretion of various solutes. • Urea is probably the most important osmotic factor, and although the remaining nephrons cannot increase the fractional excretion of urea, the GFR in the remaining nephrons does increase to a certain extent. • There may also be distortion of medullary architecture, which changes the osmotic gradient in the medullary interstitium and disrupts the counter-current mechanism. • A relative insensitivity to ADH is also postulated.
Pyelonephritis	• Pyelonephritis is an under-recognised cause of PU/PD. • It causes PU/PD because interstitial inflammation in the kidney prevents the maintenance of the medullary concentrating gradient. • The infective agent (particularly if it is *E. coli*) may also impair ADH function as occurs in patients with pyometra. • Thus this is an example of a structural *and* functional mechanism causing impaired urine concentration. • The severity of PU/PD can be marked. • It is important to realise that patients with pyelonephritis can have PU/PD without becoming azotaemic, so they do not have renal failure per se. • Impaired urine concentration is fully reversible when the infection resolves. • It is also important to recognise that urinary tract infection limited to the lower urinary tract (i.e. an uncomplicated cystitis case) may result in pollakiuria and urgency but does not cause PU/PD.

Azotaemia

It is impossible to discuss the pathophysiology of PU/PD and interpretation of urine SG without also understanding how to interpret azotaemia.

Azotaemia is defined as increased concentrations of non-protein nitrogenous wastes, measured as either serum creatinine, urea or BUN. The blood concentration of these substances increases if there is a significant decrease in the GFR. Decreased GFR is caused by underperfusion of the glomeruli or a lack of adequate numbers of functional glomeruli.

- *Decreased glomerular perfusion (sometimes referred to as pre-renal azotaemia)* occurs when renal perfusion is compromised, for example, by
  - Dehydration
  - Hypovolaemia
  - Cardiac failure
  - Shock
- *Decreased numbers of functioning glomeruli (sometimes referred to as renal azotaemia)* occurs as a result of decreased filtration through the glomerulus by one of the following mechanisms:
  - Constriction of the afferent glomerular arteriole
  - Impaired filtration at the glomerulus
  - Substantially reduced numbers of nephrons (loss of more than 75%)
- *Post-renal azotemia* occurs when there is failure of urine output
  - Ureteral, sphincter or urethral obstruction
  - Bladder rupture.

Azotaemia and impaired urine-concentrating ability often occur together in various disorders but, except in structural renal disease, the mechanisms for each differ.

The pathophysiological principles and diagnostic approach that follow in this chapter therefore apply to three problems, which may or may not occur concurrently:

- Confirmed polydipsia
- Inappropriately dilute urine in a dehydrated patient
- Inappropriately dilute urine in an azotaemic patient.

Table 13.2 summarises how different disorders cause azotaemia and impaired urine concentration.

Table 13.2 Summary of mechanisms for azotaemia and impaired urine concentration.

Disorder	Reason for decreased GFR resulting in azotaemia	Reason for impaired urine concentration
Chronic kidney disease	Decreased number of functional nephrons	Decreased number of functional nephrons
Hypercalcaemia	Constricted afferent arteriole +/– decreased renal perfusion if patient dehydrated	ADH dysfunction
Hyponatraemia	Hypovolaemia due to reduced blood volume associated with decreased serum sodium +/– additional decreased renal perfusion if patient dehydrated	Decreased medullary hypertonicity Impaired ADH release in dehydration
Dehydrated patient with normal renal function	Decreased renal perfusion	Urine concentration not impaired
Dehydrated patient with polyuric disorder	Decreased renal perfusion	Reduced medullary hypertonicity or ADH dysfunction or osmotic diuresis
Glomerular disease	Decreased rate of flow through glomerulus	Not impaired unless some form of concurrent more generalized tubular pathology develops

Diagnostic approach to the patient with PU/PD or impaired urine concentration

 Define and refine the system

It is apparent when reviewing the previous section and tables that PU/PD can occur due to a wide range of disorders that affect renal function. The key question thus becomes, *Has renal function been altered because of a structural problem or functionally?*

As discussed, persistent polyuria is due to either *primary polydipsia* (effectively a behavioural abnormality) or *primary polyuria* – a failure to concentrate urine appropriately. Primary polyuria may be the result of a *structural renal abnormality* (i.e. primary renal disease) or a *functional renal abnormality* (extra-renal disease).

A functional (extra-renal) abnormality occurs when urine concentration is impaired as a result of altered extra-renal factors that impinge on renal function. For example:

- Reduced renal medullary hypertonicity (as occurs with hyponatraemia)
- Diminished ADH function (as occurs with ADH deficiency and impaired ADH function secondary to other disorders such as hypercalcaemia, pyometra and hypokalaemia).

In other words, the primary location of pathology does not lie within the kidney but elsewhere – the kidney is merely the 'messenger'.

If the urine is very dilute (hyposthenuria), there are a limited number of diagnostic possibilities (see Table 13.2), and differentiation of the possible causes is relatively straightforward. Structural renal disease resulting in substantial (>75%) destruction of nephrons can be *ruled out* because active dilution of urine into the hyposthenuric range requires the presence of adequate numbers of nephrons to create appropriate medullary hypertonicity and thus to substantially dilute the tubular filtrate by the time it gets to the nephron's distal convoluted tubule.

Pyelonephritis poses a conceptual challenge because there are structural changes in the kidney (inflammation), but the mechanism for PU/PD involves alteration of the interstitial concentration gradient (as well as ADH dysfunction), *not* brought about by an absolute *reduction in the number* of nephrons as in CKD but by impaired *function* of the otherwise adequate number of nephrons present.

If the urine SG is between 1.008 and 1.030, the first consideration is whether the urine is inappropriately dilute for the hydration status of the patient. If a patient is dehydrated and renal function is normal, the urine SG should be greater than 1.030 (dog) or 1.035 (cat). If it is not, then renal dysfunction *must* be present – this can be due to either a structural or a functional renal abnormality.

If the urine is adequately concentrated, the patient was either *not* polyuric at the time of urine collection (which may occur in cases of primary polydipsia) or, if it is definitely polyuric at the time of collection, there must be an osmotic solute in the urine that is creating polyuria – the most common of these would be glucose.

Review Table 13.2, which summarises the mechanisms by which azotaemia and impaired urine concentration occur in various disorders.

Table 13.3 outlines the differential diagnoses for PU/PD or impaired urine concentration and outlines the key tests helpful for this purpose.

 ## Define the lesion

Table 13.3 Differential diagnosis of *confirmed* polyuria/polydipsia or impaired urine concentration.

Urine concentration	Differential diagnosis	Useful tests	Comments
Hyposthenuria Urine SG <1.008	Psychogenic polydipsia	Altered environment Water deprivation	• Water deprivation test really only used to differentiate from diabetes insipidus
	Diabetes insipidus*	Water deprivation/ ADH response test	• To differentiate from psychogenic polydipsia
	Hypercalcaemia	Serum Ca^{2+} (total and ionised)	• Other clinical signs will usually be present, though dogs with primary hyperparathyroidism can seem surprisingly well
	Hyperadrenocorticism	Low-dose dexamethasone suppression test or the less sensitive ACTH stimulation test	• Do not perform the suppression test if the patient is systemically unwell due to a concurrent non-adrenal disease

(Continued)

Table 13.3   (Continued)

Urine concentration	Differential diagnosis	Useful tests	Comments
	Pyometra	Leukogram and abdominal imaging	
	Pyelonephritis	Urinalysis, urine culture and sensitivity	• Urinalysis may have clues that a urinary tract infection is present, but they can be subtle or absent • The absence of haematuria or proteinuria does *not* preclude the diagnosis. • Urine culture and sensitivity are strongly recommended in any patient with PU/PD if an explanation has not been found from appropriate blood tests.
	Hepatic disease	ALT, ALP, bile acids and albumin	• Liver enzymes are markers of cellular damage or cholestasis, but levels do not correlate with hepatic function • Bile acids are often abnormal, but false positives and false negatives occur • Hypoalbuminaemia only occurs when 80% of hepatic function is lost

Table 13.3 (Continued)

Urine concentration	Differential diagnosis	Useful tests	Comments
	Hypokalaemia	Serum K^+	
	Hypoadrenocorticism (usually associated with isosthenuria or hypersthenuria but occasionally can cause hyposthenuria)	Leukogram, serum Na^{2+}, Na^+:K^+ ratio, basal cortisol and ACTH stimulation test	
Lack of appropriate concentration	CKD	Creatinine, urea, SDMA, phosphate, iohexol	
Urine SG 1.008–1.030	Hypercalcaemia	Serum Ca^{2+} (total and ionised)	
	Hyperadrenocorticism	Low-dose dexamethasone suppression test and ACTH stimulation test	• See previous comment
	Hepatic disease	ALT, ALP and bile acids	• See previous comment
	Diabetes mellitus	Blood and urine glucose	
	Pyometra	Leukogram and abdominal imaging	
	Pyelonephritis	Urinalysis, urine culture and sensitivity	• See previous comment
	Hyponatraemia	Serum Na^{2+}, Na^+:K^+ ratio, resting cortisol and ACTH stimulation test	• Profound hyponatraemia can occur in gut disease and other disorders
	Hypokalaemia	Serum K^+	
Concentrated Urine SG >1.030	Diabetes mellitus	Urine and blood glucose	
	Renal glucosuria	Urine and blood glucose	

Further comments related to Table 13.3

- *Animals with partial central diabetes insipidus (low but not total lack of ADH) can have isosthenuric urine *if* they are dehydrated.
- Animals with partial diabetes insipidus (central or nephrogenic) may on occasion have both hyposthenuria and isosthenuria.
- Other disorders that may be associated with polyuria/polydipsia and SG values ranging from hyposthenuric to concentrated include *hyperthyroidism, polycythaemia, pheocromocytoma, multiple myeloma*.
- Polyuria will occur in the diuretic phase of acute renal failure and post-urinary tract obstruction.
- Dogs with *internal haemorrhage*, for example, due to splenic haemangiosarcoma, can present with profound PU/PD and hyposthenuria. This is paradoxical because haemorrhage is a potent stimulus for ADH release, as ADH at high doses has a vasopressor function (hence its other name, vasopressin). This should cause increased urine concentration and hemodilution due to water retention. The observed polyuria and hyposthenuria is a compensatory measure stimulated by the initial haemodilution (excretion of excess water) compounded by the stimulation of the thirst mechanism by hypovolaemia due to profound blood loss.

Urinary Incontinence

 Define the problem

Urinary incontinence is a relatively common problem, especially in older female dogs. The owner may notice that the dog's bed is wet or that the dog seems to dribble urine unconsciously.

Urinary incontinence is essentially a result of either abnormal structure or impaired function of the lower urinary tract. Abnormal structure of the lower urinary tract resulting in incontinence is most commonly associated with congenital malformations and hence is a primary problem, while incontinence due to abnormal function may be associated with either a primary disorder or secondary to abnormalities in other body systems.

For example, an animal with otherwise subclinical impaired urethral sphincter incompetence may present with incontinence if it develops a disorder that results in PU/PD and thus an increase in urinary volume. Therefore, it is essential to ascertain if polyuria may be the cause of incontinence.

This is particularly important for the older female dog that presents with incontinence. Although sphincter incompetence is a common problem in these patients, the onset of polyuria due to renal disease, Cushing's syndrome or other disorders causing PU/PD may be the triggering factor for the incontinence. It is therefore important to do a urinalysis on all older female dogs presented for incontinence. If the urine SG is >1.030, there is no evidence of urinary tract inflammation and there is no history of other clinical problems including polydipsia, then empirical treatment for incontinence may be justified. If there *is* evidence for impaired urine concentration, this should be investigated if possible before instituting empirical treatment.

It is also important to distinguish urinary incontinence from inappropriate urination. The latter may reflect urinary tract pathology (pollakiuria, dysuria) or can be behavioural (urination in inappropriate places).

The type of incontinence and the animal's behaviour provide important clues to narrowing down the potential causes.

It is therefore important to *refine the problem* and determine whether the animal is showing:
- Intermittent incontinence, normal urination at other times
- Constant incontinence, no normal urination initiated
- Unsuccessful attempts to urinate.

 ## Define and refine the system and location

Urogenital vs. neurological
Urinary incontinence may be due to *local* lesions involving the urogenital tract or to *neurological* lesions involving the peripheral nerves and spinal cord.

Close observation and assessment of the characteristics of the animal's micturition pattern will assist in localising the appropriate system.

Questions that should be addressed are:

Does the animal ever urinate normally, that is, is it incontinent constantly or only intermittently?
If the animal can *squat and urinate normally* this indicates that detrusor function is relatively normal – that is, that the animal can sense a full bladder and initiate micturition appropriately.

If the animal *attempts to urinate but minimal volumes of urine are passed*, one can assume that the sensory and motor functions of the bladder are normal (i.e. the animal can feel its bladder filling and attempts to initiate micturition) but that there is an obstruction to outflow – this may be structural or functional.

If the animal is *never seen to initiate micturition*, particularly if it can be demonstrated that even when the bladder is full there is no attempt to urinate, one can assume that detrusor function is impaired. This may be due to neurogenic causes (spinal or peripheral nerve lesions) or local causes (e.g. disruption due to chronic distension of the stretch receptor and smooth muscle units in the bladder wall).

If the animal does attempt to urinate, what occurs?
Unsuccessful attempts to urinate indicate an obstruction of urine outflow, either at the neck of the bladder or in the urethra. The obstruction may be functional or structural.

Local lesions will involve the ureters, bladder, prostate or urethra.

Neurogenic lesions may be localised to the brain and spinal cord or peripheral nerves that innervate the bladder.
- Neurogenic lesions are usually the result of trauma, but neoplasia, intervertebral disc disease and degenerative conditions may also result in incontinence and disordered micturition.
- Upper motor neuron vs lower motor neuron lesions
  o The major differentiating feature is that *upper motor neuron* disorders cause increased urethral tone (thus functional obstruction) because of increased sympathetic discharge.
  o *Lower motor neuron* lesions (lumbo-sacral spinal cord and/or pelvic nerves) cause a flaccid bladder with reduced urethral tone.

Define the lesion

Intermittent incontinence, normal urination at other times
- Sphincter incompetence – hormone or adrenergic agonist responsive
- Urge incontinence – lower urinary tract infection/inflammation
- Reduced bladder capacity – cystitis, neoplasia, calculi
- Ectopic ureter – male (unilateral or bilateral), female (unilateral). Consider age and breed
- Prostatic disease.

Constant incontinence, no normal urination initiated
- Neurogenic
  - Bladder atony due to neurological deficits – spinal cord or peripheral nerves
- Local – urinary tract
  - Local destruction of stretch receptors and smooth muscle units in bladder wall secondary to severe and chronic distension
  - Total failure of urethral sphincter function – neoplasia, calculi (very large), neurological
  - Bilateral ectopic ureters (female).

Unsuccessful attempts to urinate
- Physical obstruction – neck of bladder or urethra – calculi, neoplasia
- Functional urethral obstruction
  - Reflex dyssynergia
    - Failure of urethral sphincter to relax appropriately when micturition is initiated
    - Differentiate from physical obstruction by catheterisation
      - There is usually no impedance to catheterisation with reflex dyssynergia
  - Upper motor neuron lesion causing increased uretheral tone.

In conclusion

Assessment of the patient with PU/PD can be relatively simple and straightforward for common disorders but more complex in other cases. Although referring to a list of differential diagnoses such as Table 13.3 can be helpful in assessing PU/PD cases, an understanding of the pathophysiological basis for impaired urine concentration assists enormously in the rational interpretation of appropriate diagnostic tests so that the diagnosis can be reached expediently and safely.

Defining and refining the problem is the real key to assessment of urinary incontinence.

Key points

As a result of reading this chapter you should be able to:
- Appreciate the difference between primary polydipsia and primary polyuria
- Recognise that primary polyuria may be due to structural renal disorders or functional, extra-renal disorders
- Recognise that determination of urine specific gravity can be important in the diagnostic work-up of the patient with polyuria/polydipsia
- Understand the similarities, but most importantly the differences, in the mechanisms by which impaired urine concentration and azotaemia occur
- Identify and recognise the significance of impaired urine concentration in a dehydrated or azotaemic patient
- Develop a logical and prioritised list of differential diagnoses for polyuria/polydipsia and how the urine SG may facilitate this process
- Develop a rational approach to the diagnosis of urinary incontinence.

Questions for review

- Briefly explain the basis for azotaemia and impaired urine concentration in chronic renal failure, hypercalcaemia, hyponatraemia and diabetes insipidus.
- What causes of polyuria/polydipsia can be *excluded* if the patient has the following urinalysis result: SG 1.002, -ve glucose, -ve protein, -ve bilirubin, -ve blood?
- A dog has confirmed PU/PD and is clinically dehydrated. It has a urea concentration of 30 mmol/L (reference range 5–10), creatinine of 250 µmol/L (reference range 55–100) and a urine SG of 1.010. What disorders are possible?
- A dog has confirmed PU/PD but is NOT clinically dehydrated. It has a urea concentration of 30 mmol/L (reference range 5–10), creatinine of 250 µmol/L (reference range 55–100) and a urine SG of 1.010. What disorders are possible?

Case example

'Bailey' is a male neutered, Labrador cross dog aged 7 years weighing 40 kg.

He was presented for annual vaccination. During the history taking the owner advised that over the past 3 weeks Bailey has had an increase in water intake. The owner reports that he usually drinks about 3L/day but this has now increased to around 4-5 L/day.

The owner has also noticed that he appears to be urinating more. There is no straining or discomfort on urination nor discolouration of the urine.

Otherwise, Bailey appears normal. His appetite is normal, and he is bright and active at home. No vomiting or diarrhoea has been reported, and he has not lost any weight since his last visit. There has been no change in diet, no change in exercise routine and no travel history. He is up to date with vaccinations and parasite control.

The problem list

1. PU/PD.

Define the problem

Bailey is drinking at least 100 mL/kg per day so polydipsia is confirmed. Increased urination has also been noted. So the problem is defined as PU/PD.

Define the system

The key question is whether Bailey has primary polydipsia or primary polyuria.

The first piece of information that will help with this assessment is a urine SG, which was 1.004 = hyposthenuria. All dipstick tests were negative, and there was no sediment.

Hyposthenuria can be due to primary polydipsia (possible as Bailey is very well otherwise) or primary polyuria. If he has primary polyuria then it must be due to extra-renal dysfunction; that is, structural renal disease causing substantial loss of nephrons (>75%) can be excluded.

Diagnostic results

Relevant blood results from the biochemistry profile were:
Total calcium 3.83 mmol/L (1.98–3.00)
Phosphate 0.90 mmol/L (0.81–2.2).
All other biochemical parameters were within the reference range.

Revised problem list and assessment

1. PU/PD – hyposthenuria
2. Hypercalcaemia

Define the lesion

The primary disorders that will cause hypercalcaemia (assuming it is repeatable) associated with a low normal serum phosphate and normal electrolytes are anything that results in an uncontrolled increase in parathyroid hormone (PTH) or something with PTH-like activity including:
- Primary hyperparathyroidism
- Malignancies elaborating PTH or PTH-like compounds such as lymphoma, anal sac adenocarcinoma.

Further diagnostics and case outcome

Diagnostic plans were to:
- Request a repeat serum calcium and phosphate and, where applicable and the result is likely to be reliable, an ionised calcium
- Repeat physical exam paying particular attention to the lymph nodes and include a rectal examination
- Do abdominal and thoracic imaging to investigate lymphoma or other neoplasms if indicated
- Consider, if indicated, cervical ultrasonography and PTH and PTrH testing.

Results
- The repeat serum calcium and phosphate were 3.9 and 0.89 while the ionised calcium was 1.8 mmol/L (1.18–1.37 mmol/L)
- On rectal examination an anal gland mass was found
- Abdominal ultrasound was performed and sublumbar lymph nodes were enlarged.

Outcome

Bailey was referred to a specialist surgeon to remove the anal gland mass and sublumbar lymph nodes. Histopathology confirmed anal gland adenocarcinoma.

CHAPTER 14

Gait abnormalities

Holger A. Volk[1], Elvin R. Kulendra[2] and Richard L. Meeson[3]

[1]Department of Small Animal Medicine and Surgery, University of Veterinary Medicine Hannover, Hannover, Germany

[2]North Downs Specialists Referrals, Bletchingley, UK

[3]Department of Clinical Science and Services, The Royal Veterinary College, London, UK

The why

- Any abnormality in locomotion would be considered a gait abnormality and may be attributable to a wide range of neurological and/or orthopaedic problems.
- Differentiating between causes of gait abnormalities in practice can be challenging. By initially defining the problem and the system involved, a list of further appropriate diagnostic tests can be performed.
- Although a 'lameness' is a type of gait abnormality where there is a reduced weight bearing of a limb, and is most commonly orthopaedic in origin, it is important to recognise that neurological disorders can have similar presentations.
- Lameness is a clinical interpretation of a change in gait, where a decreased weight bearing of the affected limb is seen, and animals may shift their weight on to their other limbs to compensate.
- Neurological disorders will more commonly present as decreased voluntary movement (paresis) usually paired with ataxia or lack of voluntary movement (plegia).
- The neurological and orthopaedic examinations remain the foundation of localising and characterising the lesion and are critical prior to any more involved tests.

Clinical Reasoning in Veterinary Practice: Problem Solved!, Second Edition.
Edited by Jill E. Maddison, Holger A. Volk and David B. Church.
© 2022 John Wiley & Sons Ltd. Published 2022 by John Wiley & Sons Ltd.

- Once the location of the lesion has been defined, a list of differential diagnoses can be formulated based on signalment, onset, clinical course and clinical features such as pain and asymmetry of clinical signs.
- Each individual case has its own challenges, and any purely rule-based system is likely to result in mistakes.

 ## Define the problem

Defining the problem for an animal with a gait abnormality primarily involves information given by the owner and observation by the clinician. Therefore, a detailed history is essential as well as focused observation.

History
- What is the clinical onset and chronological progression of the gait abnormality?
- Progression of the gait abnormality – is it deteriorating, stable or improving?
- Is it worse after exercise/after rising from recumbency?
- Any history of lameness in other limbs?
- Response to medication/rest?
- Any changes in behaviour or mentation?
- Any history of back pain?
- Has there been a history of pyrexia?
- Has there been any weight loss?

General observations
- Is the patient lame on one or more legs?
- Is there a shifting lameness?
- Is there a change in stride length?
- Is there a sign of sensory deficit and/or ataxia?
- Is the gait stilted?
- Is the patient stiff (and if so where and when)?
- Is leg movement abnormal (e.g. bunny hopping or skipping)?
- Does the animal appear 'weak'?

These observations are all important in progressing understanding of the abnormality present and the likely differential diagnoses.

Figure 14.1 provides guidance on the clinical reasoning steps that assist in identifying the problem in animals with gait abnormalities.

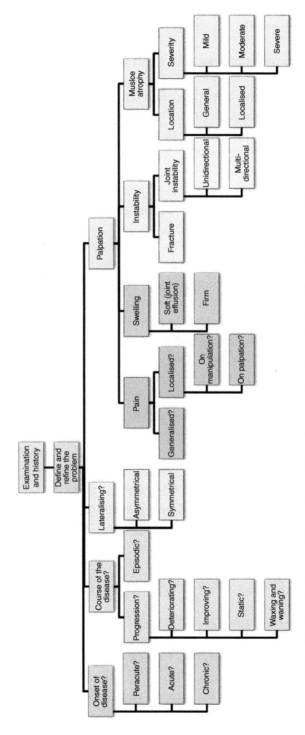

Figure 14.1   Factors to be considered for refining the problem in patients with gait abnormalities.

Define and refine the system

Differentiating musculoskeletal from neurological gait abnormalities

The majority of patients who present with gait abnormalities will have an underlying orthopaedic and/or neurological disorder. The problem may be due to a structural or functional disease process, and both can lead to 'weakness', difficulty rising, collapse and gait alterations.

A *primary structural* problem can involve the musculoskeletal system or nervous system (neuromuscular/peripheral nervous system [PNS] or central nervous system [CNS]).

A *functional abnormality* can be caused by derangements of the cardiovascular, respiratory or metabolic systems that have a secondary effect on the nervous or musculoskeletal system, for example, hypoglycaemia secondary to an insulinoma. Typically, functional abnormalities that result in alteration of the gait will have concurrent clinical signs that may be related to other body systems. For example, it would not be unusual for a dog with a pancreatic islet cell tumour ('insulinoma') to present with seizures as well as inter-ictal weakness.

Those patients who have structural abnormalities in multiple locations, for example, musculoskeletal as well as the nervous system, can prove to be a challenge, as it can be difficult to identify which is the most clinically significant problem. However, a thorough scrutiny of the history and physical examination may give the clinician clues.

Abnormalities of any of the following systems can result in clinical signs of weakness (Chapter 7), collapse (Chapter 8) or gait abnormalities.

- Primary structural
  - Musculoskeletal – muscles, bones, ligaments, tendons and joints
  - Nervous – CNS and neuromuscular system
- Secondary functional
  - Cardiovascular – heart, vascular structures and blood

- o Metabolic – electrolytes, for example, potassium/sodium and glucose
- o Respiratory – upper or lower airways, pleural space and thoracic wall
- o Inflammatory arthropathies due to systemic disease – idiopathic, infectious diseases, gastrointestinal/hepatic disease and neoplasia
  - ▪ Note that while there are clearly structural changes in inflammatory arthropathies due to systemic disease, the cause of these changes is outside of the joint, that is, the joint is just 'the messenger'. Hence the classification as secondary.

The presence of concurrent clinical signs, history and laboratory work will generally allow the clinician to prioritise the body systems in order of clinical significance. The diagnostic approach to weakness and collapse is discussed elsewhere (Chapters 7 and 8).

The majority of patients who present with gait abnormalities will have abnormalities that primarily and structurally affect either the musculoskeletal or the nervous systems. There is no simple laboratory or diagnostic test that can be performed to differentiate between the nervous and musculoskeletal body systems – the differentiation between the two systems is based on the clinician's physical examination.

Usually, myopathies present as weakness; they are discussed in Chapter 7. An example of a myopathy that may present as 'lameness' would be myotonia (e.g. in Chows or dogs with hyperadrenocortcisim) causing a stilted gait.

Figure 14.2 can be used as an aid to help identify whether the clinical signs identified are to be more likely associated with musculoskeletal (orthopaedic) or nervous system (neurological) disease.

Most animals with neurological disorders will present with *paresis and ataxia*, while those with orthopaedic disorders will present with *lameness*. It can be challenging to differentiate lameness *(inability to move)* and paresis *(inability to create movement)*. It is not

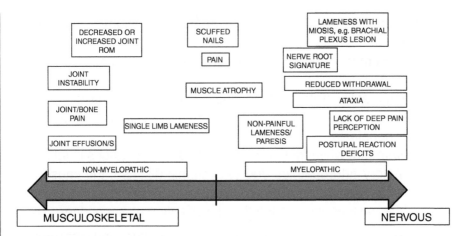

Figure 14.2 Clinical deficits to help differentiate between musculoskeletal and nervous system disorders. ROM, range of movement.

uncommon for patients with bilateral orthopaedic disease, for example, bilateral cruciate disease, to present in a similar manner to those with neurological disorders. However, the most challenging cases involve patients where both orthopaedic and neurological disorders coexist.

 Define the location

The location of the problem can be identified by a systematic and thorough orthopaedic and neurological examination. Following the examination, the clinician will hopefully be able to localise the lesion.

If the orthopaedic system is involved, structures affected include the long bones, joints, muscles, tendons or ligamentous structures. However, if the lesion involves the neurological system, the lesion may affect the CNS and PNS. Most parts of the nervous system (brain, spinal cord or neuromuscular system) can be associated with gait abnormalities (also see Chapter 7).

CNS dysfunction can involve the forebrain ('initiation of movement'), cerebellum ('fine-tuning of movement') or brainstem ('motor coordination and long fibre tracts passing to the target muscles'). Lesions affecting these brain structures can usually be easily differentiated from orthopaedic gait abnormalities, as they are accompanied by other brain-specific deficits such as behaviour and mentation changes, cranial nerve deficits and/or vestibular deficits (Chapter 8).

Deficits of the neuromuscular system or the spinal cord, however, can be more difficult to differentiate from orthopaedic problems.

History
As discussed earlier, a general history regarding the animal's overall systemic health should be obtained before focusing on more specific questions regarding the gait.

Once a history has been obtained, a general examination should be performed to identify any other concurrent conditions that may be significant. This is especially important after trauma, as it helps to identify life-threatening injuries that should be addressed before treatment of the animal's orthopaedic or neurological injuries.

Orthopaedic examination
The orthopaedic examination is the key to identify the location of the lesion. It can be divided into three parts:
- Distant examination
- Gait analysis
- Palpation/manipulation.

Distant examination
Examination should begin with observation of the animal standing or sitting, and consider:
- Evidence of muscle atrophy – most evident over the proximal thigh muscles in the pelvic limbs and over the spine of the scapula in the thoracic limbs.
- The weight distributed through the individual thoracic and pelvic limbs. Is weight distribution symmetrical? Observing the animal rising to standing from lying down may demonstrate that it favours one particular limb when rising. Evidence of exacerbation of the lameness ascending or descending stairs.
- Any evidence of limb malalignment as the animal stands straight, for example, carpal varus/valgus, antebrachial growth deformities.

Gait analysis

Following distant examination, the animal should be observed walking and trotting, ideally in a well-lit relatively long corridor or an outdoor road:

- Lead walk the dog, ensuring sufficient slack that the head is free to nod.
- Initially walk slowly up and down the corridor.
- When turning it is important that the animal is kept on the inside of the dog walker so that the gait can be assessed during this phase of the examination.
- The speed is gradually increased to a trot and potentially a run.
- For cats, observation should be performed in the examination room.
- Often it is worthwhile asking owners to make video recordings of their animals at home to help inform the assessment.
- Certain lameness can also be exacerbated when the animal is walked on hard surfaces and becomes easily identifiable from the transition from grass to concrete, for example, digital corns.

The presence of a head nod in the thoracic limb is consistent with a thoracic limb lameness. When the lame leg hits the ground, the head will rise, and when the sound leg hits the ground, the leg will sink ('SSS: sink on sound side'). Stride length should also be assessed, as animals with bilateral lameness will have shortened stride lengths present. Nails should be assessed for any evidence of scuffing, and the animal should also be assessed for evidence of ataxia (incoordination).

It is common to grade the severity of a lameness using systems of 0–10 or 0–5. Lameness grading is most useful as a subjective measure of lameness during follow-up examinations when performed by the same observer.

Palpation/manipulation

The distant examination and gait analysis would hopefully have allowed localisation of the lameness to a particular limb. The subsequent orthopaedic examination is intended to identify the source of the lameness and potentially its severity, and *hence* the patient should be examined conscious wherever possible. Small dogs are most easily examined on the table-top, but larger dogs are often examined on the floor. It is recommended to examine the affected limb last, as this is most likely to cause a reaction.

With the animal standing:

- Palpate for signs of asymmetry in muscle mass between paired limbs from distal to proximal.
  - The muscles of the proximal thigh in the pelvic limb and the supraspinatus and infraspinatus in the thoracic limbs can be used to assess muscle atrophy.
- Apply pressure to the palmar/plantar aspect of the carpus or tarsus to assess the degree of weight bearing of each limb.
  - It is important to make sure that the dog is standing square at this point.
- Flex and extend the neck dorsally, ventrally and laterally and then palpate the cervical, thoracic and lumbar spine.
  - Animals with lumbosacral pain often react when the tail is elevated dorsally.
  - If abnormalities are detected, a full neurological examination is warranted.

With the animal moved into lateral recumbency if tolerated or remaining standing:

- Examine all four limbs starting from the toes and moving proximally.
- Each joint should be examined for any evidence of swelling, restriction in range of movement, pain, signs of instability and crepitus.
- Long bones should be palpated for signs of pain or swelling, for example, neoplasia or panosteitis or fracture.

Cranial drawer and tibial thrust

Cranial drawer and tibial thrust are specific tests that are used to assess the integrity of the cranial cruciate ligament. Cruciate ligament instability is a very common cause of pelvic limb lameness in dogs and should be included in an orthopaedic examination.

Cranial drawer is performed by:

- *Stabilising* the femur with one hand and the proximal tibia with the other.
  - The thumb and index finger over the lateral fabella and patella.

- ○ The other hand stabilizes the tibia with the index finger over the tibial tuberosity and the thumb over the fibula head.
  - ○ When both hands are in position, the tips of the placed fingers and thumbs appear as the four corners of a square.
- The femur should be maintained in a fixed position while the tibia is moved in a cranial direction.
- The test should be performed in flexion and extension, as partial ruptures of the cranial cruciate ligament may only be detectable in flexion.
- Full extension of the stifle may result in a false-negative result, as the collateral ligaments remain taut in extension, preventing cranial translation of the tibia. It is also important to avoid twisting the stifle as the draw test is performed.

Tibial thrust is dynamic test of the integrity of the cruciate ligament and is often easier to perform in the conscious animal and in large/giant breed dogs.

- The test is performed by stabilising the cranial aspect of the distal femur with one hand and placing that hand's index finger over the tibial tuberosity.
- The other hand grasps the metatarsus.
- The stifle is maintained at a fixed angle and the hock is slowly flexed several times.
- Cruciate deficient stifles will result in cranial translation of the tibial tuberosity as the hock is flexed.
- The manoeuvre should be performed at various angles of flexion and extension.

Based on physical examination findings, Figure 14.3 can be used as a guide to identify the appropriate diagnostic step(s) in the investigation.

Neurological examination

It is important to perform the neurological examination in a way that the animal feels most comfortable, otherwise the exam, and in particular proprioceptive tests, can result in false positives.

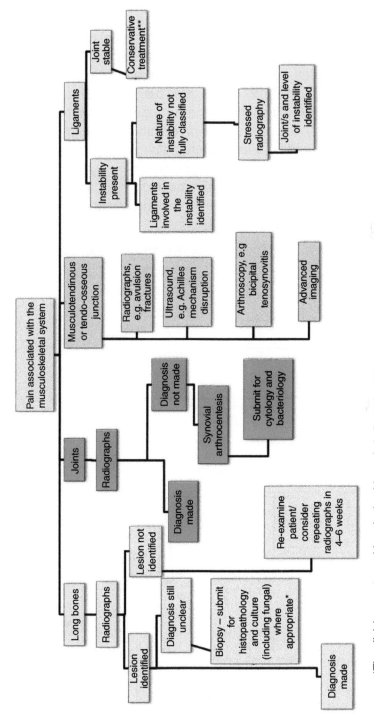

*The clinician must consider whether biopsy in indicated and the possible morbidity associated with the procedure.

** If the ligamentous injury is the result of a degenerative process it is likely to progress to joint instability.

Figure 14.3   Diagnostic work-up for the musculoskeletal system.

- General observations (mentation, posture and gait) should be completed first, and assessments with the potential to cause pain (palpation and nociception) should be left until last.
  - Ideally, a complete neurological examination is performed, but in some patients, this may not be possible.
- The order of the examination can be arranged so that tests that are more clinically relevant to the presenting complaint can be evaluated earlier (and hopefully before patient compliance is lost).
- In cases where one is uncertain about the neurological localisation, repeating the neurological examination may increase the likelihood of recognising subtle abnormalities. It may also reveal trends in the progression of clinical signs.

Figure 14.4 provides a flowchart of defining the location of the neurological lesion.

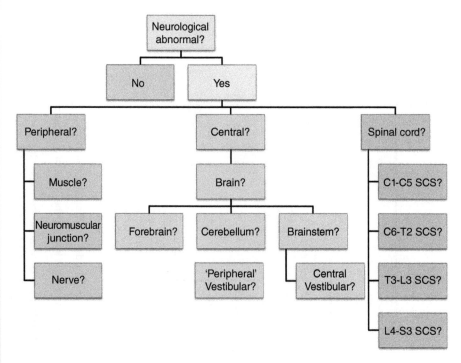

Figure 14.4 Neuroanatomical localisations. SCS, spinal cord segments.

Two questions should be asked after every neurological examination:

1 Is the animal neurologically normal or abnormal?

2 If abnormal, where is the location of the lesion?

Spinal diseases can be roughly divided into two disease categories, *myelopathic* or *non-myelopathic*. Animals that present with back pain should be differentiated between myelopathic and non-myelopathic. Animals with concurrent neurological deficits are myelopathic, whereas those that present without neurological deficits are non-myelopathic.

Spinal diseases that are accompanied by pain usually affect the meninges, spinal nerve root(s), vertebrae and/or their articulations (facet joint and intervertebral disc).

Similarly to the orthopaedic examination, the neurological examination can be divided into parts as follows:

- Hands-off examination – observation
  - Mentation and behaviour
  - Posture
  - Gait
  - Identification of abnormal involuntary movements
- Hands-on examination
  - Postural reaction testing
  - Cranial nerves assessment
  - Spinal reflexes, muscle tone and size
  - Sensory evaluation.

Once the location and distribution (focal, multifocal or diffuse) of the lesion within the nervous or muscular system is determined (Table 14.1; Figures 14.2 and 14.4), a list of differential diagnoses can be constructed (taking into account signalment, history, pain involvement and, most importantly, the onset and progression of clinical signs). Only then can a structured plan for further investigations and treatment be established.

Table 14.1 Neuroanatomical localisations and their most common deficits.

Thoracic limbs (gait affected)	Thoracic limbs' reflexes	Pelvic limbs (gait affected)	Pelvic limbs' reflexes	Postural reactions in affected limbs	Other	Neuroanatomical localisation
Yes	Intact to increased	Yes	Intact to increased	*Reduced to absent*		C1-C5 SCS (C1-C4 vertebrae)
Yes	*Reduced to absent*	Yes	Intact to increased	*Reduced to absent*		C6-T2 SCS – cervical intumescence (C5-T1/2 vertebrae)
No	Intact	Yes	Intact to increased	*Reduced to absent*		T3-L3 SCS (T2/3–L2/3 vertebrae)
No	Intact	Yes	*Reduced to absent*	*Reduced to absent*	Possibility of a Schiff–Sherington posture	L4-S3 SCS – lumbar intumescence
Possible	*Reduced to absent*	Possible	*Reduced to absent*	*Reduced to absent*		Neuromuscular system – *Nerve**
Possible	Intact (reduced)	Yes	Intact (reduced)	Intact (unless too weak)	Exercise intolerance	Neuromuscular system – *Neuromuscular Junction**
Possible	Intact	Possible	Intact	Intact (unless too weak)	Exercise intolerance	Neuromuscular system – *Muscle**

SCS, spinal cord segments (note: spinal cord is shorter than vertebral column). Intumescence = origin of the nerves for the specific limbs.

* See Chapter 8 for more details.

Define the lesion

Musculoskeletal disorders

Once the location of the lesion has been identified, the next step is to define the pathology of the disease process as well. The pathology of the disease process is likely to fall under one of a number of categories. The DAMNIT-V scheme can be used as a helpful reminder for the different type of pathological processes that can occur (Table 14.2).

Clinical progression and pattern of disease, in combination with patient signalment, help the focus on differentials. For example, a lameness with associate focal bone pain is more likely to be panosteitis in a young large breed dog, whereas it is more likely to be a primary bone neoplasm in an older large breed dog.

The differential list can subsequently be prioritised based on signalment, onset of clinical signs, duration, travel history, severity of clinical signs, number of limbs affected and whether it affects a single bone or joint or multiple bones or joints.

Neurological disorders

Once the location of a problem within a body system is identified as the nervous system, the next key question is, *What is it?* That is, you need to define the pathology. As with orthopaedic disease, it can be helpful to remember the types of pathology that can occur on broad terms using the DAMNIT-V scheme (see details mentioned previously).

Note that the list of differentials in an animal with a neurological gait abnormality relevant to a metabolic and nutritional disorder is small. The type of pathology most likely responsible for the clinical signs depends not only on the clinical course of the disease, presentation, symmetry of the deficits and pain involvement but also on the signalment of the patient (species, breed, age, sex etc.), the geographic location of the patient and what is common in that population (Figure 14.4).

Using the five-finger ('neuro-hand rule' [onset, clinical course, pain, lateralisation and neuroanatomical localisation – see also Chapter 8]) rule can be very helpful in clinical reasoning. After you have determined the problem by using your five-finger rule, use the signalment and see if it can help you refine it even further.

Table 14.2 Differentials to be considered for musculoskeletal disorders.

Category	Thoracic limb	Age	Pain	Onset	Pathological fracture	Pelvic limb	Age	Pain	Onset	Pathological fracture
Primary, structural disorders										
Degenerative						Cruciate disease	Y, A	P	G, A	
						Achilles tendon rupture, for example, Dobermans**	A	P	G, A	
						Plantar ligament degeneration	A	P	G	
Developmental	Elbow dysplasia	Y, A	P	G		Hip dysplasia	Y	P	G	
	Osteochondrosis dissecans	Y	P	G		Patellar luxation	Y	P	G, A	
	Retained cartilaginous core	Y		G		Osteochondrosis dissecans	Y	P	G	
	Angular limb deformities†	Y, A	P	G		Angular limb deformities†	Y, A	P	G	
Anomalous	Panosteitis	Y	P	A		Panosteitis	Y	P	A	
	Hypertrophic osteopathy	A	P	G		Hypertrophic osteopathy	A	P	G	
Neoplastic	Primary bone tumour	Y, A	P	G, A	Path	Primary bone tumour	Y, A	P	G, A	Path
Inflammatory/ infectious	Immune-mediated polyarthritis	Y, A	P	G, A		Immune-mediated polyarthritis	Y, A	P	G, A	
Traumatic	Septic arthritis	Y, A	P	A		Septic arthritis	Y, A	P	A	
	Fractures	Y, A	P	A		Fractures	Y, A	P	A	
	Luxations	Y, A	P	A		Luxations	Y, A	P	A	
	Ligamentous injuries	Y, A	P	A		Ligamentous injuries	Y, A	P	A	
	Tendon injuries	Y, A	P	A		Tendon injuries	Y, A	P	A	
	Muscle contracture†	Y, A	P	A		Muscle contracture†	Y, A	P	A	

Category	Thoracic limb	Age	Pain	Onset	Pathological fracture	Pelvic limb	Age	Pain	Onset	Pathological fracture
Vascular	Bone infarct*	A		A		Bone infarct*	A		A	
						Legg Calves Perthes disease	Y	P	A, G	Path
Secondary, functional or systemic disorders										
Metabolic	Hypertrophic osteodystrophy	Y	P	A		Hypertrophic osteodystrophy	Y	P	A	
	Renal hyperparathyroidism	A	(P)	G, A	Path	Renal hyperparathyroidism	A	(P)	G, A	Path
Neoplastic	Metastatic bone tumour	A	P	G, A	Path	Metastatic bone tumour	A	P	G, A	Path
Nutritional	Nutritional hyperparathyroidism	Y	(P)	A	Path	Nutritional hyperparathyroidism	Y	(P)	A	Path
	Hypervitaminosis A	Y, A	P	G		Hypervitaminosis A	Y, A	P	G	
	Vitamin D deficiency	Y, A	(P)	G, A	Path	Vitamin D deficiency	Y, A	(P)	G, A	Path
Inflammatory	Reactive immune-mediated polyarthritis due to neoplastic, infectious or parasitic disease	Y, A	P	G, A		Reactive immune-mediated polyarthritis due to neoplastic, infectious or parasitic disease	Y, A	P	G, A	

* Bone infarcts – long-term outcome following medullary infarction is limited, but it has been associated with total hip arthroplasty and neoplasia.
** An acute on chronic presentation may be appreciated with Dobermans with a degenerative achilles tendonopathy.
† Condition may or may not be associated with pain.

Age: A, adult and aged dog; Y, young dog. Pain: P, can be associated with pain; (P), pain associated with pathological fracture. Onset: G, gradual onset; A, acute onset. Pathological fracture: Path, can cause pathological fractures.

Painful non-myelopathic spinal diseases

- Animals that solely present with back pain and do not show neurological deficits need to have a thorough orthopaedic examination, as discospondylitis, or more rarely polyarthritis, may present with back pain.
- Other differentials are inflammatory, infectious and neoplastic diseases.
- If the animal presents with a history of trauma, luxation and fractures need to be considered.
- Syringomyelia is an exception and can present as a painful condition without causing neurological deficits.
  - Syringomyelia and steroid-responsive meningitis arteritis (SRMA) can appear at first similar in presentation (painful cervical spine – non-myelopathic); however, considering the clinical history, they can be differentiated.
    - Syringomyelia has a chronic-progressive history, whereas SRMA has an acute history associated often with pyrexia.
    - Note that SRMA can be cyclic, and some animals might have experienced pain episodes in the past.
    - If you then take into account breed (syringomyelia occurs in small brachycephalic breeds and SRMA usually in beagles, border collies, boxers, whippets, Jack Russell terriers and Weimaraners) and age (SRMA usually in younger animals), you have a very high chance of differentiating the two conditions.
    - A cerebrospinal fluid (CSF) sample can then verify the presumptive diagnosis of SRMA (depending in which part of the world you live you might need to consider infectious diseases) or a magnetic resonance imaging (MRI) scan to confirm the diagnosis of syringomyelia.

Myelopathic spinal diseases

The five-finger rule (onset, clinical course, pain, lateralisation and neuroanatomical localisation) can be used to effectively differentiate between myelopathies (Table 14.3).

Table 14.3 Differentials to be considered for myelopathies.

Category	Acute non-progressive	Acute progressive	Chronic progressive
Degenerative		Type-I disc disease (P, AS, A, Y)	Cervical spondylomyelopathy (P, AS, A, Y)
			Type-II disk disease (P, AS, A)
			Degenerative myelopathy (AS, A)
			Demyelinating diseases (Y)
			Axonopathies and neuronopathies (Y)
			Subarachnoid diverticulum (AS, Y, A)
			Breed-specific myelopathies (such as Afghan hound myelopathy) (Y)
			Storage disease (Y)
Anomalous			Chiari-like malformation and syringomyelia (Y, A)
			Vertebral anomalies (Y)
			Atlantoaxial (sub-)luxation (Y)
			Spinal dysraphisms (Y)
Neoplastic		Primary (AS, A)	Nephroblastoma (AS, Y)
		Metastatic (AS, A)	Primary (AS, A)
		Skeletal (P, AS, A)	Metastatic (AS, A)
			Skeletal (P, AS, A)
Nutritional			*Hypervitaminosis A (Y, A)*

(Continued)

Table 14.3 (Continued)

Category	Acute non-progressive	Acute progressive	Chronic progressive
Inflammatory/ infectious		Distemper (P, AS, Y, A)	Distemper (P, AS, Y, A)
		FIP (P, AS, Y)	FIP (P, AS, Y)
		Protozoal (P, AS, Y)	Protozoal (P, AS, Y)
		MUA (P, AS, A)	MUA (P, AS, A)
		Discospondylitis (P, AS, Y, A)	
		ANNPE (AS, Y, A)	
Traumatic	*Fractures (P, AS, Y, A)*		
	Luxations (P, AS, Y, A)		
	Contusions (AS, Y, A)		
	ANNPE (AS, Y, A)		
Vascular	Infarction (FCE; AS, Y, A)		
	Haemorrhage (AS, Y, A)		
	Vascular malformations (AS, Y)		

A, adult and aged dog; Y, young dog; P, can be associated with pain; AS, can be asymmetrical in presentation (one side more affected than the other); ANNPE, acute non-compressive nucleus pulposus extrusion; FIP, feline infectious peritonitis; MUA, meningomyelitis of unknown aetiology . Diseases that can also present with spinal pain without causing neurological signs are in italics.

Common examples

- Patients who present with peracute, non-progressive or improving, largely non-painful and lateralised neurological deficits (most often in T3-L3 spinal cord segments) have a 98% chance of having:
  - An ischaemic myelopathy such as fibrocartilaginous embolism (FCE)
  - or high-velocity but low-volume disc prolapse (acute noncompressive nucleus pulposus extrusion [ANNPE]).
- Hansen type-I disc disease (intervertebral disc extrusion) is best characterised as an acute onset, deteriorating, painful and occasionally lateralised myelopathy (often at T3-L3 spinal cord segments). Ninety percent of patients presenting with these clinical signs will have Hansen type-I disease.
  - In contrast, Hansen type-II (intervertebral disc protrusion) has a more chronic onset, is often stable and can be painful.
- Meningo(encephalo)myelitis of unknown aetiology (MUA) can present with an acute onset, deteriorating painful myelopathy.
  - MUA is four times more likely to present as a multifocal neuroanatomical localisation (multiple spinal cord segments and/or brain).
  - Many of the animals will also have mentation changes and cranial nerve deficits.

These examples demonstrate that thinking pathophysiologically and using the five-finger rule can refine the differential list significantly. If you then also take demographics and signalment into account, you have a very high chance of identifying the most likely diagnosis before embarking on diagnostics. Many of the neurological conditions will require advanced imaging and/or CSF analysis, but funds are limited, and the aforementioned approach can provide you with the framework to narrow down diagnostics to the most essential or provide the owner with a presumptive diagnosis.

Diagnostic tools for assessment of gait abnormalities

Lesion localised to the musculoskeletal system

Following lesion localisation, the area in question is interrogated further with the most appropriate diagnostic test (most often an imaging modality, and most commonly radiography).

- Bone pathology (focal discomfort, swellings etc.) should be initially evaluated with orthogonal radiographs of the affected area.
    - o It is usually advisable to also radiograph the contralateral limb to help determine whether the changes seen are pathological, normal or normal variant.
- Joint pathology (pain, crepitus, swelling, instability), again would normally have a first-line evaluation with plain radiographs.
    - o Joint effusions may be visible such as in cases of cruciate disease where cranial displacement of the infrapatellar fat pad is often present.
- In certain situations, 2D plain radiography is not able to provide a more definitive diagnosis, and contrast radiography or 3D imaging such as CT or direct arthroscopic visualization may be necessary, such as for certain types of shoulder and elbow disease.
- Stressed radiographs are indicated if there is joint instability present clinically or the cause of the pain is not apparent on the plain radiographs.
    - o Stressed radiography is commonly used to identify ligamentous injuries in the distal limbs, for example, the tarsus and carpus, but it can also be used in the more proximal joints as well.
    - o Stresses can be applied in flexion, extension, valgus and varus. The joints involved and the direction of any instability will play an important role in determining the most appropriate treatment.
    - o Stressed radiography is not always required following detection of joint instability and will depend on the clinician's clinical judgement; for example, the diagnosis of cruciate disease is often inferred following detection of cranial drawer or tibial thrust in the stifle.
- Injuries involving the musculotendinous or tendo-osseous junction or muscles may be best imaged using ultrasound or advanced 3D imaging techniques.

- Synovial arthrocentesis, although not routinely performed, may help to identify inflammatory or infectious disease processes when subtle or no abnormalities are detected on survey radiographs, yet there is clinical suspicion of pathology and joint pain.

Lesion localised to the nervous system

As in lesions localised to musculoskeletal system disease, the most appropriate diagnostic test is used to characterize the lesion further.

- Radiography is a widely available and relatively inexpensive tool allowing the rapid screening for obvious bony abnormalities. The soft tissues of the spine and nervous tissue parenchyma are not directly discernable in radiographs. Survey spinal radiographs may detect vertebral malformations, vertebral fractures and sub-luxations, bony lysis (associated with neoplasms or infectious disease processes) and narrowed intervertebral disc spaces. Correct patient positioning without rotation is important, which usually requires general anaesthesia. The only exception is spinal trauma patients, where it needs to be considered that anaesthesia can reduce muscle tone and therefore increase instability.
- Computed tomography provides far better spatial resolution and bone detail of the vertebral column and provides further certainty than plain radiographs, but it is not readily available in most practices.
- Myelography remains a useful technique to identify space-occupying lesions and remains an important diagnostic in dogs with suspected intervertebral disc herniation. Myelography is con-traindicated for animals with increased intracranial pressure and has been associated with more adverse effects when used for cervical imaging.
- Most cases require, however, more advanced imaging modalities, with MRI being the gold standard for nervous system lesions, as the nervous system can be directly visualized and therefore pathologies better characterised.
- If infectious or non-infectious inflammatory CNS disease is suspected, CSF examination is to be performed. CSF analysis is a sensitive but not a specific test. Other degenerative diseases like intervertebral disc disease, metabolic, neoplastic, traumatic or vascular diseases of the CNS may also alter CSF composition. Thus, this test needs to be evaluated together with the imaging findings.

In conclusion

The patient presenting with a gait abnormality may have orthopaedic disease, neurological disease or both. A detailed history and the orthopaedic and neurological examinations are the key diagnostic tools that will enable the clinician to formulate a rational differential list and plan appropriate diagnostic procedures to confirm the diagnosis.

Key points

As a result of reading this chapter you should be able to:
- Appreciate that gait abnormalities can be caused by disorders of the neurological system, musculoskeletal system or both. However, it is usually relatively straightforward to determine whether it is an orthopaedic lameness or a neurological gait abnormality in most cases
- Recognise the importance of obtaining a detailed history and performing a thorough orthopaedic or neurological examination prior to performing further tests such as diagnostic imaging
- Ensure your examination and diagnostics include assessment of common causes of lameness, such as stifle stability tests for cranial cruciate ligament stability assessment.
- Most orthopaedic conditions can be diagnosed using plain radiography, and more advanced imaging is only needed in select cases.

Questions for review

- What key differences do you observe between a dog with a lameness vs. neurological paresis?
- When would you consider advanced imaging for diagnosing orthopaedic or nervous system disease?

CHAPTER 15

Pruritus, scaling and otitis

Andrea Volk

Lecturer in Veterinary Dermatology, University of Veterinary Medicine Hannover, Hannover, Germany

The why

- Pruritus, scaling and otitis are the most common skin complaints in companion animals, particularly dogs.
- There are many causes of these clinical signs, and the purpose of this chapter is not to discuss the details of specific skin diseases but to give some background to the pathogenesis of pruritus, scaling and otitis and provide a structured approach to the assessment of the patient with these three conditions.

PRURITIS

Pathophysiology

Pruritus is an unpleasant sensation of the skin provoking the urge to scratch. The physiological rationale for pruritus is to eliminate parasites. Pruritus is an autonomous, pain-independent sensation, which is transmitted to the thalamus via itch-specific neuronal pathways. Recognition of pruritus leads to scratching, which induces pain over-riding the itch sensation. Pruritus-related projections to the thalamus are actively inhibited by pain-processing neurons and vice versa; once these pain neurons are suppressed, the itch sensation may increase. An example is seen in humans receiving morphine treatment. We need to remember that in animals we are only able to observe the scratching, which we interpret as a behavioural response to itch.

Clinical Reasoning in Veterinary Practice: Problem Solved!, Second Edition.
Edited by Jill E. Maddison, Holger A. Volk and David B. Church.
© 2022 John Wiley & Sons Ltd. Published 2022 by John Wiley & Sons Ltd.

An understanding of the pathophysiology of pruritus improves the clinician's appreciation of the rationale for anti-pruritic management strategies.

Pruriceptors

Pruriceptors are specific free nerve endings in the epidermis, dermo-epidermal junction and dermis. After stimulation via mediators (see next paragraph), the pruritic sensation is transmitted via afferent, slow-conducting C-fibres to the dorsal horn of the spinal cord and via central itch-specific neuronal pathways to the thalamus.

Pruritic mediators

The cytokine IL-31 has been identified as the major pruritic cytokine in people, canines and felines, predominantly produced by T_H2 cells. Other mediators stimulating pruriceptors are IL-2 (IL-6, IL-8 presumed) predominantly from T cells and mast cells, neuropeptides from keratinocytes, kinins (including bradykinin), amines (including histamine), proteases (produced by, e.g. neutrophils, bacteria, fungal organism, mast cells, other inflammatory cells), prostaglandins, leukotrienes, neurophins and substance P. Interestingly, not every mediator induces in every species or even every dog breed itch or even the same level of itch; the specific mechanisms to explain these differences in detail are still to be elucidated.

Presence of pruritic mediators in cutaneous inflammation will lead to a vicious cycle perpetuating itch and inflammation. Chronic stimulation of keratinocytes, Merkel cells, mast cells and Langerhans cells has been shown to produce nerve growth factor (NGF). This leads to an increasing number of itch fibres in the epidermis and dermis. This is one of the likely underlying mechanisms that explains the increasing difficulties that can occur in controlling chronic itch, particularly when appropriate therapy has not been started in an earlier phase.

Central factors

The itch threshold in humans has been shown to be reduced in the following circumstances:

- At night
- By increased skin temperatures
- By decreased skin hydration
- With increased psychic stress.

Stressful situations may potentiate pruritus through release of various opioid peptides. Competing cutaneous sensations (pain, touch, heat, cold) can magnify or reduce the sensation of pruritus. Thus, the sensation of pruritus is often increased at night, as other sensory input is low.

 Define the problem

Owners may not always recognise that their pet's behaviour is occurring because the pet is pruritic. It is therefore important to make owners aware of signs of itch other than obvious scratching, such as:
- Rolling
- Rubbing
- Chewing
- Scooting
- Head shaking
- Licking.

There is a validated visual analogue scale of pruritus available (Hill et al, Vet Dermatol 2007 18(5):301-8) to objectify owners' subjective perception of pruritus, and this can also be useful in monitoring the effect of treatment on the level of itch. It can be helpful to enquire whether, if there is a low level of pruritus, the owner feels the animal has a good quality of life despite the itch, as, for example, allergic patients will never be itch-free. These discussions will aid in putting the owner's expectations in a realistic light, which is very important for the management of chronic pruritic cases.

 Define and refine the system

In pruritus, the skin is the primary system affected. The initiating cause may originate from within the skin (primary skin disease) or less commonly be secondarily affected due to systemic disorders (such as biliary, renal disorders), neuropathic (Chapter 13) or compulsive behaviour disorders (Chapter 8).

 Define the location

Distribution
The distribution of pruritus is a very important guide for the differential diagnoses list (see Figure 15.1). Ectoparasites, such as scabies, are seen predominantly on lesser haired areas on pinnal margins and

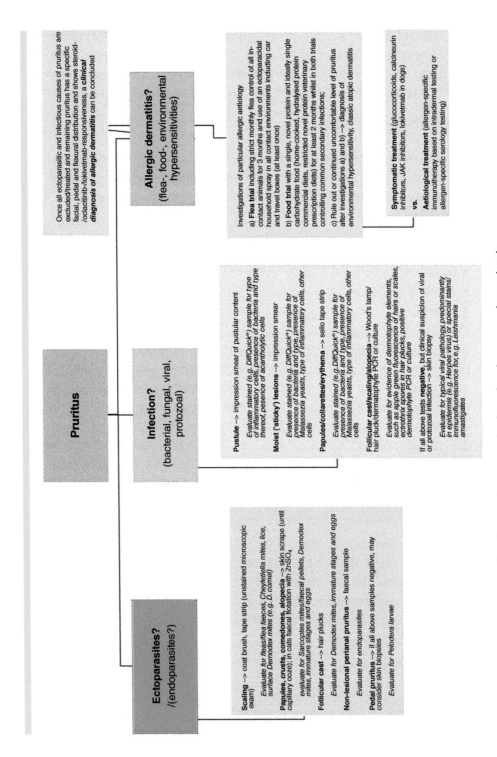

Figure 15.1   Flow diagram to the diagnostic approach of pruritus in companion animals.

extensor areas of elbow and tarsus; demodicosis is mostly found in a facial and pedal distribution; fleas and *Cheyletiella* commonly cause pruritus primarily on the dorsal rump. In contrast, allergic dogs and cats predominantly have pruritus on the flexural areas of the body and medio-ventral aspects of the body, respectively.

Define the lesion

Major causes
Many skin diseases will cause pruritus, but the major ones are:
- Ectoparasites (and endoparasites)
- Infection (bacterial, fungal, viral, protozoal)
- Allergic skin disease (flea, food, environmental hypersensitivities.

Primary skin lesions
It is important for the clinician to identify primary skin lesions and differentiate them from secondary ones. For example, the presence of follicular pustules will narrow the differential list (pyoderma, pustular dermatophytosis; pemphigus foliaceus, further sterile pustular diseases) and guide you to the correct diagnostic test (impression smear of pustular content) to either confirm the diagnosis or lead to the next diagnostic test. In comparison, identification of papules would lead to the consideration of scabies, other ectoparasites, early pyoderma (if follicular) or allergic dermatitis. Skin scrapings would be the appropriate test in these cases.

Should the skin look completely normal, but the animal is pruritic, allergic skin disease should be considered (pruritus *sine materia,* i.e. clinically normal with pruritus) as well as systemic disorders (in particular renal and biliary disorders), neuropathic disorders (ear/neck phantom scratching in dogs with syringomyelia) and compulsive behaviour disorders.

Secondary skin lesions
Secondary lesions, such as excoriations, lichenifications, scars, fissures, callus and necrosis, may not be very helpful in leading to a diagnosis. They can, however, indicate to the clinician the level of pruritus and chronicity of the disease. Other secondary lesions such as collarettes, erosions and ulcers may have some diagnostic value and may be the only lesion observed when the primary lesion is fragile, such as vesicles or pustules in autoimmune diseases.

Rate of onset

A rapid onset of pruritus is most often associated with acute secondary superficial pyoderma, *Malassezia* dermatitis, ectoparasite infestation, particularly *Sarcoptes*, *Cheyletiella* or fleas or ingestion of an ingredient to which the patient is hypersensitive. In patients with environmental hypersensitivities, there is more likely a gradual increase in pruritus when entering their allergy season. Another cause of acute pruritus can be onset of a completely new disease process, for example, a chronic mildly atopic patient developing epitheliotropic lymphoma.

Seasonality

If the pruritus recurs only in a particular season, it may suggest a likely triggering factor. For example:
* Flea-related pruritus is more common in the summer months.
* Grass hypersensitivity is more likely in spring and summer months.
* House dust/storage mite hypersensitivity is more likely to show pronounced flares from October until January/February.

Perennial itch could be related to food hypersensitivity and/or house dust/storage mite hypersensitivity. In addition, itch can increase due to psychogenic causes as a result of certain activities within the home environment (e.g. stress of visitors, building works, moving home, new animals, beloved owners in hospital).

Secondary infections

Secondary infections of the skin are a frequent complication of many pruritic disorders and will be in themselves pruritic. Thus, once infection has been identified that needs antimicrobial treatment, it is best to avoid glucocorticoids in the first instance. Pruritus and skin lesions will be re-assessed upon resolution of the infectious process and will then provide further clues as to the aetiology of the pruritus. However, a subset of allergic dogs presents with recurrent pyoderma as the only clinical sign and may be itch-free once the pyoderma has been treated and in between episodes.

Self-trauma

Unfortunately, self-trauma subsequent to pruritus will result in release of more mediators of pruritus, and hence a vicious itch–scratch cycle is initiated, even though the original inciting cause may have resolved. Increased numbers of itch fibres will further enhance pruritus, and hyperaesthesia of the skin will develop over time.

SCALING

 ### Define the problem

Most scaling disorders in human medicine are associated with increased and changed sebum production, hence the clinical descriptive term seborrhoea. Seborrhoea used in the veterinary context is a misnomer. Seborrhoea translates into 'flow of grease'. In the veterinary patient, equally dry (previously termed 'seborrhoea sicca') and greasy ('seborrhoea oleosa') *keratinisation disorders* are recognised. As a result, in the last two decades the nomenclature has been changed to keratinisation/cornification disorder, an aetiological term.

The terms keratinisation and cornification are often used interchangeably, although strictly speaking, keratinisation is only a part of the cornification process. Keratinisation is the differentiation and aggregation of intermediate filaments within the keratinocyte. Further processes involved in cornification are formation of the lipid and cornified envelope (cross linking of proteins), dissolution of nucleus and all cell organelles, and desquamation.

The clinical presentation of a patient with a keratinisation disorder will include increased scaling and, in addition, may include the following:
- Greasiness and/or malodour of the coat
- Further coat, claw or footpad changes such as
  o Dull, brittle hair or claws
  o Thickening with or without fissures on the footpads.

 ### Define and refine the system

In keratinisation disorders, the skin is the primary system. However, the underlying trigger may not originate from the skin but be an endocrinopathy (e.g. hypothyroidism, hyperadrenocorticism, sex hormone imbalances), nutritional or systemic neoplasia. Thus, when a keratinisation disorder is observed, it is very important to determine whether it is a primary (i.e. idiopathic/genetic) or secondary (metabolic, nutritional, neoplastic) disorder.

In secondary disorders, if the cause has been identified and if successful treatment is possible, the keratinisation disorder may be cured. However, primary keratinisation disorders are usually not curable, and life-long management will likely be necessary to achieve an acceptable quality of life for patient and owner.

Important clues
Primary keratinisation disorders manifest more commonly in young animals, either as focal or generalised process. Certain breeds have been recognised to be more likely affected. A primary disease is also more likely in an otherwise healthy animal, whereby not only the skin but also coat, claws and footpads are affected in a generalised manner.

Secondary keratinisation disorders should be suspected if the clinician is presented with a middle-aged to older animal with either first-time skin scaling or the scaling is a new presentation. An underlying cause must be investigated. As the patient is of middle to older age, full physical examination and history taken including any preceding drug exposure is imperative. In these cases, presence or absence of pruritus will help narrow down the differential list.

Classification
Clinically, the main feature is increased scale production, which may be associated with thickening (lichenification) of the skin, excess grease production and inflammation with or without secondary infection (bacterial/fungal). The visible scales derive from the *stratum corneum*, the upper layer of the epidermis. They are either just a cell shell without any organelles (orthokeratotic corneocyte) or they contain a retained nucleus (parakeratotic corneocyte). The latter type often clinically appears thicker.

Define the lesion

Primary scaling disorders
Generalised
- Ichthyosis
  - Epidermolytic (with epidermal loosening towards vesicle/bulla formation) in the Norfolk terrier

- o Non-epidermolytic (without epidermal loosening, epidermal retention) in the golden retriever, Jack Russell terrier, cavalier King Charles spaniel and other breeds
- Altered zinc metabolism
  - o Zinc-responsive dermatosis syndrome I in Nordic dog breeds
  - o Lethal acrodermatitis in English bull terrier.

Focal
- Ear margin dermatosis in dachshunds
- Nasal parakeratosis in Labradors
- Nasodigital hyperkeratosis in Dogues de Bordeaux, Irish terriers, Labradors
- Idiopathic facial dermatosis in the Persian cat
- Stud tail, most prevalent in longhaired cats
- Feline chin acne.

Secondary scaling disorders
Focal or generalized depending on the cause
- Ectoparasites – in particular
  - o *Cheyletiella*
  - o *Sarcoptes*
  - o Fleas
  - o *Demodex*
- Infection
  - o Pyoderma
  - o Dermatophytosis
  - o Leishmaniasis
  - o Feline leukaemia virus (FeLV)
  - o Associated giant cell dermatosis
- Endocrinopathies – for example,
  - o Hypothyroidism
  - o Hyperadrenocorticism
  - o Sex hormone imbalances
- Autoimmune diseases – for example,
  - o Sebaceous adenitis
  - o Lupus erythematosus
  - o Pemphigus foliaceus

- o Erythema multiforme
- Cutaneous adverse drug reactions
- Neoplastic
  - o Primary cutaneous neoplasm
    - For example, epitheliotropic T cell lymphoma
  - o Cutaneous paraneoplastic syndrome
    - For example, secondary to thymoma
- Nutrition
  - o Zinc-responsive dermatosis syndrome II in large breed dogs with a zinc-Deficient or phytate-rich diet
  - o Vitamin A deficiency
- Metabolic
  - o Superficial necrolytic dermatitis ('hepatocutaneous syndrome').

Diagnostic approach

Diagnostic tools for assessment of the patient with scaling include those that assess local cutaneous disorders such as ectoparasites and infection (skin scrapes, cytology, culture) and those that assess systemic causes of keratinisation disorders (see Figure 15.2). The presence of pruritus is a clue that may guide choice of tests, though absence of pruritus does not rule out local disorders. For example, most ectoparasitic infestations are pruritic; however, demodicosis can be non-pruritic. Most infectious processes within the skin are pruritic, but dermatophytosis and leishmaniasis can be non-pruritic. Note that an underlying endocrinopathy such as hyperadrenocorticism may alter the sensation of an otherwise pruritic disorder.

Thus, if the patient is not pruritic and/or has other clinical signs suggestive of a systemic disorder, haematology and biochemistry profiles should be evaluated and total serum thyroxine levels (and TSH if indicated) should be measured while keeping in mind the possibility of sick euthyroid syndrome. If hyperadrenocorticism is a feasible diagnosis when the signalment of the patient is considered (e.g. middle-aged

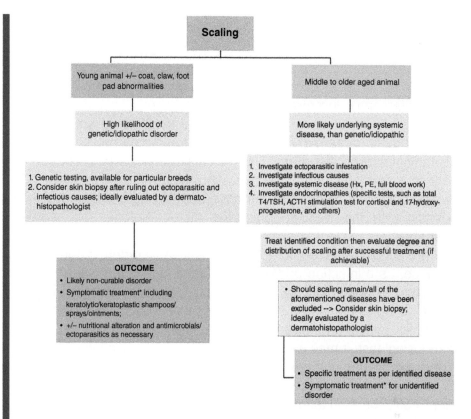

Figure 15.2 Flow diagram to the diagnostic approach of scaling presentation in companion animals.

to older dogs or cats with uncontrolled diabetes mellitus), a urine cortisol/creatinine ratio can be measured. The urine sample must be collected at home in a stress-free environment. If negative this rules out hyperadrenocorticism, if positive provocative testing of the adrenal gland such as an ACTH stimulation test or a low-dose dexamethasone suppression test is needed. To investigate potential sexual hormone imbalances, evaluating 17-hydroxy-progesterone levels in an ACTH stimulation test would be useful.

Skin biopsy
Once ectoparasitic, infectious and systemic causes of scaling such as endocrinopathies have been ruled out, skin biopsies may be

useful. Skin biopsies should be taken from affected skin, including all three layers (epidermis, dermis and subcutis) without prior manipulation of the skin (no cleaning, no scrubbing, no antiseptics) and as 'large' as possible depending on the body site (ideally 8 mm diameter). Interpreting histopathology of skin biopsies is not easy – it requires time (usually triple the time of any other organ sample to read) and special interest of the pathologist, particularly in scaling disorders. Thus, ideally the biopsies should be sent to a dermatohistopathologist, who might also be interested in seeing clinical pictures of the case and having a detailed discussion with the clinician once the histopathology has been described.

Care should be taken *not* to biopsy scaling disorders in the first instance, as if infection and/or ectoparasite infestation is/are present, the histopathology will only reflect that, even though there might be an underlying sebaceous adenitis. In addition, owners should always be prepared that histopathology is not a 'for definite diagnosing' test; it may well be non-diagnostic. In cases where the biopsy seems non-diagnostic, the histopathology could be reviewed by another pathologist/dermatologist or the effect of a trial treatment could be evaluated, depending on the clinician's strongest clinical suspicion.

OTITIS

 Define the problem

Otitis, an inflammation of the ear canal with or without pinnal involvement, is essentially an inflammation of the skin lining the ear canal and covering the pinna. As such, it's important to not just think *otitis* but instead *otitis/dermatitis*, demanding a full dermatological examination of the patient.

Patients may present with either of the following or a combination of:
- Head shaking
- Aural haematoma

- Aural discharge
- Malodour from the ear(s)
- Aural pruritus
- Aural pain
- Hearing impairment with or without obvious neurological deficits.

Thorough history taking – as always in dermatology – will help to differentiate:

- Acute vs. chronic
- Single episode, but never resolved vs. recurrent episodes with healthy ears between episodes
- Seasonality (allergic, grass seeds, swimming)
- Age of onset
- Development (extra-ear involvement).

 ## Define the system

In ear disease, if it is a primary otitis externa, the skin is the system involved. However, in cats (and often in brachycephalic dogs) the middle ear is the primary problem, which leads to the upper respiratory system being the affected system.

In cats or in long-standing canine ear disease, a neurological examination (cranial nerves) should be performed; thus, the neurological system might also be involved.

 ## Define the location

Importantly, it should be established whether there is a predominantly medial pinnal problem, or just the ear canal affected, or possibly the margins of the pinna and/or the tip, or possibly just the lateral aspect of the pinna. Either will lead to different differential diagnoses.

In addition, it is very important to examine the whole patient for further skin and mucocutaneous lesions; these may at times more obviously lead to specific differential diagnoses.

Define the lesion

As with any dermatological problem, it is important to identify the specific lesion involved (primary vs. secondary lesions). There may be:

- Macular-papular erythema on the medial pinna and auditory meatus with excoriations on the lateral aspect of the pinna (a typical sign of an allergic aetiology)
- Black mucoid material pouring out of an ear canal of a dog with pain when ears being approached (a typical sign of an ulcerative, often a bacterial, otitis with Gram-negative organisms)
- Pustules, yellow crusts on the medial pinna, point towards possible pemphigus foliaceous (thorough examination of the whole patient including mucocutaneous junctions for further pustular lesions)
- Marked scaling and crusting of the distal third of the pinnae, often medial and lateral aspects with high-grade pruritus rather point towards Sarcoptes mange
- Alopecic pinnal margins with hyperpigmentation, easily epilated fur can be a sign of hypothyroidism, sebaceous adenitis and vasculopathies.

Canine otitis

In younger dogs, otitis/aural pruritus might be related to ectoparasitic, infectious and/or allergic aetiology, whereas the middle-aged to older patient may have an underlying endocrinopathy leading to otitis. Thus, when dealing with a canine otitis externa it is useful to break down the various contributing factors to its pathogenesis into primary, secondary, predisposing and perpetuating (PSPP) factors.

- *Primary factors (can cause otitis alone)* – for example,
  - Foreign bodies (especially grass seeds)
  - *Otodectes cyanotis*/*Demodex* infestation
  - Allergic dermatitis (particularly aural atopics)
  - Keratinisation disorder ('seborrhoea')
  - Endocrinopathy
  - Immune-mediated diseases.

  Consider age, lifestyle, breed and further skin involvement.

- *Secondary factors* – infectious agents such as:
  - ○ Bacteria (coccoid- vs. rod-shaped) and/or
  - ○ Yeasts (Malassezia, Candida)
  - ○ Rarely other fungi like Aspergillus.

  Therefore, a sample of the otic material for cytology is prudent to differentiate the above, whereby a sample for culture/sensitivity is rarely needed as a first evaluation.

  Cytology (commonly stained with one of the fast Romanowsky stains, like DiffQuick® – can be done in-house or sent as an air-dried unstained smear to a clinical pathologist) shows shape and numbers of the organism as well as type of inflammatory cells.

  Both results will quickly guide the clinician as to what treatment to use as a start and which further, more specific tests might be necessary.

- *Predisposing factors (increased risk of development)*. Consider:
  - ○ Anatomy
    - ▪ Pendulous pinnae
    - ▪ Hairy ears
    - ▪ Excess cerumen production
    - ▪ Breed-specific long ear canals
  - ○ Excessive moisture
    - ▪ Regular visits to a groomer
    - ▪ Regular bathing
    - ▪ Swimming
    - ▪ Too-frequent ear cleaning
    - ▪ High environmental humidity
  - ○ Tumour
  - ○ Polyp.

- *Perpetuating factors (prevent resolution)*
  - ○ Progressive pathological changes due to chronic ear inflammation (hyperplastic, folded to stenosed ear canals), which may prevent effective topical therapy.
  - ○ Otitis media representing a nidus of infection in the middle ear, potentially protected from the action of topical treatment by the tympanic membrane, if intact.

○ And one further, and major, factor – owner compliance
  ▪ Is treatment actually administered as prescribed?
  ▪ How well is the cleaning of ears performed?
  ▪ Does the owner return for rechecks as requested?

Recurrent otitis externa problems – mostly in canine patients – might lead to otitis media at a later stage. The middle ear – important to remember – is lined with respiratory epithelium including mucin-producing cells. Also, do take a moment to remember the nerves surrounding the middle ear, which potentially can be affected in otitis media patients. Cranial nerve assessment important in patients with chronic (>4 weeks) history of ear problems.

Feline otitis

The pathogenesis of feline patients with otitis externa is different – as it is for some brachycephalic canines where the differential diagnosis can be primary secretory otitis media or 'glue ear'.

Cats often develop middle ear disease secondary to upper respiratory or oral inflammatory/infectious diseases. Over time, long-standing middle ear disease will lead to tympanic membrane rupture, allowing material to pour into the external ear canal, frequently the first sign the owner might notice of the problem.

As there is always an exception to the rule, a small proportion of allergic cats may have otitis externa (but nearly always together with other skin areas of the body being affected), or kittens/young adult cats might present with an immune-mediated disorder of the auditory meatus/vertical ear canal, called proliferative necrotising otitis externa.

Diagnostic approach to otitis

Visual observation
- Pinnal carriage
- Head carriage
- Gait (vestibular problems?)
- Signs of facial nerve paresis/paralysis
- Horner's syndrome
- Nystagmus.

Palpation

Is pain elicitable by:

- Stroking over the head
- Opening the jaws
- Palpating ear canals (vertical part)?

  Is palpation of vertical canal cartilage normal (calcification in chronic cases)?

Otoscopy

Handheld otoscope with ideally metal cones to inspect lining of the ear canal (vertical and horizontal part), degree of stenosis, erythema and material present; at last inspection of tympanic membrane (appearance and integrity).

Sampling

Lesion-specific from pinna (see Figure 15.1) and from the external ear canal for cytology (clean, not necessarily sterile swab inserted into the external ear canal until the end of the vertical part, twisted by 180 degrees, taken out and rolled out on a slide). Pathology that may be observed (Figure 15.3):

- Infectious agents
  - Bacteria? If so, coccoid- or rod-shaped ones?
  - Yeasts?
- Inflammatory cells on cytology – if so, what kind?
  - Will provide a guidance as to how chronic the problem is and/or any hypersensitivities against organism involved (e.g. Malassezia yeasts).
- Unusual/atypical cells like acantholytic keratinocytes, parakeratotic keratinocytes, other atypical epithelial – or round cells, which might guide the clinician further towards aetiologies or may lead to further investigations (e.g. biopsy).

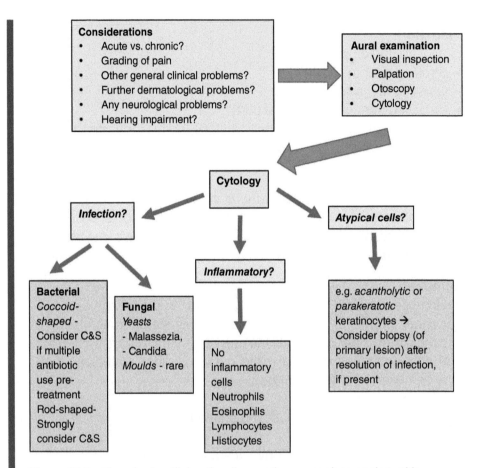

Figure 15.3   Flowchart outlining the diagnostic approach to canine otitis.

In conclusion

Pruritus, scaling and otitis are common clinical signs in small animals that reflect myriad causes. The keys to reaching a rational differential list and confirming the diagnosis where possible lie in careful examination of the patient to document the specific type and distribution of lesions, the recognition of primary and secondary skin lesions and appreciation that all three presentations can be caused by systemic disorders, not just local disease.

Most importantly, the key to success with otitis – as much as it is in our hands as vets – is to re-examine affected cases until resolution has been achieved (clinically and cytologically).

Key points

As a result of reading this chapter you should be able to:
- Understand the basic pathophysiology of pruritus
- Understand the difference between primary and secondary skin lesions causing pruritus
- Recognise the common causes of pruritus
- Appreciate the difference between primary and secondary keratinisation disorders and their causes
- Understand the importance of the fours factors in assessing the patient with otitis – primary factors, secondary factors, predisposing factors and perpetuating factors
- Appreciate the difference in the pathogenesis of canine and feline otitis.

Questions for review

- What are the three factors involved in the pathophysiology of pruritus?
- What are examples of primary keratinisation disorders?
- What are examples of secondary keratinisation disorders?
- Give examples for each the following factors relevant in otitis – primary, secondary, predisposing and perpetuating.

CHAPTER 16

Problem-based approach to problems of the eye

Charlotte Dawson

Department of Clinical Science and Services, The Royal Veterinary College, London, UK

The why

- Veterinarians commonly assess and manage animals with eye problems in small, equine, farm and exotic animal general practice.
- A logical approach to their assessment by ensuring a methodical ophthalmic examination to locate and define the lesion can greatly improve understanding of the disease process.
- Intimate understanding of ocular anatomy and physiology along with knowledge of ophthalmic therapeutics enhances visual outcomes for patients.

Introduction and classification

Problems regarding the eye(s) are common presenting clinical signs in animals presented to veterinarians in general practice. Most owners will be able to recognise that the eyes are the problem, but sometimes it can be difficult for the veterinarian to pinpoint exactly what the problem is.

For example, when describing what they perceive the animal's problem to be, owners will often refer to the eyes as being 'sore' when they actually mean they are red. When owners describe the eyes as being closed or 'blinking/winking', most of the time the eye is painful, though the owner often will not recognise this. When owners

Clinical Reasoning in Veterinary Practice: Problem Solved!, Second Edition.
Edited by Jill E. Maddison, Holger A. Volk and David B. Church.
© 2022 John Wiley & Sons Ltd. Published 2022 by John Wiley & Sons Ltd.

describe eyes as 'runny' this could mean anything from tearing (epiphora) to different types of ocular discharge. Owners may also describe their pets as 'bumping into things' or even just mild behavioral changes that are in fact visual disturbances or even blindness. And, just to complicate matters, it is not unusual for owners to present their pet because the eye just appears different to them, but they cannot identify exactly why that is.

It is therefore vital to gain a true understanding of what brought the owners to the practice that day, how long it has been going on for and how it has progressed over time. This chapter is an overarching problem-based and logical approach to ocular disease, irrespective of species. Some peculiarities will be highlighted; however, this approach can be extrapolated across different species being cared for.

Most presenting complaints can be categorised into at least one of the following six groups, and of course there will be overlap of diseases between groups.

Classification of eye problems
1 Red eye
2 Abnormal-sized pupil
3 Opaque eye
4 Wet eye
5 Blind eye
6 Abnormal-sized eye.

Define and refine the problem

It is often quite tricky to get to the bottom of what the client perceives as the problem when it comes to the eye. So, a careful history and a detailed and logical ophthalmic examination will help to define and refine the problem.

Red eye
When owners describe their pet's eye to be 'sore' quite often it becomes clear with further questioning that they actually mean the eye is red. It is important to establish which part of the eye is red in the owner's opinion and then to define and refine that from your detailed ophthalmic examination.

One key question is whether the redness is due to blood or inflammation. Could this be a normal variant (is the patient albinotic/subalbinotic)?

Albino patients lack pigment altogether. It is very rare in cats, dogs and horse but is common in exotic species such as rodents and rabbits. This is where the layers of the eye that would usually have pigment do not have any. Therefore, the uvea (vascular layers) are more obvious, leading to a red appearance to the iris and retina.

Subalbinotic patients have a blue iris and lack pigment in the retinal pigmented epithelium (RPE), hence why they have a red tapetal reflection and the blood vessels of the choroid can be seen on retinal examination in the non-tapetal fundus.

Abnormal-sized pupil

With regards to an abnormal-sized or -shaped pupil, it is vital to establish exactly what the problem is – that is, refine the problem.

- Does the patient have anisocoria (different-sized pupils compared to each other)?
  - If there is anisocoria present, the important question to answer is which eye is abnormal, meaning which pupil is dilated or which pupil is constricted?
  - There is a simple test that can help determine which eye is abnormal – the dim light test.
    - With an abnormally large pupil, when you dim the lights in the consult room the anisocoria becomes less obvious in the dark.
    - With an abnormally small pupil, the anisocoria becomes more obvious in the dark.
- Does the patient have an abnormal-shaped pupil (dyscoria)?
  - Remember that in different species the pupil is normally different shapes. For example, in a cat the pupil is a slit shape, in a horse the pupil is a horizontal oval shape.
- Or is there bilateral mydriasis (large pupils) or bilateral miosis (small pupils)?

Opaque eye

Often with an opaque eye, the owner will present the patient because the eye 'looks different'. Usually this is a color change of the cornea.

The cornea can change colour for several different reasons, and it is good to have an idea of what the colour change can indicate.

Refine the problem: there are four corneal colour categories (red/pink, white/yellow, blue and brown/black). These will be discussed further later in the chapter.

An opaque eye could also be due to colour change within the eye such as:
- Aqueous humour colour changes
  o Hyphaema (blood)
  o Hypopyon (white blood cells and fibrin/protein)
  o Uveal cysts (black/brown or clear cysts).
- Lens opacity
  o True cataract
    ▪ An opacity of the lens that the fundus cannot be visualised through
  o Nuclear sclerosis
    ▪ Aging, bluish change to the lens that the fundus can be visualised through
- Vitreal opacities
  o Haemorrhage
  o Inflammation (vitritis)
  o Age-related degeneration
  o Asteroid hyalosis
    ▪ White deposits floating in the vitreous consisting of calcium and phospholipids
  o Synchysis scintillans
    ▪ Small focal opacities in the vitreous consisting of cholesterol.

Wet eye
When an animal presents with a wet eye, it is important to distinguish between epiphora (tearing) and ocular discharge.

Refine the problem:
- If it is ocular discharge, what is the colour? Consistency? Where is it? Is there nasal discharge?
- If it is epiphora, is it over-production of tears (due to a painful or irritated eye), or is there a blockage of the nasolacrimal duct?

If there is over-production of tears, the Schirmer tear test that quantifies tear production will be elevated. If it is a nasolacrimal duct

blockage the Jones test will be negative. The Jones test is when fluorescein is applied to the eye and can be visualised at the nares or on the tongue. The passage of tears is from the eye via the nasolacrimal duct to the nose or pharynx.
• Or is this aqueous leakage from a corneal perforation?

Blind eye
In this case, owners present their pet to you with a history of blindness or bumping into things. Often working individuals (dogs, horses, for example) may be presented earlier, and specific behavioral changes have been noted by the owner.

Refine the problem: behavioural changes associated with blindness can be confused with other clinical problems. Ascertaining if the patient is blind or ataxic or there is a true behavioral change unrelated to changes in sight may be tricky at times. If the eye or eyes are blind, it is then important to determine if this is a primary ocular complaint or a neurological/systemic cause of blindness (define the system).

Abnormal-sized eye
This category is possibly the most difficult to define. Often the owner will present the patient because the eye 'looks different'.

Refine the problem: from a detailed ophthalmic examination certain questions are good to have in the examiner's mind:
• Is there facial or ocular asymmetry?
• Could this be exophthalmos (bulging of the eye anteriorly out of the orbit)?
• Could this be proptosis?

Proptosis is the entrapment of the eyelids behind the equator of the globe and is a true ophthalmic emergency. This is different to exophthalmos as exophthalmos is where there is a space-occupying lesion in the orbit pushing the eye forwards. The eyelid margins can be visualised in exophthalmos whereas in proptosis they are hidden behind the globe and just the haired eyelid skin can be seen adjacent to the globe.

If one eye is a different size, which eye is bigger or smaller? Taking photographs can be very helpful in answering some of these questions.

Define and refine the system

For ophthalmic problems it is obvious that the eye is the organ and system involved. However, the key question is, *How is it involved?* It can sometimes be challenging to determine if there is a primary eye problem where the pathology is localised to the eye (i.e. only the eye is involved) or if the eye problem is secondary to an underlying systemic or neurological disease.

Generally speaking, obtaining a full patient history and performing a thorough physical as well as ophthalmic examination will often flag concerns that systemic or neurological disease is present.

In cases where the history, physical and ophthalmic examination findings suggest a potential underlying systemic or neurological disease process, the eyes should be managed alongside further diagnostic investigations. This is vital for the patient's quality of life as consequences of poorly managed ocular disease can be vision threatening and uncomfortable.

For example, in cases of uveitis, where there is an extensive list of differential diagnoses – local and systemic – topical medications should be initiated pending the results of any further tests. This is because sequalae to uncontrolled uveitis such as synechia (adhesions between adjacent structures in the eye), glaucoma (increased intra-ocular pressure) and retinal detachment can cause blindness, are painful and are usually irreversible.

Systemic causes of ocular disease include the following. These are examples and this is not an exhaustive list:

- Neurological disorders affecting the:
  - Optic nerve
  - Optic chiasma
  - Lateral geniculate nucleus
  - The visual cortex
- Systemic inflammatory disease
  - Immune-mediated disease such as immune-mediated thrombocytopenia
  - Neoplastic disease such as lymphoma
  - Sterile inflammatory disease such as hepatitis
- Systemic infectious disease
  - Septic disease processes such as pyometra, septic arthritis, septic biliary mucocele

- o Viral disease such as feline infectious peritonitis, hepadenovirus, herpesvirus
- o Bacterial disease such as brucellosis
- o Fungal disease such as aspergillosis
- o Parasitic disease such as *Angiostrongylus vasorum*
- o Protozoal disease such as toxoplasmosis
- Systemic hypertension
  - o Renal disease
  - o Hyperthyroidism
  - o Hypercalcaemia
  - o Pheochromocytoma
  - o Idiopathic.

 ## Define the lesion

Of course, due to the intimate nature of ocular anatomy some of these presenting problems and their causes can overlap.

Tables 16.1–16.6 are not an extensive differential list but cover the most common causes of these ocular abnormalities. It is out of the scope of this chapter to discuss neurological diseases, so the overarching themes are listed here but not detailed. The tables summarise the causes of each of the presenting complaints.

Table 16.1   Causes of the red eye.

Location	Sublocation	Ophthalmic diagnoses
Eyelid	• Red eyelids • Red third eyelid	• Periocular dermatitis (primary ocular or dermatological) • Meibomian gland disease • Prolapsed gland of the third eyelid • Third eyelid protrusion
Ocular surface	• Conjunctival hyperaemia	• Follicular conjunctivitis • Conjunctivitis • Keratoconjunctivitis sicca (KCS) • Corneal disease • Irritation (distichia/ectopic cilia/burns) • Corneal vascularisation

(Continued)

Table 16.1 (Continued)

Location	Sublocation	Ophthalmic diagnoses
Intra-ocular	• Episcleral congestion	• Uveitis • Glaucoma • Intra-ocular disease
	• Subconjunctival hemorrhage	• Clotting disorders • Ocular trauma • *Angiostrongylus vasorum* • Immune-mediated thrombocytopenia
	• Iris hyperaemia	• Uveitis • Neoplasia
	• Hyphema	• Trauma (penetrating or blunt) • Intra-ocular neoplasia • Retinal detachment • Systemic hypertension

Table 16.2 Causes of the abnormal-sized pupil.

Location	Sublocation	Ophthalmic diagnosis
Ophthalmic	• Iris	• Iris coloboma • Persistent pupillary membranes (PPMs) • Uveal cyst • Iris atrophy • Posterior synechia • Iris melanoma/melanosis
	• Lens	• Anterior lens luxation • Cataract and second
	• Retina	• Sudden acquired retinal degeneration syndrome (SARDS) • Retinal detachment • Progressive retinal atrophy (PRA) • Optic nerve hypoplasia (ONH)hypoplasia/coloboma • Optic neuritis
	• Miosis/mydriasis	• Uveitis • Horner's syndrome • Glaucoma (primary or secondary) • Dysautonomia • Fear • Central blindness

Table 16.2   (Continued)

Location	Sublocation	Ophthalmic diagnosis
Neurological	• Miosis/ mydriasis	• Neurological disorders affecting visual or PLR pathway • Middle cranial fossa syndrome • Horner's syndrome • Dysautonomia • Central blindness (see Chapter 8 for more detail)
	• Visual/PLR pathway	• Pre-chiasmal lesions • Focal optic tract lesion (see Chapter 8 for more detail)

Table 16.3   Causes of the opaque eye.

Location	Sublocation	Ophthalmic diagnosis
Cornea	• Red/pink	Neovascularization • Irritants • KCS • Eosinophilic keratitis (EK) • Lymphocytic plasmacytic keratitis (LK or pannus) • Corneal ulcer • Granulation tissue • Neoplasia
	• White/yellow	Deposit/infiltrate • Lipid • Calcium • White blood cells • Scar • EK • LPI
	• Blue	Oedema • Corneal ulcer • Vascularization • Intra-ocular disease (corneal endothelial damage)
	• Brown/black	Pigment • Sequestrum • Neoplasia • Foreign body • Iris prolapse

(Continued)

Table 16.3 (Continued)

Location	Sublocation	Ophthalmic diagnosis
Anterior chamber	• Flare • Hypopyon • Hyphema	• Uveitis • Trauma (blunt or penetrating) • Systemic hypertension • Coagulopathy

Lens	• Cataract
	• Nuclear sclerosis
		Causes of cataract
		• Primary ocular
		  ○ Congenital
		  ○ Inherited
		  ○ Ocular trauma
		  ○ Secondary to uveitis or glaucoma
		• Systemic disease
		  ○ For example, diabetes mellitus
		• Aging change

Vitreous	• Haemorrhage • Vitritis • Persistent hyaloid • Asteriod hyalosis	• Uveitis • Systemic hypertension • Retinal detachment • Coagulopathy • Developmental • Aging change
Retina	• Retinal detachment	• Rhegmatogenous (retinal tear leads to fluid accumulation between the retinal pigmented epithelium and the neurosensory retina) • Exudative (fluid accumulation between the retinal pigmented epithelium and the neurosensory retina due to systemic disease)

Table 16.4 Causes of the wet eye.

Location	Sublocation	Ophthalmic diagnosis
Tearing	• Eyelid abnormality	• Distichiasis • Trichiasis • Ectopic cilium • Entropion • Ectropion • Eyelid mass • Eyelid agenesis
	• Conjunctiva	• Tear film abnormality • Foreign body • Conjunctival neoplasia

Table 16.4   (Continued)

Location	Sublocation	Ophthalmic diagnosis
Abnormal drainage	• Cornea	• Pain (corneal ulcer) • Tear film abnormality • Foreign body
	• Intra-ocular	• Uveitis • Glaucoma • Trauma (blunt or penetrating)
	• Third eyelid gland prolapse	• Prolapsed gland of the third eyelid • Scrolled cartilage • Third eyelid neoplasia
	• Eyelid abnormality • Blockage of the nasolacrimal duct	• Entropion • Ectropion • Exophthalmos • Proptosis • Dacryocystitis • Foreign body

Table 16.5   Causes of the blind eye.

Location	Sublocation	Ophthalmic diagnosis
Ophthalmic	• Cornea	• Symblepharon • Keratitis

	• Lens	• Cataract
		  ○ Primary ocular
		    ■ Congenital
		    ■ Inherited
		    ■ Ocular trauma
		    ■ Secondary to uveitis or glaucoma
		  ○ Systemic disease
		    ■ For example, diabetes mellitus
		• Lens luxation

	• Uvea	• PPMs • Uveitis • Hypopyon • Hyphema • Synechia • Intra-ocular neoplasia

(Continued)

Table 16.5 (Continued)

Location	Sublocation	Ophthalmic diagnosis
	• Retina	• Systemic hypertension
		• Retinal detachment
		• PRA
		• SARDS
		• Retinal dysplasia
		• Enrofloxacin toxicity in cats
	• Glaucoma	• Congenital
		• Primary
		• Secondary glaucoma (chronic uveitis, hyphemia, post-cataract surgery, post-corneal perforation repair, chronic lens-induced uveitis)
Neurological/central	• See Chapter 8 or more detail	

Table 16.6 Causes of the abnormal-sized eye.

Location	Sublocation	Ophthalmic diagnosis
Eye	• Microphthalmos	• Microphthalmia
		• Phthysis bulbi (chronic shrunken end-stage eye due to long-term damage and untreated disease, e.g. uveitis and glaucoma)
	• Buphthalmos	• Glaucoma
	• Enopthalmos	• Ocular pain
		• Loss of orbital fat
Orbit	• Exophthalmos	• Retrobulbar abscess
		• Retrobulbar mass
	• Proptosis	• Traumatic

Diagnostic approach

Defining and refining the ophthalmic problem usually involves defining the location of the problem further within the eye. The ophthalmic examination and some ancillary tests are the most useful aids in this process.

The ophthalmic examination

- Moving around the patient and the eye to appreciate different angles is very important.
- Looking at the anterior chamber from the side with the light being shone from the front is very helpful. The examiner can assess anterior chamber depth, assess aqueous flare and see any lesions in a more three-dimensional aspect as opposed to straight on.
- Also, when trying to assess the tapetal reflection with distant direct ophthalmoscopy and moving onto indirect or close direct ophthalmoscopy to assess the retina, the examiner must be slightly lower or at least in line with the patient's eye to elicit the tapetal reflection. The reason for this is that the tapetum (in species and individuals that have them) is dorsal, therefore if the examiner is higher than the eye, the reflection will be dark as the light is aimed at the non-tapetal aspect of the retina.
- It is also possible to define where an opacity is within the eye with regards to it being anterior or posterior to the lens.
- When performing distant direct ophthalmoscopy, once the tapetal reflex is elicited, if the examiner moves from left to right, then an opacity anterior to the lens (in the cornea, anterior chamber) will move in the opposite direction to the examiner. An opacity in the posterior to the lens (vitreous) will move in the same direction as (with) the examiner. An opacity in the lens will not move at all.

Ancillary tests

Ancillary tests can also help to define the location of the problem.

Schirmer tear test

- Measures tear production and is performed using small calibrated paper strips that are placed in the lateral third of the lower eyelids and remain in place for 1 minute.
- Tear readings are very helpful in determining if there is adequate tear production.
- This test should be performed at the beginning of the examination, as manipulation of the eyes/eyelids and shining lights into the eyes can lead to an artificially elevated reading.
- Equally, if the strip is not correctly positioned in the lateral lower eyelid and in contact with the tear film an artificially low reading can be obtained.

- Tear readings should be taken in light of clinical signs. For example, if the tear reading is within the normal range but the eye is painful, this means there is probably a low tear reading because with a painful eye the reading should be higher than normal.
- Keratoconjunctivitis sicca (KCS) results in low tear production, and increased tearing can be related to pain, irritation or aqueous leakage.

Tonometry

- Measures intra-ocular pressure and is performed using a tonometer. There are several types of tonometer, but two are commonly used in veterinary species: applanation (Tonopen) and rebound (Tonovet). The applanation tonometer requires topical local anesthesia and needs the user to gently touch the tip of the machine to the patient's cornea. Rebound tonometry does not require local anesthesia and the probe is fired from the machine and gently touches the patient's cornea.
- Falsely elevated readings are very easy to obtain accidentally. This is because any pressure on the neck, eyelids, globe and/or in a patient lying down or the head not being in a natural position can increase intra-ocular pressure transiently and give the examiner a false reading.
- Therefore, it is important that the patient is in a sitting or standing position with the head in a neutral position (looking forward) and there is no lead or collar placed tightly around the neck/jugulars.
- Equally with horses and exotic species, the head should not be elevated or lowered or pulled out (chelonians in particular).
- High intra-ocular pressures are indicative of glaucoma and low intra-ocular pressures are indicative of uveitis.

Fluorescein staining

- This is performed by applying a drop of stain to the conjunctiva. If using a strip it must be wet first with sterile saline or water for injection, and the dry strip should not be directly placed onto the eye. The eye is then flushed with sterile saline until the fluid is clear. A cobalt blue light should be shone onto the eye and the cornea assessed for uptake of stain.

- Fluorescein is a useful vital dye as it can help to diagnose the presence of corneal ulcerative disease but also can confirm the patency of the nasolacrimal duct via the Jones test (which is where stain is visualised at the nares or on the tongue if the nasolacrimal duct is patent).
- It can also be used to identify leakage of aqueous from a ruptured eye via the Seidel test. The Seidel test is where stain is applied to the eye and not flushed. If there is a penetrating corneal lesion, then a 'river' of clear fluid (aqueous) can be seen running through the dye.

Cytology
- Corneal cytology samples can be safely and effectively obtained with a cytobrush and topical local anaesthesia. Topical local can be used once when a corneal ulcer is present for sampling reasons but should not be continued as a treatment.
- Confirmation of the presence and type of bacteria (cocci or rods) from sampling a corneal ulcer is helpful to determine logical empirical antibiotic usage whilst awaiting culture and sensitivity results.

Culture and sensitivity
- Samples for culture and sensitivity can be obtained from the corneal ulcer by gently running the tip of the swab over the ulcer (if it is close to perforation then sample the sides of the ulcer and not the ulcer bed).
- It is often necessary to start empirical treatment for corneal ulcers. However, if there is bacterial resistance to the empirical treatment chosen, the antibiotic may still be ineffective. It is therefore helpful to obtain a sample from the ulcer for culture and sensitivity and to change the antibiotic if necessary, once the results are obtained.

Nasolacrimal duct flush
- This is performed by inserting a lacrimal canular into the upper, then the lower canulicui and gently flushing with a small volume of sterile saline. In species where there is a lower and upper punctum occluding the one that the canular is not in, it is required to flush the saline down the nasolacrimal duct and not just out the puncta.

- This is a vital step in patients with epiphora and a negative Jones test because it helps to determine if the blockage can be freed or if further imaging and potential surgery are indicated.

Gonioscopy
- Gonioscopy is the visualisation of the iridocorneal angle and is done by placing a goniolens onto the cornea and visualising the angle with a slit lamp.
- This allows the examiner to visualise the iridocorneal angle and helps to differentiate between primary and secondary glaucomas.

Electroretinogram (ERG)
- ERG is a technique usually only performed in specialist practice.
- If a patient presents with visual disturbances or blindness and on examination the cause is located to the retina or visual pathways, then an ERG will aid in defining the location (retinal vs. visual pathway/brain).

Imaging
- Imaging of the eye, particularly ultrasound, is useful in cases where the cornea or anterior chamber is opaque and the inside of the eye cannot be visualised. This can be performed in general and specialty practice.
- For example, if there is marked corneal oedema and the pressure is high but it is not clear as to the location of the lens (is this a lens luxation or primary glaucoma?).
- It can also help to determine if there is an intra-ocular mass or a retinal detachment.
- Advanced imaging (computed tomography [CT] and magnetic resonance imaging [MRI]) is helpful in cases of exophthalmos, blocked nasolacrimal ducts, non-ocular causes of blindness and for metastasis assessment for ocular/periocular or orbital neoplasia.

Visual testing
- Can be performed by using maze testing and observing the patient navigating in different light levels. Maze testing can be performed by placing an obstacle course in the consult room or stables for the patient to navigate in different levels of light. If the visual disturbance is thought to be unilateral, then the 'visual' eye can be covered and the process repeated.

- Maze testing is vital to help identify and further define blindness and visual disturbances.
- For example, with progressive retinal atrophy (PRA), patients can navigate well in bright lights but appear blind or have worse vision in dim lights.
- Conversely, horses with a granular iridica cyst that is affecting vision might struggle in bright light because the pupil is smaller, and the cyst occupies more of the visual field.

The management of the wide variety of ophthalmic disorders discussed in this chapter is beyond its scope. Relevant resources and guidance are available from other textbooks.

Key points

As a result of reading this chapter you should be able to:
- Appreciate the importance of defining and refining the presenting ocular problem
  - Red eye
  - Abnormal-sized pupil
  - Opaque eye
  - Wet eye
  - Blind eye
  - Abnormal-sized eye
- Identify the causes of the different presentations of ocular disease
- Develop a rational approach to the investigation of the different presentations of ocular disease.

Questions for review

- What are the key questions to ask when defining and refining each of these ocular problems:
  - Red eye
  - Abnormal-sized pupil
  - Opaque eye

- o Wet eye
- o Blind eye
- o Abnormal-sized eye?
- What are potential systemic causes of ophthalmic abnormalities?
- How many primary ocular causes of the following can you remember?
  - o Red eye
  - o Abnormal-sized pupil
  - o Opaque eye
  - o Wet eye
  - o Blind eye
  - o Abnormal-sized eye.

CHAPTER 17

Problem-based approach to small mammals – rabbits, rodents and ferrets

Joanna Hedley

Department of Clinical Science and Services, The Royal Veterinary College, London, UK

The why

- Small mammals may be presented to the veterinary practice for many different reasons, and the variety of species, each with their own anatomical, physiological and behavioural differences, can be daunting. Often the species may be unfamiliar or their presentation novel.
- Applying a structured problem-solving approach can help the veterinarian work his/her way through these cases logically, whether dealing with a rabbit or more exotic small mammal or a new or previously encountered presentation.

Introduction and classification

Veterinarians have their own preferred methods of dealing with the cases that are presented to them. Often in general practice, when working with commonly seen species such as dogs and cats, similar presentations are seen repeatedly. The experienced clinician may therefore be able to quickly 'match' the presentation with the most likely diagnosis and treat appropriately. As discussed in Chapter 2, this pattern recognition approach, however, relies on having encountered this presentation previously, in addition to having reached a

Clinical Reasoning in Veterinary Practice: Problem Solved!, Second Edition.
Edited by Jill E. Maddison, Holger A. Volk and David B. Church.
© 2022 John Wiley & Sons Ltd. Published 2022 by John Wiley & Sons Ltd.

correct diagnosis every time. This can consequently be an error-prone method for the less experienced clinician or for animals presented with multiple disorders. There is also a natural tendency to attempt to fit the clinical signs or information with what is perceived to be the most likely disease (confirmation bias), potentially missing a serious alternative.

When dealing with species that are less frequently presented, a pattern recognition approach can become even more flawed, as even an experienced clinician cannot be expected to be familiar with all of the presentations that may occur in all of these different species. Many conditions have not even yet been reported in the small mammal literature, although logic dictates that each small mammal species would be susceptible to the same range of pathologies as any domestic animal.

When presented with a small mammal patient, the clinician is therefore faced with a few alternatives. The first is to *perform routine diagnostic tests* such as haematology and biochemistry to screen for any abnormalities. If lucky, test results may reveal an obvious pattern of abnormalities that can help guide the clinician to the diagnosis. Unfortunately, the situation is not always so straightforward. An added challenge when working with small mammals is that reliable reference ranges for haematology and biochemistry are lacking for many species. Consequently, if a parameter is out with the reference range, this could be interpreted as indicating an underlying problem, or it could be normal for that animal. Equally, all results being completely 'normal' may not indicate systemic health.

An additional challenge when working with many small mammals is how to actually obtain a blood sample. Whilst a diagnostic sample can be obtained relatively easily from most rabbits, the veins of many other small mammals are either too small to obtain a useful sample or inaccessible in the conscious animal. General anaesthesia or at least sedation is usually required to safely access larger vessels and obtain a sufficient sample for analysis, but debilitated patients may be at high risk of anaesthetic complications.

The benefit of anaesthetising or sedating a small mammal therefore needs to be weighed against the risks, and it is worth considering the following questions:

- Is this test likely to provide useful results that will help us reach a diagnosis and ultimately change the treatment plan for this patient?
- What diagnostic samples are needed to reach a diagnosis?
- Would any other diagnostics requiring sedation (e.g. imaging) also be of benefit in reaching a diagnosis? If so, what location needs to be imaged and which imaging method will be most useful?

Repeat sedations or anaesthetic events should be avoided if possible, so having an idea of exactly what diagnostic question is being asked is vital to ensure that the most helpful information can be obtained at one time.

Alternatively, another option is performing a *treatment trial*. Many clients prefer this approach initially as it often appears a cheaper option than diagnostics. But again, success relies on the clinician having previous experience or knowledge of this presentation to select the most appropriate treatment. If lucky, the problem is resolved, either due to, or in spite of, treatment. But if unlucky, this approach will potentially delay more appropriate diagnostics or treatment. This delay can be particularly significant for small mammals, as the majority are prey species, adept at hiding signs of disease. Conditions are therefore often advanced by the time owners recognise clinical signs and animals are presented to the veterinary clinic.

The third alternative is to apply *problem-based clinical reasoning* principles to assist the clinician in reaching an appropriately prioritised differential list and allow rational selection of diagnostic tests or treatment. The principle of problem-based inductive clinical reasoning is that each of the patient's problems are assessed separately in a structured way before then deciding if they relate to the same underlying cause. Although small mammals or 'exotic animals' are considered to fall into a separate field of medicine, there is no reason why this approach cannot be applied to these species in practice, just as with more familiar animals. Applying the same approach across species can increase confidence and competence, as there is no need to panic that this is an unfamiliar situation. Whilst species-specific knowledge is always helpful, the same stages of problem-solving can be applied as follows.

Define and refine the problem

At this first stage, presenting problems should be identified and then may be prioritised. Most patients will present with multiple problems, and often it is easiest to start by assessing the most specific problem.

For example, if presented with a lethargic, inappetent, sneezing rabbit, sneezing is the most specific clinical problem to investigate, so it becomes the 'diagnostic hook' that is most likely to lead the clinician to successful diagnosis of the underlying disease.

In some cases, all problems can be related to the one underlying disease, but care should be taken to assess each problem separately, before then assessing if they relate to each other in case multiple disease processes are involved. This is particularly common in small mammals, due to their tendency to hide signs of disease for as long as possible. Once they can no longer hide signs, multiple disorders often become apparent.

- For example, the guinea pig presenting with inappetence and weight loss may have dental abnormalities on examination but also subclinical renal disease, which may be harder to detect.

This is also the time to clarify the exact nature of the problem. Sometimes this is obvious, but often the clinical history can be misleading.

- For example, it is not uncommon for owners to present a rabbit for diarrhoea, whereas in reality what they are presuming as diarrhoea is actually uneaten caecotrophs.
- There are some very different underlying causes for these two problems and appropriate history taking and a thorough clinical examination at an early stage is vital to accurately define the problem and so avoid inappropriate treatment or diagnostics.

Signalment is often discussed as a predisposing factor for various diseases in dogs and cats, and the same principles apply to small mammals too. In addition, inadequacies in husbandry and diet may also be relevant issues (potentially major problems in their own right) that will influence differentials and ultimately the treatment plan for each patient. A full husbandry and diet history is therefore vital to help both define the problem and prioritise differentials.

Developing a problem list ensures that no issues are missed, no matter how irrelevant they initially appear, and problems can subsequently be prioritised. From a diagnostic viewpoint, the priority is the most specific problem, as this will provide a diagnostic hook for the clinical reasoning process.

In contrast, from a treatment viewpoint, the problem list may be prioritised in a different order. For example, a lethargic rabbit with an enlarged stomach on examination may be severely hypothermic on presentation. Hypothermia is not the most specific problem in this scenario but is an important prognostic indicator, and addressing this is a vital part of the treatment plan, otherwise the rabbit may not survive diagnostics or any surgery needed to relieve the cause of the enlarged stomach.

 Define the system

Clinical signs are often associated with an obvious body system, but this is the stage to determine whether signs are due to a *primary* disease of that system or whether signs could be occurring *secondary* to other disease.

Sometimes this may be obvious on history and clinical examination.

- For example, sneezing in a rabbit implies that the animal has primary respiratory disease.

Alternatively, some presentations may need further diagnostics to determine the system involved.

- For example, dyspnoea in a rabbit could be due to primary respiratory disease or secondary to cardiac or other non-respiratory issues.

If performing diagnostics at this point, they can be targeted to answer a set question (e.g. *Is this a respiratory or non-respiratory problem?*), and we can select the most appropriate diagnostic test rather than needing to perform a full diagnostic work-up for every case.

Define the location

Having determined the body system involved, the next stage is to determine the location of the lesion within that body system. For the dyspnoeic rabbit, this may be determining whether a respiratory problem involves the upper or lower respiratory system or both. This may be obvious on history and clinical examination; if the animal is also sneezing it is likely that the upper respiratory tract is involved.

Alternatively, further diagnostics may be necessary, but localising the lesion helps targeted use of diagnostics. For example, taking a deep nasal swab may be helpful if upper respiratory pathology is suspected but is unlikely to yield useful information if this is primarily lower respiratory disease. An additional consideration is that sedation or anaesthesia is likely to be required to obtain samples.

Whilst a rabbit with mild upper respiratory tract disease may be considered a low anaesthetic risk, a rabbit with pneumonia is likely to be at a much higher risk of complications. For the latter case, diagnostics may need to be delayed whilst the animal is stabilised and treatment plan and client expectations adjusted accordingly.

 ## Define the lesion

Once the location of a problem is determined, the final stage is to identify the underlying pathological lesion. Types of pathology can be remembered by using the DAMNIT-V acronym to create a list of differentials. Having localised the problem, the differential list is generally much shorter than if we had started listing every possible differential for every presenting problem.

Based on the most likely differentials at this stage, the appropriate resources can now be used to logically identify the final underlying cause or combination of causes. We may not always achieve a full histopathological diagnosis in every case but should be able to reach an understanding of the most likely cause based on more than random guesswork.

Common small mammal clinical scenarios

The rabbit with 'gut stasis'

Reduced faecal output is one of the most common reasons for a pet rabbit to be presented in practice and is often described as the animal being in 'gut stasis'. In fact, reduced faecal output may occur due to a reduction in motility anywhere along the gastrointestinal (GI) tract, but for the purposes of this chapter the term 'gut stasis' will be used.

It is important to appreciate that gut stasis in a rabbit is only a clinical sign, not a diagnosis, and occurs as a consequence of underlying disease. Common causes include stress, pain, dietary change and foreign body ingestion to name but a few (Table 17.1). To understand how these causes contribute to reduced faecal output, it is important to have some understanding of how GI motility is controlled in a rabbit.

Relevant physiology and management

The digestive process
The rabbit's digestive system is adapted for processing large volumes of high-fibre food. Ingesta passes forwards through the stomach, small intestine and into the large intestine, where peristaltic movements retropulse small fibre particles into the caecum where they can be fermented. Large undigestible fibre particles continue their journey forwards through the large intestine and are expelled as regular faecal pellets. Caecal material is expelled as soft mucus-covered caecotrophs at regular intervals, which are usually directly re-ingested. Although described in stages, rabbits spend the majority of their active time eating, so ongoing movement of the GI tract is vital to ensure that food can be continuously processed.

The role of diet
Food type is a major factor affecting intestinal motility, especially amount of fibre in the diet. Diets containing large amounts of indigestible fibre will stimulate gut motility by stretching the colon as fibre

particles pass through. In contrast, a low-fibre diet will reduce intestinal motility both directly and indirectly by encouraging increased production of butyrate in the caecum, which inhibits gut movement.

High-carbohydrate diets will also reduce gut motility by inhibiting the release of motilin, a hormone produced in the small intestine that stimulates GI smooth muscle. Gut movement is regulated by the fusi coli, an area of colon that initiates peristaltic waves and is often referred to as the 'pacemaker' of the gut. The fusus coli is controlled by the autonomic nervous system, in addition to stimulation by hormones such as aldosterone and prostaglandins. Increased stress causing adrenergic stimulation will therefore inhibit gut motility. These are just some of the mechanisms influencing GI motility, a complex and multifactorial process.

Therefore, in presentations such as a rabbit with gut stasis, a logical problem-solving approach is particularly useful to help the clinician sift through the large number of possible causes and concentrate on the most likely differentials.

 ## Define and refine the problems

- Is faecal output reduced or completely absent?
- Are there any changes in appetite, and if so, was it the reduced faecal output or reduced appetite that occurred first, or were they both noticed simultaneously?
- Are there any gut sounds present?
  - Auscultation of gut sounds can be used to assess degree of gut stasis but are an unreliable indicator of the problem.
  - Many small herbivores examined in the veterinary clinic after a stressful journey will have little to no gut sounds audible, despite the owner reporting that they had normal faecal output at home and going home to continue normal faecal output.
    - This is usually just a case of transient reduction in gut motility and would only be considered as a problem if accompanied by ongoing reduced faecal output.
  - Gut sounds may, however, be a helpful indicator of recovery, as they are often found to increase along with faecal output once treatment has been implemented and stress levels have reduced.

- Are there any signs of complete GI obstruction?
  - A large distended stomach can usually be palpated on examination, and the rabbit is often extremely lethargic and collapsed. These animals are critical patients and likely to need intensive medical and surgical management so should be identified at an early stage.

Define the system

Primary GI disease as a cause of gut stasis should be strongly suspected if:
- There is history of a low-fibre, high-carbohydrate diet or recent dietary change
- An abnormality is palpable in the gut
- There is history of a recent or ongoing moult (especially in a long-haired animal)
- The onset of gut stasis preceded any development of signs of malaise – depression and/or anorexia.

Secondary GI disease as a cause of gut stasis may be suspected if there is:
- History of stress
- An obvious source of pain, for example, dental disease
- A variety of other clinical signs, for example, polyuria/polydipsia (PU/PD).

Considering that gut motility is influenced by multiple factors, primary and secondary causes may overlap.
- A rabbit undergoing a heavy moult may be ingesting significant hair that is building up and leading to a partial or complete GI obstruction. This could be interpreted as a primary GI problem, but a healthy rabbit with a standard coat type should be able to tolerate hair passing through its GI system.
- Certain breeds may be more susceptible to trichobezoar formation due to their long or dense fur types, but could there actually be other factors involved, such as a recent stressful event that has slowed gut motility and resulted in hair building up rather than passing through?

- We may not be able to answer this question in every case, but starting to differentiate primary from secondary GI disease is important to help us decide on the most appropriate diagnostic plan.

Define the location

If a primary GI problem is suspected, the next stage is determining which part of the GI tract is primarily affected. This may be by abdominal palpation alone or confirmed by imaging (usually radiography).

If a secondary GI problem is suspected, imaging may still be indicated, but tests that can be performed in a conscious animal such as haematology and biochemistry are more likely to help us progress towards a diagnosis, unlike in primary GI disease.

Define the lesion

Ideally at this point, the problem will have been localised and the lesion can be identified. Dental lesions, for example, can often be easily localised on clinical examination.

In some cases, however, confirming a definitive diagnosis would require exploratory surgery, which may not be possible and definitely would not be considered desirable for every rabbit in gut stasis. In these cases, it is more important to work through the logical steps to exclude all except the most likely cause or causes in this multifactorial problem.

Table 17.1 Causes of gut stasis in rabbits.

Primary GI causes
- Low-fibre/high-carbohydrate diet
- Reduction in food intake
- Recent dietary change
- Foreign body/excessive hair ingestion (particularly in longhaired breeds)
- Infection
- Inflammation
- Neoplasia

Table 17.1   (Continued)

Secondary causes
- Stress
- Dental disease
- Pain anywhere in the body
- Renal disease
- Hepatic disease (e.g. liver lobe torsion)
- Toxicity (e.g. lead)
- Certain pharmacological agents (e.g. opioids)

When to investigate?

Not every rabbit presenting with gut stasis will need a full investigation at every presentation, and a pragmatic approach should be taken to deciding when further diagnostics are required.

If this is the first time that this animal has been seen with gut stasis, but the animal is bright, vital parameters (temperature, heart rate, respiratory rate and effort and mucous membrane colour) are within normal limits and a GI obstruction is not suspected based on clinical examination, symptomatic treatment is often the most appropriate initial approach. In fact, performing diagnostics in every rabbit with gut stasis is likely to increase their stress levels or require sedation, which will potentially further reduce gut motility.

If there is a recent history of stress, dietary change or increased moulting in this rabbit (or its companion), pursuing a full diagnostic approach is probably not necessary at this stage. It is, however, still important to narrow down whether the problem is most likely due to a primary or secondary GI cause to focus on most likely differentials in case repeat episodes occur or the patient deteriorates.

For patients being managed symptomatically, it is vital that clinical status is re-evaluated regularly to ensure that they are responding to treatment as expected and that underlying pathology has not progressed, as changes in clinical condition can happen rapidly in small mammals. A common example would be hair building up within the GI tract progressing from a partial to complete obstruction. The treatment plan needs to change quickly in this case, as surgical intervention will be needed to resolve this problem.

Investigations are also recommended for:

- Rabbits presenting with repeated episodes of gut stasis where cause is unknown
- Those not responding to symptomatic treatment (e.g. warmth, fluids, nutritional support, analgesia, prokinetics) within 1–2 days
- Those with a suspected GI obstruction
- Those with pale mucous membranes or other presenting problems.

The chinchilla with weight loss

Reduced weight is one of the most common findings in pet chinchillas seen in practice and is often accompanied by reduced appetite +/- some degree of 'gut stasis'. Some chinchillas may be weighed regularly by their owners at home and weight loss detected at an early stage, but in many cases the problem is only detected once significant weight loss has occurred. Many chinchillas are not presented routinely for veterinary health checks, so a baseline weight may not be available and body condition scoring is important to quantify the problem. Unfortunately, there are no validated body condition scoring systems for chinchillas, but palpation of the spine, pelvis and ribs can help subjectively determine body condition and provide a clue whether this animal is thinner than expected, indicating that the condition is more chronic.

 ## Define and refine the problems

Weight loss can be defined objectively by a change in recorded weight or subjectively by a low body condition score. Usually associated with an underlying disease process, it is also important to consider whether the animal being fed appropriately to maintain weight.

Initially, a thorough husbandry and in particular diet history is vital to establish any deficits that could account directly for the weight loss (e.g. by inadequate nutrition) or indirectly by predisposing to specific disease processes (e.g. dental disease). Hay should make up the majority of a small herbivore's diet, and if good quality, minimal supplementary food may be needed. Often, however, a small amount of chinchilla-specific pelleted food is necessary to maintain weight, especially if hay quality is variable or animals are young, geriatric, reproductively active or affected by underlying disease. Social structure should also be considered to rule out any influence of bullying that may be restricting access to food.

If this weight loss truly appears an individual problem, approach is similar to that of other animals. The key question is whether this is *weight loss due to a decreased appetite* or *weight loss in spite of a normal or even increased appetite*. It can be surprisingly difficult to ascertain how much a chinchilla is actually eating as many will pick up food and 'play' with it, but not actually ingest what their owner thinks they are.

Faecal output can be similarly difficult to ascertain if the chinchilla is kept with others. However, defining this problem clearly is vital to prioritise differentials. If in doubt, a short period of isolation (or at least separation during feeding time) is recommended so that individual food intake and faecal output can be properly monitored. Although the amount of hay eaten can be difficult to quantify, a pre-measured quantity of pelleted food can be weighed in and the remainder weighed out at the end of the isolation period to properly quantify food intake.

Can't eat?

If appetite is decreased, is the animal still keen to eat but struggling to prehend food, or is there reduced interest in eating? An inability to eat is a fairly specific diagnostic hook. It often indicates underlying dental disease or another oro-facial lesion. It is also worth considering that chinchillas prehend their food in a different way to some other small mammals, often by picking it up and grasping it in their forepaws to eat in an upright position rather than lowering their head to eat directly off the ground. Injuries or other pathology to the limbs should therefore be ruled out by clinical examination if the chinchilla appears to be having problems prehending food.

Won't eat?

In contrast, a reluctance to eat has many more potential causes and is a fairly non-specific diagnostic hook. A thorough history and clinical examination is required to identify if there are any more specific problems.

Unlike in dogs or cats, a 'wait and see' approach is not appropriate for a small mammal, as even a short period of anorexia can result in gut stasis, hypoglycaemia or potentially hepatic lipidosis in a previously overweight individual. At minimum, nutritional support needs to be provided at an early stage, usually by means of syringe feeding.

Define the system

Weight loss with a reduced or absent appetite
Oral/dental disease should be strongly suspected if:
- The animal shows interest in food but struggles to prehend
- Drooling is seen
- The animal is rubbing at the face
- Dental abnormalities are detected on clinical examination
- Ocular discharges or blepharospasm are present (due to elongated tooth roots impinging on the globe and nasolacrimal duct)
- There is a history of previous dental disease in this individual or in other related chinchillas.
  Other disease may be suspected if:
- The animal has no interest in food
- Other clinical signs are present, for example, dyspnoea.

If in doubt, dental disease should be considered a key differential until proven otherwise, as some animals with dental disease will have no interest in food by time of presentation, and some may have other clinical signs from concurrent disease.

Weight loss with a normal or increased appetite
As discussed in Chapter 5, weight loss can be due to maldigestion, malabsorption and/or malutilisation.

In chinchillas, weight loss due to malassimilation (maldigestion or malabsorption) can be suspected if diarrhoea or large soft faecal pellets are present. In these animals, primary GI disease is most likely, although secondary GI disease can sometimes occur. For example, hepatic disease may result in maldigestion and malabsorption, but other clinical signs would be expected in these cases.

Weight loss due to malutilisation can be suspected if the animal is eating normally with normal faeces (as established by weighing food in and out and collecting faeces passed), and in these cases, a range of body systems could be involved including:

- Cardiac
- Renal
- Liver
- Thyroid
- Neoplasia
- Pancreas.

Pathology affecting each of these systems would be expected to have other clinical signs, so weight loss is unlikely to be the diagnostic hook in these cases.

 ## Define the location

If a primary oral or dental problem is suspected, a full oral examination will be required to determine the location of the problem. Full examination can only be performed under deep sedation or general anaesthesia due to the narrow gape of the chinchilla's oral cavity. Imaging (usually skull radiography) should be performed at the same time to identify any dental root pathology or other lesions.

If a primary GI problem is suspected, faecal analysis can be a helpful start to rule in or out infectious causes. Imaging (radiography and abdominal ultrasound) would be the next stage in investigations, and blood sampling should also be considered under the same sedation or anaesthesia if a systemic cause of disease is suspected.

 ## Define the lesion

Some lesions may be relatively easily defined by the diagnostics already discussed, but if the clinical signs do not completely fit the disease process, re-evaluate.

- A chinchilla with weight loss, drooling and a marginally increased respiratory rate may just be breathing faster due to stress or pain from dental disease.

- Dental lesions can usually be easily identified through a full dental examination and imaging and subsequently managed.

Having a full overview of any other problems and predisposing factors will, however, be vital in formulating a long-term plan. Most dental problems are chronic in nature and will require multiple general anaesthetics for dental treatment. If the increased respiratory rate actually reflects an underlying cardiac or respiratory problem, this could have a serious impact on the prognosis for this patient. Each clinical finding needs to be evaluated as a separate problem to ensure we really do have a full overview of our patient's condition.

The dyspnoeic rat

Rats are commonly presented in practice for dyspnoea, sneezing or snuffling. The situation is often complicated by the fact that the majority of pet rats are kept with at least one companion, so whilst a logical problem-solving approach is useful to help the clinician concentrate on the most likely causes of signs for the individual, a population approach may also need to be considered if an infectious cause is suspected. Rats are obligate nasal breathers, so open-mouth breathing is an absolute emergency and immediate oxygen supplementation is vital in these cases prior to a full examination.

 ## Define and refine the problems

It is rare for dyspnoea to be the only clinical sign seen.
- Is the animal also sneezing?
- Are there ocular or nasal discharges?
  - If so, what is their appearance, and are they unilateral or bilateral?
  - As obligate nasal breathers, rats rarely allow nasal discharges to accumulate but will use their front paws to clean these away. Staining or matting of the fur on these paws will therefore provide a helpful clue that discharges have been present.
  - Discharges can often be red due to porphyrin pigments, which are released from the Harderian gland at times of stress (chromodacryorrhea). Owners may confuse these red discharges with epistaxis, but porphyrin pigments are much more common,

and microscopic examination of discharges will confirm a lack of red blood cells.

- Are there respiratory noises, either audible from a distance or on auscultation?
  - ◦ If so, what is their nature?
  - ◦ Coughing as seen in dogs and cats is rarely observed in rats, but owners often present their rat for other suspected respiratory noises such as clicking.
  - ◦ Unfortunately, these cannot always be detected on examination at the clinic. It can be helpful to ask the owner to record videos of any respiratory noise and keep a diary of the pattern of noises, to determine the character of the problem and to help track changes in the animal's condition.

 Define the system

Primary respiratory disease is the most common cause of dyspnoea in pet rats and is indicated if:
Sneezing, snuffling, ocular or nasal discharges are present.
   Non-respiratory disease is less common but may be suspected if:

- Dyspnoea has not improved with oxygen therapy
- An obvious source of pain is located
- Abdominal distension is present
- Other clinical signs are present, for example, cold extremities.

 Define the location

If clinical signs suggest primary respiratory disease, the next stage is determining which part of the respiratory tract is primarily affected. This may be obvious on clinical examination.

- Rats with *upper respiratory disease* are classically sneezing, snuffling and present with ocular or nasal discharges on examination, although they are often still bright and active.
- Rats with *lower respiratory disease* are more commonly depressed, inappetent and may have lost weight, although signs are often only seen when a large proportion of the lungs has been compromised.

- Wheezing may be audible on auscultation, although some animals may have both upper and lower tract disease, and referred upper respiratory noise can compromise auscultation of the lungs.
- Alternatively, if lung consolidation has occurred, lung sounds may be quieter than expected. Imaging (usually radiography) can be used to confirm location and extent of disease, although this will require general anaesthesia so is not generally performed on first presentation.

If clinical signs suggest a non-respiratory cause of dyspnoea, imaging is much more important to establish the location of the problem. Radiography, computed tomography (CT) and echocardiography may all be used successfully to define the location of a problem in a dyspnoeic rat.

 ## Define the lesion

Usually at this point, the lesion would be defined and a definitive diagnosis would be confirmed. Common causes of dyspnoea in rats include bacterial infections and viral infections (Table 17.2), although mycoplasmosis is almost always involved, especially in chronic respiratory disease. Bacterial infections may be identified by a deep nasal swab or BAL, whilst PCR testing can be used to confirm viral infections or mycoplasmosis.

In reality, in dyspnoeic small mammals, definitively defining the lesion is not always possible or even desirable in many cases, as confirmation would likely require general anaesthesia and sampling, which could carry high risks in a dyspnoeic rat.

A positive result also does not always indicate causality, as discussed below. As for the rabbit with 'gut stasis', it is more important to work through a logical thought process, in this case to determine if disease is respiratory or non-respiratory and particularly location involved, as this will influence treatment protocol and prognosis. In most rats, this can be determined by thorough history taking and clinical examination. Imaging, however, may be useful as a prognostic indicator to establish severity and extent of disease for chronic problems and is important if a non-respiratory cause of dyspnoea is suspected.

Table 17.2   Causes of dyspnoea in rats.

Primary respiratory causes
- Bacterial respiratory infections
  - *Mycoplasma pulmonis*
  - *Streptococcus pneumonia*
  - *Corynebacterium kutscheri*
  - *Cilia-associated-respiratory (CAR) bacillus*
  - *Haemophilus* spp.
  - *Klebsiella pneumoniae*
  - *Pasteurella pneumotropica*
- Viral respiratory infections
  - Sendai virus (a paramyxovirus)
  - Sialodacryoadenitis virus (a coronavirus)
  - Rat respiratory virus (a hantavirus)
  - Pneumonia-virus-of-mice (a paramyxovirus)
- Pulmonary neoplasia

Non-respiratory causes
- Cardiac disease
- Mediastinal neoplasia
- Pain
- Diaphragmatic hernia
- Enlarged stomach or other abdominal structure pressing on diaphragm

Chronic respiratory disease (CRD) in rats

CRD is almost always a consequence of *Mycoplasma pulmonis* infection in rats, although other bacterial and viral infections may also be co-pathogens. *Mycoplasma* is known to be widespread in the pet rat population, but presence of clinical signs depends on environmental and individual factors.

- High ammonia levels, irritant bedding, cigarette smoke, cooking fumes, stress from inappropriate social grouping, nutritional deficiencies and concurrent infections may all be predisposing factors.
- Clinical signs include sneezing, snuffling, dyspnoea and sometimes a head tilt if infection ascends to the middle ear to cause otitis media.
- Alternatively, rats may live with an asymptomatic infection, although signs are more common with increasing age.

- Diagnosis is usually based on clinical suspicion rather than definitively proven by diagnostic testing.
  - PCR testing can be used to confirm from either a nasal or oral swab and serological testing is also available, but surveys indicate that the vast majority of pet rats test positive for *Mycoplasma* without necessarily having clinical signs.
  - Imaging may be helpful to determine location and extent of infection, especially if there is a poor response to treatment.

Rats may live with mycoplasmosis for several years, but flare-ups of clinical signs need to be recognised and treated promptly.

The guinea pig with alopecia

Skin problems are another very common reason why small mammals are presented in veterinary practice, no doubt at least partly because by their nature they cannot be hidden from an observant owner, unlike the majority of other conditions. Similar to respiratory disease, many of the disease processes that result in alopecia may affect multiple animals in a group, so approach to diagnostics and treatment within a population is important.

Define and refine the problems

When defining this problem, unlike in more familiar species, the first question to ask is whether the alopecia is really a problem.
- For example, it is normal for a guinea pig to have hairless patches just caudal to the pinna, in addition to over the medial aspect of the carpus and a large scent gland on the rump that produces a sebaceous discharge.
- In other species, different locations of normal anatomical structures such as scent glands or significant changes in coat condition at time of moult may also be misconstrued by owners as a problem.

Clinical examination and history taking should be able to establish whether alopecia is in a normal or abnormal location for the animal and season.

Is pruritus present?

If truly abnormal alopecia, the next question to ask is whether alopecia is accompanied by pruritus. If so, this leads us down a completely different diagnostic path compared to that taken for those animals with non-pruritic alopecia.

Pruritus should be easily noticed by owners as manifested by excessive scratching, grooming behaviour or head shaking. This does, however, depend on how much the animal is being observed by the owner, and for animals kept outside this may be more difficult to determine.

Alternatively, some animals with excessive pruritus may be presented for seizure-like behaviour. This appears particularly common in guinea pigs with severe *Trixacarus caviae* mite infestation. These animals can be incredibly sensitive to being touched, and clinical examination may be limited.

 ## Define the system

Primary dermatological disease should be strongly suspected if:
- There is pruritus present (although certain conditions such as dermatophytosis often present without pruritus)
- No other abnormalities are detected on systemic examination
- Companion animals (or people in contact) are showing similar signs
- There has been a recent change in environment (e.g. bedding), diet or social structure.

Secondary dermatological disease may be suspected if:
- No pruritus is present
- Other clinical signs are present, e.g. weight loss.

In this case, other clinical signs may provide a more specific problem to be the diagnostic hook

 ## Define the location

The distribution of skin lesions can often help determine the cause of signs. For example, dermatophytosis lesions are often found in guinea pigs around the face and pinna, whereas endocrine causes of alopecia usually manifest as flank alopecia. Lesions should be measured and photos taken for future comparison so that disease progress or resolution can be objectively tracked.

Define the lesion

At this stage, the most appropriate diagnostic plan can be implemented depending if primary dermatological disease or a secondary cause is suspected. Common causes of alopecia are listed in Tables 17.3 and 17.4.

Table 17.3   Causes of pruritic alopecia in a guinea pig.

Ectoparasites
• Mites *(especially Trixacarus caviae, Demodex caviae, Chirodiscoides caviae)*
• Lice *(Gliricola porcelli, Gyropus ovalis)*
Bacterial (or fungal) skin infection – often a secondary problem
Allergic dermatitis – not well defined in guinea pigs

Table 17.4   Causes of non-pruritic alopecia in a guinea pig.

Primary dermatological cause
• Dermatophytosis
Secondary causes
• Normal variation towards end of pregnancy
• Cystic ovarian disease
• Hyperthyroidism
• Hyperadrenocorticism

Diagnostic approach

Primary dermatologic disorders
• If a primary cause is suspected, then sampling such as skin scrapes, hair plucks (for microscopy and fungal culture) and potentially skin biopsies are likely to be necessary to determine the definitive cause.
• Skin scrapes and hair plucks can usually be performed conscious in all but the most hyperaesthetic patients so usually form the first stage of the diagnostic approach.
• Further investigations such as skin biopsies can be performed under anaesthesia at a later stage if initial testing is unrewarding.

- A common approach to pruritic skin problems in small mammals is often to start with a treatment trial with ivermectin or a similar ectoparasiticide treatment.
  - This can be a successful approach in an otherwise systemically healthy animal as long as companion animals and the environment are also treated.
  - Unfortunately, however, whilst a response to treatment implies that ectoparasites were present, an incomplete response to treatment does not rule out ectoparasites.
- Equally it is not uncommon for an animal to present with multiple skin disorders.
  - The classic example would be a young guinea pig recently obtained from a pet shop with both ectoparasites infestation and dermatophytosis.
  - By just performing a treatment trial for ectoparasites some improvement in the animal's clinical condition may be seen, but the concurrent zoonotic infection is ignored.
  - The risks of this approach should therefore be discussed with owners. A treatment trial is not appropriate for an animal showing systemic signs of disease.

If alopecia is considered most likely to be secondary to systemic disease, more appropriate diagnostics can be selected depending on the most likely disease process.

Secondary dermatologic disorders
Cystic ovarian disease
- Ovarian cysts can be found in the majority of female entire guinea pigs with prevalence increasing with age.
- Cysts can be unilateral or bilateral, hormone producing or non-hormone producing.
- Those that produce hormones result in bilateral symmetrical alopecia extending over the flank and rump.
- Other clinical signs include behavioural changes, abdominal distension and potentially weight gain despite reduced body condition.
- If large, cysts may eventually lead to inappetence.
- Cysts may be suspected on abdominal palpation and confirmed with abdominal ultrasound.

Hyperthyroidism
- A difficult condition to definitively diagnose in guinea pigs, clinical signs of hyperthyroidism include bilateral symmetrical flank alopecia, polyphagia, PU/PD and weight loss.
- A goitre may be palpated, but presence is not always associated with clinical signs.
- Hyperthyroidism can be diagnosed by an elevated TT4 level in the blood, but a low or normal TT4 level does not rule out disease, as concurrent disease conditions are common in guinea pigs, resulting in a reduction in TT4.
- If hyperthyroidism is suspected, full haematology, biochemistry and imaging is necessary to rule out other underlying conditions.

Hyperadrenocorticism
- Similar to the presentation in dogs, hyperadrenocorticism in guinea pigs can result in PU/PD, a pot-bellied appearance and bilateral symmetrical flank alopecia.
- Adrenal gland ultrasonography may be performed, but adrenal size can be highly variable even in normal guinea pigs.
- Alternatively, measurement of basal salivary cortisol levels and ACTH stimulation testing is possible, although testing is not standardly offered by most laboratories.
- Diagnosis is usually based on clinical suspicion in these cases.

The ferret with hindlimb weakness

Hindlimb weakness is a common presentation in ferrets but can occur for a wide variety of reasons (Table 17.5). Both primary neurological and secondary causes may result in similar presentations of weakness, so a logical approach is important to identify the most likely causes.

Define and refine the problems

This can be challenging, as weakness can at first appear to be a vague non-specific sign and relies on thorough history taking and clinical examination.

- First, it is important to establish whether the animal is persistently weak or just having transient episodes of weakness.
  - A ferret with an insulinoma may appear weak after a period of fasting but be able to ambulate normally after eating.
- Is this true weakness, or could the problem actually be inability to move due to a musculoskeletal cause?
- Finally, are there any other clinical signs or abnormalities on examination, which could be a more specific diagnostic hook?

 ## Define the system

Hindlimb weakness can be due to neurological or musculoskeletal disease (discussed in greater detail in Chapters 7 and 14).

Primary causes of neurological disease may be suspected if:

- A full neurological examination reveals neurological deficits. Unfortunately, prolonged handling and examination is not tolerated by many ferrets, so neurological assessment often needs to be staged unless the animal is collapsed.

Secondary causes of neurological disease may be suspected if:

- There are other clinical signs or abnormalities present, for example, PU/PD, dyspnoea
- There is a history of potential toxin exposure

  Musculoskeletal disease may be suspected if:

- An area of pain or crepitus is detected on orthopaedic examination. Response to pain can, however, be unreliable in ferrets, so an underlying painful process cannot be ruled out on examination alone. Also as previously mentioned, many ferrets are intolerant of prolonged clinical examination, so the process may need to be staged.
- There is a history of sudden onset perceived 'weakness' following an episode of trauma

- There is a history of potential nutritional deficits. Raw food diets may predispose to nutritional secondary hyperparathyroidism in ferrets, especially in young growing animals.

  Some animals may have skeletal pathology (e.g. a vertebral fracture) resulting in a secondary neurological problem, so these categories are not always exclusive.

Define the location

- If a primary neurological cause is suspected, neurological examination should localise which part of the neurological system is affected
- If a musculoskeletal problem is suspected, orthopaedic examination will also help to localise the lesion.
- If any other cause is suspected, the location of the problem is usually narrowed down by thorough history taking and clinical examination.

Define the lesion

The best method of identifying and defining the lesion will depend on the body system and location affected. In most cases, approach will be similar to that of a dog or cat.

Primary neurological problems
- Primary neurological problems are luckily rare in ferrets, and input from a specialist neurologist is advisable if suspected.
- Advanced imaging techniques such as magnetic resonance imaging (MRI) and cerebrospinal fluid (CSF) sampling may be required for definitive diagnosis.
- Usually these will only be performed if secondary causes of neurological dysfunction have been ruled out.

Secondary neurological problems

- These can generally be identified by tests performed in practice such as biochemistry if suspecting metabolic derangements, haematology if suspecting an infectious process or imaging (either radiography or ultrasound) to provide more detail on a specific organ system such as the heart or bladder.
- Unless collapsed, sedation or anaesthesia is usually required for these diagnostics, so it is a sensible approach to perform both blood sampling and imaging under one anaesthetic episode.

Musculoskeletal problems

For a musculoskeletal problem, imaging (usually radiography) can be used to identify any skeletal pathology. CT will provide more detailed information if available.

Ferret-specific diseases causing hindlimb weakness
Insulinoma

- Although insulinomas are seen in other species, in ferrets they are the third most common neoplasia seen and should be considered an important differential for transient weakness, often following a period of fasting.
- Diagnosis is based on monitoring serial blood glucose levels over a 4–6 hour period of fasting, and blood glucose levels <3.4 mmol/L are usually considered diagnostic for this condition.
- Care should be taken when using handheld glucometers as these are not specifically calibrated for ferrets, although reference ranges have been established for some specific meters.
- Plasma insulin levels may be increased but not in every case so are not considered a reliable diagnostic tool.

Aleutian disease

- Caused by a parvovirus, this disease is an immune complex-mediated condition.
- Immune complexes result in plasmacytic lymphocytic inflammation in a variety of organs including GI tract, kidneys, liver and spinal cord.

- Hindlimb weakness generally develops gradually and is accompanied by weight loss, melaena, lethargy and sometimes other neurological signs.
- Signs are usually seen in animals between 2 and 4 years old.
- Diagnosis is based on a positive faecal PCR result, but hypergammaglobulinaemia is strongly suggestive of disease.

Disseminated idiopathic myofasciitis
- A disease affecting mostly young ferrets.
- Signs include hindlimb weakness, ataxia, depression, pyrexia, pain when touched and inappetence.
- Diagnosis is based on skeletal muscle biopsy from a hindlimb, which reveals suppurative pyogranulomatous inflammation.
- Aetiology has not yet been established.

Table 17.5 Examples of causes of hindlimb weakness in ferrets.

Primary neurological
- Infectious (e.g. Aleutian disease, toxoplasmosis, sarcocystosis, distemper, rabies)
- Neoplasia (e.g. lymphoma, fibrosarcoma, chordoma)
- Myaesthenia gravis
- Congenital vertebral abnormality
- Intervertebral disc disease
- Neuronal ceroid lipofuscinosis

Secondary neurological
- Cardiovascular disease
- Pulmonary disease
- Hypokalaemia/hyperkalaemia
- Hypocalcaemia – especially if nutritional deficits or a lactating jill
- Toxins (e.g. *Clostridium botulinum* toxin, lead, organophosphates, ibuprofen)
- Hypoglycaemia – often associated with insulinoma
- Anaemia – a specific problem in itself
- Neoplasia (e.g. lymphoma with the neurological system)
- Infectious disease (e.g. heartworm)
- Systemic granulomatous inflammatory syndrome
- Pain or space-occupying lesion in abdomen (e.g. caudal abdominal mass, urolith, peritonitis)

Musculoskeletal
- Traumatic injuries
- Degenerative change
- Nutritional secondary hyperparathyroidism
- Disseminated idiopathic myositis

Can this approach be applied in every case?

Although a problem-based approach can be extremely helpful for many presentations in small mammals, it does rely on initially being able to identify a specific problem. This may be challenging if clinical signs are subtle and history is vague, as signs are often not present on initial examination at the veterinary practice.

Asking owners to supply videos of changes in behaviour at home can be a useful aid to defining the initial problem and often helps to ensure their cooperation as they realise that their concerns are being taken seriously.

There will still be times when pattern recognition is important, for example, if presented with an unvaccinated rabbit with swollen eyelids, swollen genitals, nasal discharge and pyrexia. In this situation, recognising that myxomatosis is by far the most likely differential is critical to avoid other individuals being infected and for welfare of the individual animal.

Summary

A problem-based clinical reasoning approach can be helpful for any vets dealing with small mammals. Although it may initially seem to be a long list of stages to perform, ultimately this approach can avoid wasting time and money on unnecessary diagnostics or treatment, in addition to helping both the clinician and the client understand why any selected diagnostics or treatments are being performed. Often this will result in clients being much happier to allow further investigations as they can understand how their animal may benefit from these. It can also be very helpful to vets building their confidence and experience working with unfamiliar species. Although each species will have their own individual problems, by applying the same principles of logical problem-solving to each case we should be able to deal with almost any species presented to us.

Key points

As a result of reading this chapter you should be able to:
- Understand the importance of logical clinical problem-solving in your small mammal patients
- Develop a rational approach to gut stasis in a rabbit
- Develop a rational approach to weight loss in a chinchilla
- Develop a rational approach to dyspnoea in a rat
- Develop a rational approach to alopecia in a guinea pig
- Develop a rational approach to hindlimb weakness in a ferret.

Questions for review

- When is a fuller work-up of a rabbit with gut stasis indicated as opposed to symptomatic treatment?
- What are the key questions you need to ask if you are presented with a chinchilla with weight loss?
- How would you define the location of the problem in a dyspnoeic rat?
- What clinical findings in a guinea pig with alopecia would suggest to you that alopecia is more likely to be secondary to systemic disease?
- If a ferret is presented with hindlimb weakness, what are the first key questions you need to ask?

CHAPTER 18

Problem-based clinical reasoning examples for equine practice

Michael Hewetson

Department of Clinical Science and Services, The Royal Veterinary College, London, UK

The why

- Equine practice lends itself very well to problem-based inductive clinical reasoning.
- Many of the clinical problems seen in small animal practice are recognised in the equine patient, and in most cases a similar approach can be adopted.
- There are, however, some important behavioural, physiological and anatomical differences that require you to adopt a different approach in some circumstances.
- The examples outlined in this chapter highlight some of these key differences and provide you with a framework with which to apply a problem-based clinical reasoning approach to any clinical problem that you may encounter in equine practice.

Introduction

Equine veterinary medicine has developed rapidly over the past decade, and equine practitioners now have the expertise and equipment to diagnose and treat horses at the very highest level. Because many of the clinical problems seen in small animal practice are recognised in the equine patient, in most cases a similar approach can be adopted. In fact, equine practice lends itself very well to problem-based inductive clinical reasoning. You may need to adopt an alternative approach

Clinical Reasoning in Veterinary Practice: Problem Solved!, Second Edition.
Edited by Jill E. Maddison, Holger A. Volk and David B. Church.
© 2022 John Wiley & Sons Ltd. Published 2022 by John Wiley & Sons Ltd.

in some circumstances however, as there are important behavioural, physiological and anatomical differences unique to the horse.

In this chapter, I am going to highlight some of these differences using examples of clinical problems that are commonly encountered in equine practice. This will provide you with a framework with which to apply your recently acquired skills in problem-based clinical reasoning and give you a better idea of the general approach to the equine patient. With a little practice, you should be able to use the same logical approach to tackle any problem that may walk through the door or, rather, the stable!

Throughout this chapter, your ability to approach a specific clinical problem is based on the assumption that you are competent in taking a thorough history and performing a complete physical examination. This is essential, as it provides you with the information to construct a problem list from which you are then able to apply logical clinical problem-solving. The ability to construct a problem list implies the ability to recognise normal from abnormal. Whilst certain clinical problems can easily be recognised when outside of the normal 'range' (e.g. rectal temperature), others require a deeper understanding of equine behaviour, physiology and anatomy to interpret, and there is unfortunately no substitute for experience. For example, physiological dysrhythmias are common in horses at rest due to high vagal (parasympathetic) tone. These disappear with exercise and should not be mistaken for pathological dysrhythmias.

Once a problem is recognised, interpreting its significance requires additional knowledge of the equine industry and the intended purpose of the horse. For example, a low intensity cardiac murmur suggestive of aortic valve insufficiency in an older sedentary horse is likely to be insignificant. However, the same murmur in a young sports horse will have major significance and would require an in-depth investigation to determine if that animal is safe to ride. Furthermore, whilst horses are considered companion animals, it is important to realise that they may have a monetary value, and the extent to which you undertake a diagnostic investigation may vary depending upon the perceived value of the horse and its intended use. Careful consultation with the owner and management of expectations is therefore very important.

Your ability to approach a specific clinical problem also implies competence in performing and interpreting appropriate diagnostic tests and the ability to generate a relevant differential diagnosis list. Routine diagnostic procedures are usually performed in the field, and the equipment is often quite different to that which you may be used to in small animal practice. You should familiarise yourself with which tests are available and how to interpret them. Once the location of a problem within a body system has been determined, you should be able to generate a differential diagnosis list that is specific to the horse. This implies knowledge and awareness of common equine diseases in your geographical area, consideration of the body system involved, the signalment of the patient and the clinical onset and course of the clinical signs.

In this chapter, I will primarily focus on information that is relevant to problem-based clinical reasoning in equine practice, and I encourage you to refer to the relevant chapters in this book for a more general discussion on the approach to the various body systems.

COLIC (ABDOMINAL PAIN)

Introduction

Colic is a common presenting problem and is second only to lameness as the most likely reason that you will be called out to examine a horse in equine practice.

Approximately 10% of horses will develop colic in any one year and up to 90% of these horses will respond to medical therapy. This is reassuring, as it means that the vast majority of horses with colic that you are going to examine in practice will be 'simple' colics that respond well to routine medical therapy in the field. On occasion, however, you are going to encounter cases that are not so simple, and it has been shown that up to 10% of horses with colic will require referral/surgery. These are usually horses that have compromised intestinal blood flow, leading to damage to the mucosal barrier and ultimately cardiovascular compromise secondary to absorption of endotoxin. Although this is a small proportion of cases, these are the horses that you absolutely have to identify as requiring referral because, if not, they will have little chance of recovery.

A logical problem-based approach to colic is therefore of paramount importance, as it enables you to identify the most likely pathophysiological mechanism causing the colic and helps you localise and identify the lesion. This information enables you to make a decision on whether that horse can be treated appropriately and effectively out in the field or whether it needs to be referred to a hospital for further evaluation, treatment and potentially surgical management.

Define the problem

Colic is a sign of real (or apparent) abdominal pain in the horse and, depending upon the severity, it may manifest in a variety of ways. Horses with mild colic tend to lie down more often than usual and may be seen to stretch out, flank watch, curl their upper lip or kick at their abdomen. As the severity of pain intensifies, the horse will become increasingly restless and may begin to paw at the ground and attempt to lie down repeatedly. With increasing severity, the horse will roll and will often throw itself violently onto the floor or against the wall. In such instances, sedatives may be required to facilitate the colic examination. Foals with severe colic will often lie down and roll into dorsal recumbency with their forelimbs retracted up over the head and neck. In cases of meconium impaction, foals will demonstrate tenesmus in addition to colic.

It is important to remember that horse owners may only see their horses once or twice a day. This means that in many instances, the colic may have been going on for a number of hours prior to the owner seeking veterinary assistance. The presence of abrasions over bony prominences (e.g. the orbital rim or tuber coxae) and bedding in the tail and mane in such cases should alert you to the fact that the horse has had bouts of violent colic, even if the animal is not actively painful at the time of your examination.

Define and refine the system

Colic is most commonly caused by a primary disorder of the gastro-intestinal tract (GIT). Nevertheless, on rare occasions it may be secondary to diseases affecting other body systems. In such cases it is referred to as 'false' colic.

Colic can be classified into five distinct pathophysiological mechanisms:
- Simple distension
  - Spasmodic colic
  - Gas colic
- Simple obstruction
  - Intra-luminal obstruction
  - Non-strangulating displacements or entrapment
- Strangulating obstruction/non-strangulating infarction
- Inflammatory/toxic
- Non-GIT (false) colic.

By far the most common type of colic that you will encounter in practice is caused by simple distension of the intestinal wall. Distention can be caused by gas (flatulent colic) or intestinal spasms (spasmodic colic). This type of colic is invariably mild and resolves following administration of analgesics and spasmolytics. In most cases, no abnormalities are identified on physical examination, although on occasion hypermotile borborygmi and flatulence may be appreciated. Gas colic is caused by overfermentation and is often (but not always) seen in horses on lush pasture. The exact cause of spasmodic colic is less clear, but it is thought to be related to transient intestinal spasms or uncoordinated intestinal motility.

Simple obstructions are mechanical in origin and can be divided into intra-luminal obstruction (e.g. impactions) or obstruction from adjacent compression (e.g. intestinal displacements). No compromise to the blood supply or mucosal barrier occurs, and therefore these horses respond well to medical management if identified and treated early enough. Affected horses usually present with mild to moderate colic; however, in some cases colic can be severe, particularly if there is marked gaseous or fluid distension oral to the obstruction. If left untreated, distension leads to further intra-luminal secretion and will eventually compromise capillary blood flow to the intestinal mucosa. No change is seen in the peritoneal fluid until late in the course of the disease. In such cases, medical management will no longer be effective, and these horses will require surgical intervention.

Strangulating obstructions are also mechanical in origin, but in these cases the blood supply to the affected portion of bowel is compromised. Colic caused by non-strangulating infarctions is also included in this group. Obstruction of the lumen and simultaneous reduction in blood supply to the intestine results in ischaemic injury and eventually necrosis. The mucosal barrier rapidly degenerates, resulting in transmural migration and absorption of endotoxin. Bowel necrosis is reflected by inflammatory changes in the peritoneal fluid. Affected horses present with severe colic that is minimally responsive to analgesics and signs of progressive cardiovascular compromise. This type of colic always requires surgical management.

Inflammation of the bowel can also cause colic, and depending upon the location, can be divided into colitis and small intestinal enteritis. This type of colic often causes severe pain and other clinical signs that may be difficult to distinguish from strangulating lesions. Damage to the integrity of the mucosal barrier leads to transmural absorption of endotoxin as is the case in strangulating obstructions. Furthermore, in the case of small intestinal enteritis, ileus leads to gas and fluid distension that is indistinguishable from that caused by a mechanical obstruction. Horses with inflammatory lesions of the bowel usually present with moderate to severe colic, and you may recognise additional signs that will help you differentiate them from other types of colic. For example, affected horses will often have a fever. This would be unusual in other types of colic. Additional signs that may be evident include diarrhoea in the case of colitis and profuse gastric reflux without other evidence of a strangulating lesion in the case of enteritis. Peritoneal fluid analysis is very useful for distinguishing this type of colic from strangulating obstructions requiring immediate surgical intervention.

Toxic causes of colic are rare, with grass sickness being most commonly reported. Although the cause of grass sickness is unknown, the nature of the damage to the autonomic system suggests that *Clostridium botulinum* type C toxin may be implicated. Grass sickness can be very difficult to distinguish from other causes of colic and should always be considered in any horse with colic that has access to pasture.

On occasion, a horse may demonstrate colic that is not attributable to a lesion within the GIT. A good example is a myopathy or acute laminitis. These horses will often present in an identical manner to a horse with an intestinal lesion, and differentiating them from a horse with 'true' colic can be a diagnostic challenge. Careful examination of the horse is required to identify additional clinical signs that might alert you to the fact that a different organ system is involved (e.g. a stiff gait or unwillingness to move in the case of a horse with acute laminitis).

 ## Define the location

In the majority of cases, colic can be localised to the GIT. Further localisation and characterisation of the lesion within the GIT requires assimilation of information obtained from the history, physical examination and standard diagnostic tests including abdominal ultrasonography, trans-rectal palpation and passage of a nasogastric tube. Lesions can be broadly classified into those that affect the small intestine and those that affect the large intestine.

Horses with small intestinal lesions will usually present with nasogastric reflux. On rectal examination, distended loops of small intestine will be evident. In contrast, horses with large intestinal lesions will often present with abdominal distention and will not have any appreciable nasogastric reflux. On rectal examination, gaseous distension of the large intestine, taut taenial bands and/or palpable doughy impactions will be suggestive of large intestinal displacements or obstruction. On occasion, colic may also occur due to lesions affecting the stomach (e.g. gastric impactions); however, this is uncommon. Even less commonly, colic may be caused by lesions affecting other organ systems.

 ## Define the lesion

The following tables summarise the causes of colic in adult horses and foals (Tables 18.1 and 18.2).

Table 18.1   Causes of colic in adult horses.

Simple distention	• Gas colic (e.g. horses on lush pasture)[†] • Spasmodic colic (hypermotility/intestinal spasms)[†]
Intra-luminal obstruction	• Pelvic flexure impaction[†] • Small colon impaction • Right dorsal colon impaction • Caecal impaction[†] • Ileal impaction • Gastric impaction • Transverse colon impaction • Foreign bodies (sand, enterolith, phytobezoar) • Functional ileus
Non-strangulating displacement	• Left dorsal colonic displacement[†] • Right dorsal colonic displacement[†] • Retroflexion of the colon
Strangulating obstruction/ non-strangulating infarction	• Colon volvulus[†] • Intussusceptions • Pedunculated lipoma[†] • Mesenteric rents • Hernias (inguinal, epiploic, umbilical, diaphragmatic) • Small intestinal volvulus • Strongylus vulgaris associated thromboembolism
Inflammatory/toxic	• Acute colitis[†] • Anterior enteritis[†] • Idiopathic focal eosinophilic enteritis • Grass sickness (equine dysautonomia)[†] • Grain overload • Gastric ulcers
Non-GIT colic	• Acute laminitis[†] • Exertional rhabdomyolyis[†] • Pleuritis/pleuropneumonia • Obstructive diseases of the urinary tract • Rupture of the middle uterine or utero-ovarian artery • Splenic haematoma and haemoabdomen • Intra-abdominal abscessation • Peritonitis • Intra-abdominal neoplasia • Hepatic disease

[†] Common.

Table 18.2   Causes of colic in neonates and weanling foals.

Intra-luminal obstruction	• Meconium impaction[†] • Ascarid impaction[†] • Duodenal strictures secondary to gastric ulcers • Atresia ani/coli
Strangulating obstruction	• Large colon volvulus • Intussusception[†] • Hernias (inguinal[†], umbilical[†], diaphragmatic) • Small intestinal volvulus[†]
Inflammatory	• Necrotising enterocolitis • Salmonellosis[†] • Clostridiosis (*C. perfringens* Type A, *C. difficile*)[†] • Rotavirus[†] • Gastric ulcers[†]
Non-GIT colic	• Ruptured bladder (uroperitoneum)[†]

[†] Common.

Diagnostic approach to the equine patient with colic

The diagnostic approach to colic implies your ability to assimilate and interpret information obtained from the history, physical examination and standard diagnostic tests that can be performed routinely in the field. Using this information, you should be able to determine the most likely underlying pathophysiological mechanism causing the colic and attempt to localise the lesion further within the GIT (i.e. small intestine or large intestine). This will enable you to differentiate between those horses that can be managed medically in the field and those that need prompt referral before it is too late.

When approaching a horse with colic, you should perform a basic examination including the following:
• Subjective assessment of pain and abdominal distension
• Mucous membrane colour and capillary refill time (CRT)
• Temperature, pulse and respiratory rate
• Abdominal auscultation and percussion
• Rectal examination
• Passage of a nasogastric tube.

In some cases additional diagnostic procedures may be necessary:
- Abdominal ultrasonography
- Abdominocentesis
- Additional clinical pathology (e.g. lactate and packed cell volume [PCV]).

Using the information assimilated from this initial examination, you should be able to formulate a treatment plan for the horse by taking into consideration (i) the cardiovascular status of the horse, (ii) the specific diagnosis (where possible), (iii) the need for referral and (iv) the prognosis for survival.

Colic is an emergency, and you should attend to the horse as soon as possible. The first step is to determine the horse's 'immediate needs'. This involves a rapid assessment of the horse's cardiovascular status as well as its demeanor and degree of pain. This is important because it is going to give you a quick overview of how compromised the horse is and whether or not it requires immediate therapeutic intervention. The heart rate should be determined first. Tachycardia is most commonly caused by pain and anxiety. However, it may also be a compensatory mechanism for hypovolemic or endotoxic shock. A heart rate of greater than 80 bpm in an adult horse has been shown to be associated with an increased mortality in horses with colic. This is likely due to its association with endotoxic shock, which is seen with strangulating lesions and certain types of inflammatory lesions that result in a compromised mucosal barrier and endotoxaemia.

Mucous membrane colour and CRT should be assessed next. They provide an indication of peripheral perfusion and can be assessed directly by lifting the upper lip and examining the gingiva. In a normal horse the mucous membranes should be pale pink in colour with a CRT usually less than 2 seconds. A brick red to purplish discoloration indicates poor tissue oxygenation and results from arteriovenous shunting and poor venous return. This, together with a prolonged CRT, is another indication of endotoxic shock. These horses are invariably very sick and will require prompt referral to a hospital for further management.

The severity of pain demonstrated by the horse should be assessed next. Pain has been associated with an increased risk of mortality in horses with colic. This is probably because the more painful a horse is, the more likely it is that the horse has a lesion that requires surgical intervention. The severity of pain is therefore a very useful guide as to whether or not the horse is going to require referral. Horses with moderate to severe colic can be dangerous to manage, and you have to think about your own safety and that of the handler/owner. If a horse is actively colicking when you arrive, it may be necessary to administer a short-acting analgesic to be able to complete your examination safely. The α2 agonists are a good choice, as they provide excellent short-term visceral analgesia in addition to sedation. If you do decide to use an α2 agonist, it is important to try and determine the heart rate and assess the mucous membranes prior to administration of the drug, as it will affect the cardiovascular system, thus confounding interpretation of the cardiovascular status at presentation. Longer acting analgesics (e.g. non-steroidal anti-inflammatory drugs [NSAIDs]) should be avoided until you have completed your examination and determined the most appropriate therapeutic approach.

Once you have assessed the horse's 'immediate needs', you should obtain a thorough history. The most important questions to ask include the age of the horse, any recent changes in management and feeding, deworming history, any previous history of colic, the time of onset and severity of colic signs, treatments administered and when last the horse passed faeces. The answers to these questions are extremely important because they alert you to the presence of any risk factors that may have led to the horse developing colic, thus providing you with additional information that enables you to determine the underlying pathophysiology and localise the lesion.

The next step is to complete the physical examination. The horse's demeanor should be carefully assessed. Most horses with 'simple' colic will not appear depressed. Abrasions around the head should alert you to the fact that the horse has had bouts of violent colic, even if the animal may appear to be comfortable at the time of examination. The temperature should be taken before you do a rectal exam. If the horse is febrile, an inflammatory lesion (e.g. colitis, peritonitis or enteritis) should be considered. The heart rate, mucous membrane colour and CRT should be assessed if you have not done so already, and further assessment of the cardiovascular system should include determination of jugular fill, pulse quality, distal limb temperature and skin turgor. As discussed previously, evidence of cardiovascular compromise suggests a more complicated type of colic, and referral should be considered.

An elevated respiratory rate is usually suggestive of pain and anxiety but may also be due to mechanical impairment of respiration by abdominal distension. The abdomen should be auscultated as an indirect assessment of intestinal motility. Borborygmi may be hyper-motile, normal, hypomotile or absent. In addition, the presence of a 'ping' on simultaneous auscultation and percussion suggests the presence of a gas distended viscus, most likely large intestinal in origin. This can be assessed further by examining the horse from behind and determining if there is any evidence of abdominal disten-sion. A normal horse is 'pear' shaped whereas a horse with abdomi-nal distension is 'apple' shaped. Foals with gaseous or fluid distension of their abdomen will lose their 'waist' and will appear bloated.

A rectal examination should be performed next with the aim of identifying the presence of small intestinal or large intestinal disten-sion (gas or ingesta), displacements or other abnormal structures (e.g. masses). Small intestine is not normally palpable per rectum, and therefore the presence of distended loops of small intestine (they feel like bicycle inner tubes!) is always significant.

Common abnormalities of the large intestine that are palpable per rectum include colonic displacements and impactions. Colonic dis-placements can usually be recognised by assessing the direction and tautness of the taenial bands. Impactions have a characteristic firm doughy consistency and occur most commonly in the pelvic flexure. It is important to remember, however, that you can only pal-pate approximately 20–40% of the abdomen. In many cases, you will not be able to reach a diagnosis on rectal examination alone. The rectal examination should rather be seen as an additional tool that can be used to help localise the lesion and provide more infor-mation regarding severity of the problem and the need for referral. Rectal examination is not possible in foals; however, a digital exami-nation should be performed and will often identify hard faecal con-cretions in the rectum in cases of meconium impaction.

A nasogastric tube should be passed next. This is mandatory in all horses that present with colic as they are not able to vomit and therefore are at risk of gastric rupture. Less than two litres of reflux in an adult horse is normal. Anything more than that is considered abnormal and indicates obstruction, strangulation or ileus of the small intestine.

Abdominal ultrasonography can also be performed in the field and is very useful for determining the presence of abnormal peritoneal fluid as well as evaluating the size and topography of the GIT. Fluid distension of the stomach indicates gastric reflux, and a nasogastric tube should be passed immediately! Distended small intestine suggests strangulation, obstruction or ileus. Thickened, oedematous intestinal wall suggests strangulation or inflammation. Fluid-filled large intestine suggests acute colitis. There are many more examples.

If you are concerned about a strangulating lesion, you may want to perform an abdominocentesis to guide your decision for referral and to help with prognosis. Analysis of peritoneal fluid enables assessment of bowel 'health' as compromised intestine leaks cells and protein. This results in a serosanguinous colour to the peritoneal fluid with an elevated white blood cell (WBC) count and total protein and is highly suggestive of intestinal ischaemia and necrosis. Such a case should be promptly referred.

Additional clinical pathology is not always available stall side but can be useful.

PCV and TP are useful indicators of hydration status. Lactate is a useful indicator of tissue perfusion and helpful in identifying horses with cardiovascular compromise that will likely require referral.

Putting it all together – when to treat and when to refer?

In most cases, the decision to refer a horse with colic implies that you think it requires surgical intervention; however, in some cases, it may be that you want to refer a horse for further evaluation and/or intensive medical management. This could be as simple as a horse with a stubborn impaction that requires repeated doses of enteral fluids, or it could be a horse with an inflammatory lesion (e.g. acute colitis) that is in endotoxic shock and requires intravenous fluid therapy and intensive care to survive. Thus, from the perspective of an equine practitioner examining a horse with colic in the field, determining the need for referral is paramount, and differentiating between those horses that require surgery and those that only require intensive medical management is probably less important.

The decision when to refer a horse with colic should be based upon the information assimilated from the history and from your initial examination. This may seem daunting at first, and you may find the following guidelines helpful. It is important to remember, however, that there is no single criterion that can be consistently relied upon to predict which horses require referral and which do not. These are only guidelines, and it is essential to place them in the context of the 'bigger picture'. It is equally important to remember that repeated examinations may be necessary to determine the need for referral, and keeping a record of vital signs and other measured parameters over time (e.g. lactate and PCV) is an extremely useful tool for monitoring trends.

Indications for referral
Pain
Severe unrelenting pain or recurrence of pain following administration of visceral analgesics is suggestive of a strangulating obstruction and is therefore a very important indicator of the need for referral (and surgical intervention).

Abdominal distension
Abdominal distension is associated with gas accumulation in the large colon and caecum and is suggestive of a displacement or complete obstruction. Severe distension may compromise respiration or even perfusion to the distended bowel and is therefore an important indicator for referral. The presence of a uroperitoneum secondary to a ruptured bladder should also be considered in a foal with a distended abdomen

Absent borborygmi
Absence of borborygmi or a progressive reduction in borborygmi over time suggests abnormal or absent intestinal motility and may be an indicator for referral if present in a horse demonstrating other signs consistent with a strangulating lesion.

Gastric reflux

The presence of more than 2 litres of gastric reflux is suggestive of small intestinal obstruction, strangulation or ileus and is an important indicator for referral.

Rectal examination

Rectal findings that may indicate a need for referral include:
- Distended loops of small intestine
- Gas distension of the large colon
- Taut or painful taenial bands
- Palpable masses, for example, enteroliths, tumours, hard impactions.

Abnormal peritoneal fluid

Abdominocentesis does not need to be performed in all horses with colic but may help in your decision for referral when there is a suspicion of a strangulating lesion. Indications for referral include serosanguinous peritoneal fluid with a total protein greater than 25 g/L, a total white cell count greater than 10×10^9 cells/L and a lactate concentration greater than peripheral blood. If referral is not an option, abdominocentesis will help with prognosis and can be used as a guide for when euthanasia is indicated.

Systemic deterioration

In many instances, the decision for referral is made based upon progressive deterioration in the cardiovascular status of the horse over time despite appropriate initial medical therapy in the field, for example, a horse with a heart rate that continues to rise (>60 bpm) despite analgesics and other supportive treatment. In such cases, the horse should be promptly referred unless the diagnosis is clear and you are confident that continued medical therapy in the field will resolve the problem.

DIARRHOEA

Introduction

Diarrhoea is another common presenting problem in equine practice and can be acute or chronic. Acute diarrhoea is a potentially life-threatening disorder characterised by hypersecretion of fluid, motility disturbances and an impaired mucosal barrier that results in absorption of endotoxin. The diarrhoea is usually severe and the clinical progression is rapid, making it a medical emergency. Affected horses are depressed, anorexic and may present with colic. On physical examination they are invariably febrile and demonstrate signs of endotoxic shock, including tachycardia, tachypnoea, delayed CRT and red to purple discolouration of their mucous membranes. They are often severely dehydrated and will have poor jugular filling and a prolonged skin tent. Secondary problems are common, including thrombophlebitis and acute laminitis. In contrast, horses with chronic diarrhoea are bright, alert and able to maintain their hydration without additional supportive care. The diarrhoea is usually mild and will often have persisted for months. Depending upon the underlying disease process, other clinical signs such as weight loss and dependent oedema may be evident.

In the case of foal heat diarrhoea is also common in foals, and it has been reported that 80% of foals will develop diarrhoea at some point in their first 6 months. The clinical presentation will depend upon the age of the foal and the underlying aetiology.

In the case of foal heat diarrhoea and some dietary intolerances, the foal will be asymptomatic. In other cases, affected foals may present with colic and abdominal distension. Neonatal foals are particularly susceptible to dehydration, and in cases of severe diarrhoea, they usually present with sunken eyes/entropion and a prolonged skin tent. In cases of bacterial enteritis, affected foals will often demonstrate signs of septic shock including hypo- or hyperthermia, congested mucous membranes, tachycardia and tachypnoea. It is worth noting that up to 50% of foals under the age of 30 days that present with diarrhoea will be bacteraemic, and therefore antimicrobial therapy in this age group is an essential component of initial supportive therapy. This is in contrast to adult horses, where the administration of antimicrobials is contraindicated in most cases.

Define the problem

A normal horse will defaecate a heap of formed faecal balls between 8 and 10 time per day. Diarrhoea is defined as passage of unformed faeces with increased water content and increased frequency of defaecation. The faecal consistency can range from watery to soft 'cow pat' in appearance and, in the case of chronic diarrhoea, may change in consistency from day to day. The tail and perineum of affected horses will often be stained with faeces, and in some cases staining of the stable walls may be evident. This should alert you to the presence of diarrhoea even if you do not actually see it. Foals with diarrhoea have a faecal consistency that can range from watery to pasty, and it may vary in colour from yellow to blood stained.

Some horses will be seen to pass normal faeces, but before, after or during defecation, faecal water is seen running out of the anus. This is referred to as faecal water syndrome and appears to be a distinct entity that is recognised in otherwise healthy horses. It should not be confused with diarrhoea. The cause is yet to be elucidated but is likely to be related to diet.

As is the case in small animals, it is of the utmost importance to determine from the outset if the diarrhoea is acute or chronic, as this will dictate your initial therapeutic and diagnostic approach. This is particularly important in the adult horse. Determining whether the diarrhoea is of small bowel or large bowel in origin and whether it is due to primary or secondary GI disease is less important in the horse.

 ## Define and refine the system

Diarrhoea in the horse is invariably caused by a primary disorder of the GIT, although on rare occasions other body systems may also be affected, for example, sepsis in neonatal foals. The most important pathophysiological mechanisms that should be considered include hypersecretion, malabsorption and inflammation. Osmotic diarrhoea and motility alterations are less common and seen primarily in foals. Pressure alterations (e.g. portal hypertension) are unlikely to result in diarrhoea in the horse.

Define the location

When approaching a case of diarrhoea in small animal practice, it is important to try and determine if it is small bowel or large bowel in origin. In horses, anatomical and functional differences in the GIT call for an alternative approach.

Diarrhoea in an adult horse is always a manifestation of large intestinal disease. This is why in the adult horse the term 'acute colitis' is often used to describe acute diarrhoea. Horses with small intestinal disease and normal colon function will not present with diarrhoea. This is due to the fact that the colon is the primary source of water absorption in the GIT and is thus able to compensate for excessive amounts of fluid presented to it as a result of small intestinal disease. It is only when the absorptive capacity of the colon is compromised that diarrhoea will occur. In foals, especially neonates, this is different because their diet is different. A foal's diet consists predominately of milk, which is mostly digested within the small intestine. The large colon is relatively undeveloped, and microbial digestion is not as important as in adults.

This information can help you localise the lesion within the GIT. In an adult horse with diarrhoea, it is invariably a problem in the large intestine. In contrast, diarrhoea in foals can be due to problems in both the small intestine and the large intestine. In fact, the most common causes of diarrhoea in foals predominately affect the small intestine.

Define the lesion

The following tables summarise the causes of acute and chronic diarrhoea in adult horses and foals (Tables 18.3–18.5). Differentials are organised using the DAMNIT-V classification of disease.

Table 18.3   Causes of acute diarrhoea in adult horses.

Nutritional	• Carbohydrate overload
Infection (bacterial/viral/fungal)	• Salmonellosis[†]
	• Clostridiosis (*C. perfringens* Type A, *C. difficile*) [†]
	• Equine coronavirus
Infection (parasites/protozoa)	• Larval cyathostomiasis[†]
	• Potomac horse fever (*N. risticii*)
Iatrogenic	• Antimicrobial-induced diarrhea (tetracyclines, erythromycin, cephalosporins, penicillin, sulphonamides)
Idiopathic	• Idiopathic (undiagnosed) colitis[†] aka colitis X
Toxic	• NSAID-induced ulcerative right dorsal colitis
	• Plant toxicosis (e.g. acorn poisoning)
	• Blister beetle poisoning (cantharidin)

[†]Common.

Table 18.4   Causes of chronic diarrhoea in adult horses.

Neoplasia	• Gastrointestinal neoplasia (e.g. alimentary lymphoma)
Nutritional	• Excessive grain intake
	• Lush pasture[†]
Mechanical	• Sand enteropathy[†]
Infection (bacterial/ viral/fungal)	• Chronic salmonellosis (*S. typhimurium*, *S. anatum*)
	• Intestinal tuberculosis (*M. avium* ssp. paratuberculosis; *M. avium* spp. Avium; *M. intracellulare*)
Infection (parasites/ protozoa)	• Larval cyathostomiasis[†]
Inflammatory	• Peritonitis
Immune-mediated	• Inflammatory bowel disease[†] (granulomatous, lymphocytic-plasmacytic or eosinophilic enterocolitis; multi-systemic eosinophilic epitheliotropic disease [MEED])
Idiopathic	• Idiopathic (undiagnosed) colon dysfunction[†]
Toxic	• NSAID-induced ulcerative right dorsal colitis

[†] Common.

Table 18.5 Causes of diarrhoea in neonates and weanling foals.

Nutritional	• Foal heat diarrhoea[†]
	• Dietary intolerances (e.g. milk replacer)
	• Secondary lactose intolerance
Mechanical	• Sand enteropathy
Infection (bacterial/viral/ fungal)	• Lawsonia intracellularis (proliferative enteropathy)[†]
	• Campylobacter spp.
	• Cryptosporidium spp.
	• Salmonellosis[†]
	• Clostridiosis (*C. perfringens* Type A, *C. difficile*)[†]
	• Rotavirus[†]
	• Neonatal septicaemia[†]
	• *Rhodococcus equi* colitis
Infection (parasites/ protozoa)	• Strongyloides westeri
	• Larval cyathostomiasis[†]
Inflammatory/ischemic	• Necrotising enterocolitis

[†] Common.

Diagnostic approach to the equine patient with diarrhoea

There are a large number of differentials to consider when approaching a horse or foal with diarrhoea. Unfortunately, the aetiology will often remain elusive despite your best diagnostic efforts. Furthermore, even if a diagnosis is made, the cause of the diarrhoea is rarely known at the time of onset of clinical signs or during initial therapy. The initial therapeutic approach should therefore be symptomatic, and owners should be made aware from the outset that in many cases a definitive diagnosis is not possible despite investment of substantial time, effort and cost.

Despite these limitations, I would still encourage you to try to determine the specific underlying aetiology wherever possible. The reason is twofold. Firstly, some causes of diarrhoea are contagious and can cause outbreaks of disease that may have major economic and welfare implications. A good example is an outbreak of salmonella in a veterinary hospital or rotavirus on a stud farm. Secondly, in some cases there are specific treatments that are required in addition to supportive treatment without which the horse will not improve – for example, anthelminthics in the case of larval cyathostomiasis.

The initial approach should be aimed at obtaining additional information from the signalment and history that can be used to narrow down your differential diagnosis list.

The first step is to determine the age of the animal because a number of diseases are age specific, thus enabling you to narrow down your list of differentials immediately. For example, diseases like foal heat diarrhoea, rotavirus and neonatal septicaemia are only seen in young foals. In older foals, diseases like *Rhodococcus equi*-induced colitis, intestinal parasitism and proliferative enteropathy (PE) become more likely. Other differentials should be considered in any age group, for example, salmonellosis.

The next step is to establish if the diarrhoea is acute or chronic. The causes of acute and chronic diarrhoea in adult horses are outlined in Tables 18.3 and 18.4. As you can see, there is some overlap, and it is important to remember that some diseases may cause both acute and chronic diarrhoea.

The final step is to try to determine if there are any risk factors that could help you narrow down your list further. For example, previous exposure to an individual with diarrhoea increases the risk of contagious diseases such as salmonellosis or rotavirus. Inadequate deworming is a proven risk factor for larval cyathostomiasis and should be considered in any horse with an inadequate deworming history, particularly if the diarrhoea corresponds with the emergence of hypobiotic larvae in late winter or early spring. Previous administration of antimicrobials or NSAIDs increases the risk of antimicrobial-induced diarrhoea and ulcerative right dorsal colitis, respectively. Failure of passive transfer increases the risk of neonatal septicaemia, and poor foaling hygiene has been associated with outbreaks of clostridial diarrhoea in neonatal foals. These are just a few examples, and they underscore the importance of obtaining a good history. If any aspect of the history points to a primary disease, then that particular aspect should be focused on during the physical examination.

When performing the physical examination, the main consideration is to determine if there are any other clinical signs apart from diarrhoea that may point towards a specific underlying disease process. For example, a concurrent history of progressive weight loss and peripheral oedema in a horse with chronic diarrhoea should alert you to the possibility of a protein-losing enteropathy. In this case, conditions such as cyathostomiasis, inflammatory bowel disease (IBD), ulcerative right dorsal colitis and PE should be considered. Unfortunately, many of the clinical signs associated with diarrhoea in the horse are non-specific and may overlap considerably.

If this is the case, then blood should be submitted for complete haematological and biochemical analysis. The results of these tests will help identify a specific pathophysiological process (e.g. malabsorption), determine presence of an inflammatory or infectious condition and dictate whether further laboratory tests or diagnostic procedures are indicated. For example, profound leukopenia is a consistent feature of acute salmonellosis. Conversely, leukocytosis, hyperfibrinogenemia and anaemia of chronic disease are more consistent with chronic diseases such as cyathostomiasis, intra-abdominal abscessation and PE. Hypoalbuminemia, a common feature in horses with malabsorption, will be seen in diseases that result in a protein-losing enteropathy. Blood tests are also extremely important for identifying electrolyte and acid base abnormalities, also common features of diarrhoea in the horse.

If the information obtained from the history, physical examination or laboratory tests helps to localise the disease process, then further investigation that is focused on that process should be pursued – for example, abdominal ultrasonography to determine intestinal wall thickness in the case of a protein-losing enteropathy. Based on this information, you should be able to formulate a list of differential diagnoses specific to that individual and then select appropriate diagnostic tests and imaging modalities with which to make a definitive diagnosis (i.e. define the lesion).

Some of the more commonly performed diagnostic tests include:
- Salmonellosis – faecal culture (3–5 cultures using at least 10 g faecal material is recommended). A faecal PCR is also available.
- Clostridiosis – faecal culture and demonstration of enterotoxins (ELISA toxin assay or PCR).
- Larval cyathostomiasis – faecal egg counts are often negative. Demonstration of larvae in the faeces provides circumstantial evidence. An ELISA for detecting cyathostomin-specific IgG (T) antibodies in equine serum is now available.
- Rotavirus – faecal sample for electron microscopy, ELISA or PCR.

Coughing

Introduction

It is common to be asked to examine a coughing horse in equine practice. The presenting cough may be acute or chronic and is often associated with other signs of respiratory disease such as increased respiratory effort or nasal discharge. These concomitant signs may help in further defining the aetiology. Determining the cause of the cough is important for several reasons. A cough may be caused by an underlying condition that affects performance (e.g. inflammatory airway disease [IAD]), or it may be caused by a contagious disease (e.g. equine influenza) and therefore has implications for other horses on the yard.

 ### Define the problem

A cough is a sudden expiratory release of air from the lungs through the mouth and easily recognisable in the horse. It is unlikely to be confused with any other clinical signs. The cough can be soft and productive (e.g. bacterial pleuropneumonia) or it can be dry and harsh (e.g. equine influenza). Coughing may also occur spontaneously at rest, or it may be associated with exercise. It is not unusual for horses to cough once or twice at the start of exercise; however, the cough should not persist.

 ### Define and refine the system

Coughing is a reflex activity associated with stimulation of irritant and mechanical receptors within the pharynx, larynx, trachea and bronchi, and this implies that the respiratory system is involved. In the horse, coughing is invariably caused by a primary disorder of the respiratory system. Coughing secondary to pulmonary oedema that is commonly recognised in other species as a result of left-sided heart failure is extremely rare in the horse.

Coughing may occur with large or small airway disease. Horses have few cough receptors in the oro- or nasal pharynx and larynx so a cough usually suggests localisation to the distal trachea or bronchi. This is easily demonstrable when passing a nasogastric tube in a horse, where inadvertent passage into the proximal trachea will often occur without eliciting a cough.

There are exceptions to this rule (e.g. epiglottal abnormalities), and lesions in the upper airway (oro- or nasal pharynx or larynx) should therefore not be completely discounted. It is also worth noting that there are no cough receptors on the alveoli/alveolar sacs, and therefore horses with diseases of the lung parenchyma (e.g. interstitial pneumonias) will not present with a cough unless the conducting airways (bronchi) are also affected. Neonatal foals will rarely cough, making detection of respiratory disease difficult. This is thought to be due to a delay in maturation of the irritant receptors within the airway.

Define the location

Thoracic auscultation is vital when attempting to localise a cough and can be facilitated in the adult horse by the use of a rebreathing bag. This induces an increase in respiratory rate and depth, thus enabling you to hear sounds over the entire lung field. Gently squeezing the trachea at the bifurcation of the larynx and proximal trachea can also be useful. Percussion is less useful and requires experience to interpret, nevertheless it may be of use in some cases to identify regions of dullness.

The absence of abnormalities on thoracic auscultation and a positive tracheal squeeze test suggest that the cough is likely to be associated with stimulation of receptors in the trachea and the upper airway. Further refinement can be achieved by determining if the cough is associated with feeding. Horses with pharyngeal/laryngeal paralysis and oesophageal choke will cough when fed. Other conditions of the nasopharynx that may be associated with coughing include arytenoid chondritis, epiglottal entrapments, subepiglottic cysts and pharyngitis. On rare occasions, tracheal foreign bodies may cause a horse to present with a cough without any appreciable abnormalities on thoracic auscultation. Further localisation within the requires the use of upper airway endoscopy.

Abnormalities on thoracic auscultation suggest upper airway involvement of the lungs and can be broadly divided into continuous wheezes, discontinuous crackles and ventral regions of silence. Wheezes are produced when there is narrowing/obstruction of the airways and are commonly heard in horses with diseases primarily affecting the small conduction airways (bronchi), most notably equine asthma. Crackles are produced by sudden forceful opening of small airways to equalise pressure and suggest the presence of intra-luminal exudate. Crackles are commonly heard in horses (and foals) with bronchopneumonia and pulmonary oedema. Ventral regions of silence (and dullness on percussion) are commonly appreciated in horses with pleural effusions and pulmonary abscessation. Pleural friction rubs may also be heard in horses with pleuritis and sound like creaking/rubbing of leather. Note that if the pathology is confined to the pleural space or lining coughing is not usually a clinical feature.

The presence of increased respiratory effort (dyspnoea) is an additional useful sign that can be helpful in localising the cough and has been described in detail in Chapter 9. In general, coughing accompanied by dyspnoea suggests involvement of the lower airways and is most likely due to bronchopulmonary problems (e.g. equine asthma). On rare occasions, coughing and dyspnoea may be associated with upper airway disease (e.g. epiglottal disorders or tracheal collapse). In such cases, the dyspnoea tends to be inspiratory, whereas with diseases of the lower airways, the dyspnoea tends to be expiratory or throughout inspiration and expiration.

Further localisation within the lung requires the use of thoracic ultrasonography, thoracic radiography, trans-tracheal aspirates/tracheal washes and bronchoalveolar lavage (BAL).

Define the lesion

The following tables summarise the causes of coughing in adult horses and foals (Tables 18.6 and 18.7). Differentials are organised using the DAMNIT-V classification of disease.

Table 18.6 Causes of coughing in adult horses.

Developmental	• Cricopharyngeal-laryngeal dysplasia
	• Tracheal collapse
	• Subepiglottic or pharyngeal cysts
Neoplasia	• Pulmonary granular cell tumour
Mechanical	• Epiglottal entrapment[†]
	• Oesophageal obstruction (choke)[†]
	• Tracheobronchial foreign body
	• Pulmonary oedema
	• Tracheal stenosis/stricture
	• Pharyngeal/laryngeal paralysis (guttural pouch mycosis)
Infection (bacterial/viral/ fungal)	• Viral respiratory disease[†]
	○ Equine herpesviruses 1 or 4
	○ Equine rhinitis virus A and B
	○ Equine adenovirus 1 and 2
	○ Equine coronavirus
	○ Equine influenza
	• Bacterial bronchopneumonia/pleuritis[†]
Infection (parasites/protozoa)	• Lungworm infection (*Dictyocaulus arnfieldi*)
Inflammatory	• Equine asthma (recurrent airway obstruction or inflammatory airway disease)[†]
	• Inhalation pneumonia (smoke, thermal injury, noxious gases)
	• Pharyngitis
	• Epiglottitis
	• Arytenoid chondritis[†]
Iatrogenic	• Aspiration pneumonia
	• Endotracheal tube injuries
	• Pharyngeal or laryngeal surgery

[†] Common.

Table 18.7   Causes of coughing in neonates and weanling foals.

Developmental	• Cleft palate[†]
	• Cricopharyngeal-laryngeal dysplasia
	• Megaesophagus
	• Subepiglottic or pharyngeal cysts
Infection (bacterial/ viral/fungal)	• Viral respiratory disease
	◦ Equine herpesviruses 1 or 4
	◦ Equine adenovirus 1 and 2
	◦ Equine influenza
	• Bacterial bronchopneumonia[†]
	◦ *Rhodococcus equi*
	◦ *Streptococcus equi subsp zooepidemicus*
	• Aspiration pneumonia (meconium or milk)[†]
Infection (parasites/ protozoa)	• *Parascaris equorum* migration (summer colds)[†]

[†] Common.

Diagnostic approach to the equine patient with a cough

The diagnostic approach to coughing begins with determining the signalment of the animal, obtaining a thorough history and performing a physical examination. Age is very important in creating a differential list for the patient. Coughing that has occurred since birth is likely to be secondary to congenital abnormalities, and disorders such as cleft palate, pharyngeal dysplasia and tracheal collapse should be considered. Endoscopy of the upper airways will confirm the diagnosis in most cases.

If the cough is acquired, you should establish if it is acute or chronic and if it is associated with a fever. Adult horses with an acute cough and fever most likely have viral respiratory disease. These horses will be normal on thoracic auscultation, and the index of suspicion for viral disease will increase if more than one animal is affected. The three most commonly used methods of diagnosis are virus isolation, serology and detection of viral particles/antigens by immunological techniques. Other causes of an acute cough with fever include bacterial pneumonia/pleuropneumonia and pulmonary abscessation (*Rhodococcus equi* in foals). In such cases individual animals are affected and thoracic auscultation is usually abnormal. Diagnosis is based on thoracic ultrasonography, radiography and culture of a trans-tracheal aspirate. Horses with strangles (*Streptococcus equi subsp. equi*) may cough; however, this is unusual. Causes of an acute cough without fever that should be considered include lung worm, *Parascaris equorum* migration or a tracheobronchial foreign body.

A chronic cough in an adult horse is most likely due to equine asthma. Affected animals are afebrile and, in the case of recurrent airway obstruction (RAO), the cough is associated with increased respiratory effort. Horses with IAD will have normal respiratory effort and will usually only cough during exercise. Endoscopy and a BAL/tracheal wash/trans-tracheal aspirate for cytology will confirm the diagnosis. In such cases, you will see increased mucus in the trachea. On cytology of BAL fluid, you will see inflammation with an increased percentage of neutrophils, eosinophils and/or mast cells. Bacterial culture of a tracheal wash/trans-tracheal aspirate will not yield any growth.

Less common causes of a chronic cough include pharyngeal/laryngeal dysfunction, epiglottal entrapment, epiglottitis and pulmonary neoplasia. In the case of pharyngeal/laryngeal dysfunction and epiglottal disorders, the cough is usually associated with feeding and is often accompanied by bilateral mucopurulent, food-stained nasal discharge. Further investigation should include endoscopy of the nasopharynx and assessment of the guttural pouches for mycotic plaques. Pulmonary granular cell tumours are occasionally encountered and should be suspected in older horses with a chronic cough, exercise intolerance and occasional epistaxis. LRT endoscopy and biopsy will confirm the diagnosis.

PALLOR AND ANAEMIA

Introduction

Pallor caused by anaemia is a common presenting problem in equine practice and can be challenging to investigate. It is important to remember that anaemia is a haematologic abnormality resulting from an underlying disease process and should not be considered as a diagnosis. Unfortunately, equine practitioners will often ´treat` anaemia without determining the underlying cause. This leads to therapeutic failures and frustration for the client and veterinarian involved. A problem-based clinical reasoning approach to anaemia will enable you to make a definitive diagnosis and will facilitate rational therapy aimed at the underlying disease process.

 ## Define the problem

Mucous membrane pallor is characterised by a decrease in rubor in the mucous membranes (usually appreciated in the gingiva, conjunctivae or vulva) associated with decreased oxyhemoglobin delivery. It is worth mentioning that many horses have a constitutional pallor (pale pink) to their gingival mucous membranes that is often perceived as abnormal by veterinarians that are more used to the bright pink colour of the mucous membranes seen in dogs and cats.

Potential causes of pallor include decreased perfusion (regional or systemic) and normal perfusion with decreased oxygen-carrying capacity (i.e. anaemia). In most cases, anaemia should be considered first as this is the most common cause of pallor in the horse. A simple way of differentiating the two, however, is to assess pallor in conjunction with other signs of decreased peripheral perfusion, most notably a prolonged capillary refill time (CRT).

Whilst the primary presenting clinical sign in horses with anaemia is pallor, other clinical signs directly related to decreased tissue oxygenation and the physiologic compensatory mechanisms that are initiated in an attempt to alleviate this hypoxia may be seen. Horses with mild to moderate anaemia often have no obvious clinical signs or may only have lethargy and slightly pale mucous membranes. In cases of severe anaemia, the clinical signs will vary depending upon the cause and rate at which anaemia develops. Horses with chronic anaemia are able to compensate for the reduced oxygen transport from the lung to the tissues of the body, and often the only presenting clinical sign is exercise intolerance or lethargy. With acute anaemia, the clinical signs are far more dramatic and will become evident at a much higher red cell mass, as affected horses are unable to compensate for the reduction in oxygen-carrying capacity of the blood. Affected horses present with tachycardia, tachypnoea and weakness. A systolic heart murmur can often be identified in these horses due to decreased viscosity and increased turbulence of the blood. With acute anaemia due to severe blood loss, the clinical signs are attributable to hypovolaemic shock and include tachycardia, tachypnoea, pale mucous membranes, prolonged CRT, hypothermia, muscle weakness and eventual cardiovascular collapse. Other clinical signs, including fever, icterus, haemoglobinuria, petechial haemorrhages, lymphadenopathy and weight loss may be present in anaemic horses and reflect the primary pathophysiologic process or underlying disease process involved.

 Define and refine the system

Anaemia is defined as a decrease in the circulating red blood cell (RBC) mass caused by an imbalance in the rate of loss or destruction of erythrocytes and the rate of their production in the bone marrow and, as such, localises to the haematopoietic system. Anaemia can be due to a primary disease process (e.g. haemolysis), or it can be secondary to an underlying disorder (e.g. anaemia of chronic disease).

Once anaemia is confirmed, it should be classified into one of three pathophysiological mechanisms:

- Blood loss
- Increased red cell destruction (haemolysis)
- Decreased red cell production.

Anaemia caused by blood loss or haemolysis is generally regarded as regenerative, while anaemia caused by decreased red cell production is non-regenerative. Unlike other domestic species, horses do not release immature red cells into the peripheral circulation, and therefore RBC indices such as size and morphology are not useful for differentiating between regenerative and non-regenerative anaemia.

Consequently, the initial diagnostic approach in the horse is aimed at determining if the anaemia is caused by blood loss or haemolysis. If there is no evidence of this, a bone marrow biopsy or aspirate should be obtained early in the course of the investigation to confirm decreased red cell production.

Define the location

The first step in the investigation of anaemia is to determine if the horse has blood loss. Blood loss in the horse can be broadly classified as acute or chronic and external or internal. Horses with anaemia secondary to external blood loss will often have a concomitant hypoproteinemia.

Acute blood loss is usually associated with surgery, trauma or rupture of a large vessel. If severe (>30% of blood volume), affected animals will present with signs of progressive haemorrhagic shock and require emergency medical treatment. External blood loss is visible on physical examination and is not difficult to identify. Internal blood loss presents more of a diagnostic challenge, however, as it is often insidious and may be difficult to identify. Diagnosis in these cases is facilitated by thoracic and abdominal ultrasonography, endoscopy, abdominocentesis, thoracocentesis and rectal examination. It is important to remember that the PCV and total protein in these cases will not be representative of the true volume of blood loss until approximately 24 hours after the haemorrhage has occurred. This is because of the dilutional effect caused by a net movement of fluid from the interstitial space and increased water intake to compensate for the loss in intravascular blood volume. The PCV will usually stabilise within 24 hours after the haemorrhage has been controlled and will begin to increase in 4–6 days due to a regenerative bone marrow response.

Chronic blood loss can be caused by a plethora of disorders and results in a slowly developing anaemia because the bone marrow has a chance to compensate for the lost red cells. Anaemia only occurs once the rate at which red cells are lost exceeds the rate at which they are produced in the bone marrow. Common causes of chronic blood loss in the horse include bleeding from gastrointestinal lesions, haematuria and haemostatic disorders. Diagnosis is facilitated by gastroscopy, faecal occult blood tests, urinalysis, thrombocyte counts and clotting times.

If there is no obvious source of blood loss and the horse has normal plasma protein, the next step is to determine if there is any evidence of haemolysis. This can be determined by demonstrating the presence of icterus (increase in total and indirect bilirubin), haemo-globinaemia or haemoglobinuria. The simplest of these questions to answer is to look for evidence of icterus. Icterus indicates the presence of elevated bilirubin in the blood and is manifested clinically as a yellow discolouration of the mucous membranes and sclera. Haemolysis can be extravascular or intravascular. Both cause hyperbilirubinaemia. It is important, however, to rule out other causes of hyperbilirubinaemia, including anorexia and liver disease. Also remember that haemolysis may occur without icterus if the rate of RBC destruction does not overwhelm hepatic clearance of bilirubin.

Further evidence of haemolysis can be obtained by demonstrating the presence of haemoglobinaemia or haemoglobinuria. Acute severe intravascular haemolysis causes haemoglobinaemia that is easily verified by the presence of pink plasma. Mild intravascular haemolysis may not discolour plasma but may cause an increase in mean corpuscular volume (MCV) and mean corpuscular haemoglobin concentration (MCHC). If renal threshold is reached, haemoblobinuria (red-brown discolouration of urine) will become evident. Microscopic traces of haemoglobin can be identified as a positive for blood on a urine dipstick, but remember that a urine dipstick cannot differentiate between free blood, haemoglobin and myoglobin. Free blood can be ruled out by examining a urine sediment smear for red cells, and myoglobin can be ruled out by looking at CK and AST. Extravascular haemolysis does not cause haemoglobinuria or haemoglobinaemia. In such cases damaged red cells are removed by the reticuloendothelial system, and haemoglobin is converted to unconjugated bilirubin.

If blood loss and haemolysis have been ruled out, a bone marrow aspirate or biopsy should be performed to determine if the bone marrow is responsive or not. If the myeloid:erythroid (M:E) ratio or reticulocyte count is inadequate, then the anaemia is considered to be non-regenerative, and attempts should be made to determine the underlying cause.

Define the lesion

The following tables summarise the causes of anaemia in adult horses and foals under the broad classification of blood loss, hemolysis and decreased red cell production (Tables 18.8–18.10). Differentials are organised using the DAMNIT-V classification of disease.

Table 18.8 Causes of acute and chronic blood loss in adult horses and foals.

Degenerative	• Middle uterine artery rupture in post-partum mares[†]
	• Intrathoracic aortic rupture
	• Acquired coagulopathy secondary to liver failure
Neoplasia	• Ethmoid haematoma[†]
	• Pheochromocytoma
	• Haemangiosarcoma
	• Gastric carcinoma
Mechanical	• Urolithiasis (cystic and renal calculi)
	• Exercise-induced pulmonary haemorrhage[†]
Infection (bacterial/viral/ fungal)	• Guttural pouch mycosis[†]
	• Pulmonary abscessation
Infection (parasites/ protozoa)	• Lice[†]
	• Ticks[†]
	• Large strongyles
Inflammatory	• Disseminated coagulation (DIC)[†]
	• Purpura haemorrhagica
Inherited	• Hemophilia A or other congenital factor deficiencies
Immune-mediated	• Immune-mediated thrombocytopenia (ITP)[†]
Iatrogenic	• Surgery[†]
	• Incorrect passage of a nasogastric tube[†]
	• Splenic rupture secondary to administration of phenylephrine
Idiopathic	• Urethral rents in geldings
Toxic	• Warfarin or dicoumarol toxicosis
	• Moldy sweet clover toxicosis
	• Blister beetle (cantharidin) toxicosis
	• NSAID toxicosis
Traumatic	• External trauma (e.g. laceration of a major blood vessel, haemothorax, haemoabdomen, haematuria) [†]
	• Foaling injuries (e.g. lacerated vaginal blood vessels)[†]

[†] Common.

Table 18.9 Causes of haemolysis in adult horses and foals.

Autoimmune	• Primary immune-mediated haemolytic anaemia[†] • Neonatal isoerythrolysis[†]
Infection (bacterial/viral/ fungal)	• Equine infectious anaemia
Infection (parasites/ protozoa)	• Piroplasmosis (*Babesia caballi* and *Theileria equi*)[†] • Equine granulocytic ehrlichiosis (*Anaplasma phagocytophilum*)[†]
Immune-mediated	• Secondary immune-mediated haemolytic anaemia[†]
Iatrogenic	• Incompatible blood transfusions
Toxic	• Red maple leaf toxicosis • Onion toxicosis

[†] Common.

Table 18.10 Causes of decreased red cell production in adult horses and foals.

Inflammatory	• Anaemia of chronic disease (e.g. abscessation, chronic pleuropneumonia, etc.)[†]

Neoplastic	• Myelophthisic disease
	  ○ Lymphoid leukaemia
	  ○ Myeloid leukaemia (myelomonocytic or granulocytic)
	  ○ Plasma cell myeloma

Nutritional	• Iron deficiency anaemia
Toxic	• Aplastic anaemia (e.g. administration of recombinant human erythropoietin)

[†] Common.

Diagnostic approach to the equine patient with anaemia

Anaemia should be confirmed by laboratory demonstration of reductions in packed cell volume (PCV, % or L/L), decreased RBC count and hemoglobin concentration (g/dl). There are some features unique to the equine erythron that may complicate interpretation of anaemia, and it must be remembered that the PCV should always be interpreted in light of the horse's age, breed, use and level of hydration and excitement.

The next step in the investigation of anemia is to determine if the horse has hypoproteinaemia. Horses with anaemia and concurrent hypoproteinaemia are likely to have blood loss, and every attempt should be made to try to identify the source of blood loss.

If the horse has normal plasma protein and there is no obvious source of blood loss, the next step is to determine if there is any evidence of haemolysis. As discussed, this should be determined by demonstrating the presence of icterus, haemoglobinaemia or haemoglobinuria.

If haemolysis is likely, a blood smear should be made and examined for the presence of Heinz bodies, which would be indicative of oxidative erythrocyte damage. A blood smear can also be used to identify erythrocyte or granulocyte cytoplasmic inclusions, which would be indicative of piroplasmosis or equine granulocytic ehrlichiosis, respectively. If there is a high index of suspicion for the disease in the absence of parasitaemia, then serology and/or PCR should be performed.

If there is no evidence of oxidative erythrocyte damage or parasitaemia, then haemolysis is most likely secondary to immune-mediated haemolytic anaemia (IMHA), and an EDTA blood sample should be examined for evidence of red cell agglutination. Agglutination occurs when antibodies and/or complement binds to the erythrocyte membrane; when present, it confirms a diagnosis of IMHA. Occasionally red cell agglutination can be seen with the naked eye, and this is termed autoagglutination. This finding should be interpreted with caution, however, as equine erythrocytes have a tendency for rouleaux formation, which can be misinterpreted as autoagglutination. Autoagglutination can be confirmed by performing a simple 'in-saline agglutination' test. True autoagglutination confirms IMHA, although some affected horses will not demonstrate autoagglutination and, in these cases, a direct antiglobulin test (Coombs test) should be done. The most well-recognised form of IMHA is neonatal isoerythrolysis and should be ruled out in any neonatal foal that presents with anaemia, weakness and icterus. The disease occurs when the foal ingests colostrum-containing alloantibodies directed against the foal's erythrocytes.

If blood loss and haemolysis have been ruled out, a bone marrow aspirate or biopsy should be performed. When evaluating bone marrow specimens, the clinical pathologist will usually report the M:E ratio and reticulocyte count as an indication of the regenerative response of the bone marrow. The normal M:E ratio in horses ranges from 0.5 to 1.5, and the reticulocyte count ranges from 0.5% to 2%. For the anaemia to be classified a regenerative, the M:E ratio should be <0.5 and the reticulocyte count >2%. The overall cellularity of the sample and the presence or absence of abnormal cells will also be reported, and an indirect assessment of bone marrow iron stores will be made by determining the haemosiderin content on slides stained with Prussian blue. If the M:E ratio or reticulocyte count is inadequate, then the anaemia is considered to be non-regenerative, and attempts should be made to determine the underlying cause. By far the most common cause of non-regenerative anaemia in the horse is anaemia of chronic disease, and every attempt should be made to rule this out before considering other less common causes.

Other Common Clinical Problems in Equine Practice

The examples of clinical problems outlined in this chapter are used to highlight some of the key differences between horses and other species and will provide you with a framework with which to apply a problem-based clinical reasoning approach to other clinical problems that are commonly encountered in equine practice. These include nasal discharge, epistaxis, weight loss, collapse, recumbency, pruritis, icterus, dysphagia, oedema, fever, pigmenturia, polyuria/polydipsia, poor performance, respiratory noise, stranguria, seizures, lameness, ataxia, murmurs and dysrhythmias, to name but a few!

Key points

As a result of reading this chapter you should be able to:
- Implement problem-based clinical reasoning in your approach to common problems in equine practice and recognise that the principle is similar to small animal practice
- Identify specific behavioural, physiological and anatomical differences unique to the horse that might require you to adopt a different approach in some circumstances

- Use information assimilated from the history and physical examination to formulate and refine a problem list and come up with a rational list of differential diagnoses based on plausible pathophysiological mechanisms
- Determine a definitive diagnosis by selecting the most appropriate diagnostic tests and imaging modalities, taking into account the limitations of equine practice
- Use the examples outlined in this chapter as a framework to apply a problem-based clinical reasoning approach to other clinical problems that are commonly encountered in equine practice. Practice makes perfect!

CHAPTER 19

Principles of professional reasoning and decision-making

Elizabeth Armitage-Chan

Department of Clinical Science and Services, The Royal Veterinary College, London, UK

The why

- Is gold-standard medical care always the best option for our patients?
- How do we balance the needs of our patient, client, ourselves, our colleagues, our practice, the profession and society?
- The practice of clinical veterinary medicine involves more than just the interaction between the veterinarian and the patient, and a successful outcome of a case requires more than clear clinical reasoning leading to a correct diagnosis and appropriate treatment.
- While animal welfare remains our primary focus as veterinarians, consideration of the needs of the client and other stakeholders also plays an important role in how we determine an appropriate course of action for our patient.
- In this chapter we will discuss a systematic, logical framework that you can use to support your decision-making in complex situations where there is no clear 'right or wrong' pathway that meets the needs of the key stakeholders involved.

Introduction to professional reasoning

Consider the following clinical scenario. It is a busy Saturday morning and as a recent graduate it is the first time you are the only veterinarian in the practice. You have a full appointment list and your first client brings in her elderly dog. You can see from the clinical record

Clinical Reasoning in Veterinary Practice: Problem Solved!, Second Edition.
Edited by Jill E. Maddison, Holger A. Volk and David B. Church.
© 2022 John Wiley & Sons Ltd. Published 2022 by John Wiley & Sons Ltd.

that the dog has been a patient at the practice for a long time, although without any significant medical history.

At the most recent vaccination appointment (2 years ago) the dog was described as being slightly overweight but, when you examine the dog this morning, she is markedly underweight.

The client is concerned about a swelling on the dog's mouth, which is approximately 2 cm diameter, located on the lip. The client asks you if you can remove the lump as it sometimes bleeds a little when the dog is given something to chew (a toy or treat).

The dog also seems painful and stiff when walked into the consultation room and coughs occasionally during the appointment. The client apologises for coming on a Saturday morning, which is usually reserved for emergency appointments, but says she is reliant on her daughter being able to drive her to the practice. The daughter is waiting outside in the car.

How do you proceed with this case? Throughout this book the focus has been on clinical reasoning, which is also relevant here, and would help you to medically prioritise the dog's problems and work towards diagnoses for the lesion on the mouth, the weight loss, the cough and the generalised pain and stiffness. However, as with the majority of clinical cases, there are additional elements that complicate the veterinarian's decision-making. How much diagnostic exploration is 'right' for a dog of this age? Should the mass be removed without investigating the cough? What is the dog's long-term prognosis, given the chronic pain and weight loss? How much money is the client willing to spend and how much is 'right' to spend in this situation? How will post-operative care and re-check appointments be managed if the client has limited access to transport? What is the role of the daughter in this situation?

While decisions about how to proceed are complicated by these uncertainties, experienced veterinarians will know that such cases can also lead to conflict and further complexity if the recommendations they make are either declined by or unaffordable for the client. Furthermore, such cases can be complicated further if colleagues disagree on the preferred course of action.

Many different scenarios could develop from this initial case presentation, depending on the direction and quality of the conversation, and the individual needs, preferences and values of those involved. For example, in one scenario, the veterinarian might feel he or she cannot proceed with the client's request without first identifying the nature of the mass, the cause of the cough and the reason for the chronic weight loss, requiring diagnostic steps that may be financially unaffordable for the client. Equally, the client may feel she simply doesn't want to put the dog through the additional visits and interventions required, or she may not feel the cough and weight loss are of sufficient impact on the dog's life for her to prioritise them. The veterinarian therefore reaches an impasse, feeling discomfort with the client's preferred plan but unable to implement his or her own professional preferences.

As an alternate solution, the veterinarian may feel that simple excision of the oral mass is in everyone's best interests and elects a short procedure (to minimise detrimental impact of a long anaesthetic and prolonged recumbency on the dog's painful joints and on any underlying systemic disease). This may turn out well, with the excised tissue being non-malignant and the wound healing well. Alternatively, the anaesthetic may exacerbate underlying thoracic and systemic disease, and the mass may be malignant, heal poorly and rapidly recur.

These uncertainties, about what is the 'right' way to proceed and what might happen as a consequence, present challenges to a veterinarian's decision-making that extend beyond clinical reasoning and impact significantly on wider stakeholders. Such impacts are financial, emotional and social, affecting the client, the veterinarian and the practice, as well as the quality of the future relationships between these parties.

In this chapter, the principles of this wider veterinary professional reasoning will be presented, providing veterinarians with a systematic, logical framework that they can use to support decision-making in such complex situations.

Why are professional reasoning skills just as important as clinical reasoning skills?

Many veterinarians demonstrate preferences towards what is commonly understood as 'gold standard' care: that which is most likely to result in disease resolution and has high-quality evidence supporting its use (Armitage-Chan and May 2018). Such an approach, in which solutions to clinical problems are understood as 'right or wrong' (there being a clear, preferred solution, with alternatives being substandard) is linked to veterinarians' perfectionist nature and compounded by education systems that reward single best answers to clinical questions (Cooke and Lemay 2017).

However, the strive to consistently emulate the solution associated with the greatest prognostic evidence means that veterinarians neglect in their decision-making the wealth of alternate, reasonable and appropriate actions that are available to them, their patients and their clients. In many situations, what may be conceived as 'gold standard' according to the clinical assessment may not represent the optimal solution for the client, patient or even the veterinarian.

Within human medicine, deviations from 'best-evidence' approaches are increasingly recognised as being equally valid to those afforded the 'gold standard' label, particularly if they are easier for a patient or family to manage or avoid the welfare compromise and distress of invasive surgery (Mulley, Trimble, and Elwyn 2012). In the context of veterinary medicine, there is a similar, increasing discourse expressing doubt about the inherent superiority of diagnostic and treatment interventions that are focused on disease resolution and longevity of life, particularly if these also carry significant financial consequences for the client, welfare implications for the patient (e.g. prolonged hospitalisation, painful surgery or impaired post-operative mobility) or alter the human–animal relationship from one of companionship to one of patient and carer (Grimm et al. 2018; Springer et al. 2019).

For many veterinarians, their well-being and career satisfaction is enhanced if they construct their professional priorities broadly, incorporating holistic client and patient needs, rather than focusing their goals exclusively on a patient's disease resolution (Armitage-Chan and May 2018). Placing value on these wider professional priorities enhances employability and contributes to a veterinarian's sustainability within the profession (Bell, Cake, and Mansfield 2018). However, this arguably presents a more complicated approach to problem-solving, as multiple influences must be considered to reach a balanced decision. There is greater inherent uncertainty, and as a result this can be particularly challenging for those with perfectionism traits (Crane, Phillips, and Karin 2015).

A systematic approach to logically considering the problem and those that are affected by it, then analysing one's chosen decision, can help provide tangible steps in an otherwise overwhelming situation, ensure important elements are not neglected, provide a means to manage uncertainties and reduce the influence of cognitive bias (Armitage-Chan 2020). There are multiple sources of uncertainty in these complicated, multi-stakeholder cases. Uncertainty is troubling and evokes discomfort, even amongst experienced clinicians (Ilgen et al. 2021). Uncertainty arises in not knowing whether a chosen solution will be effective clinically, and without relevant experience and evidence, any outcome is difficult to predict. Furthermore, individuals' preferences and their feelings associated with a case will not be static, and uncertainty arises for the veterinarian in how any outcome will be perceived by the client, as well as by other important stakeholders (one's colleagues, peers, role models, practice managers). As in clinical reasoning, cognitive biases will exert an effect on the veterinarian's reasoning process; while we might think we are considering the case according to the unbiased analysis of the needs of all stakeholders, innate biases orient our focus towards those stakeholder needs that align with our own preferred action, while simultaneously neglecting those that are counter to it (McKenzie 2014).

Define the problem

Figure 19.1 presents the main influences on decision-making, and those influenced by the decision, for simplicity, henceforth referred to as the stakeholders in veterinary care.

A simplified approach to identifying possible solutions is also included.

In clinical reasoning, the problem is defined by generating a prioritised problem list, and then identifying those problems that need to be refined and explored further. As we move to multi-stakeholder professional reasoning, the problem will typically be perceived differently amongst the main stakeholders. For example, a client's 'problem list' might be that he/she fears the immediate loss of the pet, is anxious about the financial consequences of pursuing treatment and is concerned about looking foolish or uncaring in the eyes of the

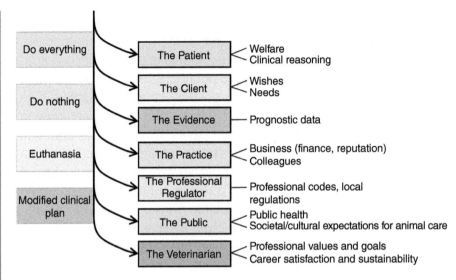

Figure 19.1 The main influences on professional reasoning and decision-making.

veterinarian. Within the same case, the veterinarian's 'problem list' might include wanting to identify and resolve the patient's disease, avoid compromising the relationship with the client, provide a clinical plan that is financially suitable for the client's needs and act in a way that is deemed acceptable to professional peers.

Analysing the problem according to each stakeholder's needs

As a first step in navigating this kind of professional dilemma, Figure 19.1 can be used to create a list of relevant stakeholders (not all stakeholders in Figure 19.1 will be relevant to every scenario), and from this, an analysis of the 'problem' (as perceived by each stakeholder), with their needs for an acceptable outcome. Next, the boxes on the left of Figure 19.1 can be used to generate initial solutions:

- *Doing everything:* Typically the steps needed to achieve a definitive diagnosis and disease resolution.
- *Doing nothing:* Is it feasible to do nothing at this stage? 'Doing nothing' can represent a useful temporary solution, providing both the veterinarian and the client with more time to make a decision about how to proceed. Such an approach is generally feasible as

long as the patient is stable and can be palliated with analgesics or minimally invasive treatments to manage clinical signs. In some cases, the disease may resolve spontaneously, or the patient may be able to continue in the short or longer term without requiring treatment.

- *Euthanasia:* A decision that might not be appropriate for all cases, but a feasible solution where there is limited long-term prognosis, or where it is not possible to ensure an acceptable level of welfare for the patient and client.
- *Modified clinical plans:* This represents the most complicated of solutions, as the deviation from best-evidence approaches leads to increased uncertainty and a range of different solutions. However, in many situations, some form of mid-way action, that is neither 'do everything', nor 'do nothing' and is formed through ongoing communication and negotiation of stakeholder needs, represents the ultimate outcome. This will be discussed further in the remainder of this chapter.

Applying this to the scenario presented at the start of this chapter yields the following initial analysis of the problem (Table 19.1).

Table 19.1   Analysis of the problem, as perceived by the stakeholders in veterinary care.

	Problem list (needs)	How stakeholder needs are met by each of the possible solutions
The patient: The elderly dog	• Alleviation of orthopaedic pain • Resolution of oral mass to prevent infection, or if it is interfering with eating/play • Identification and management of the reasons for the marked weight loss	*Do everything:* a matter of ethical debate: does this meet the dog's welfare interests? *Do nothing:* no alleviation of orthopaedic pain and oral mass may eventually cause pain, infection or compromise eating, if it isn't already *Euthanasia:* no welfare compromise and the dog would not be aware *Modified clinical plan:* a solution that addresses pain and discomfort would address the dog's needs

(Continued)

Table 19.1   (Continued)

	Problem list (needs)	How stakeholder needs are met by each of the possible solutions
The client: The dog's owner	• Concerns about the oral mass • Unable to attend frequent veterinary appointments (and may experience guilt/distress about this) • Needs veterinary care to be financially manageable • (Presumed) companionship and human–animal relationship	*Do everything:* challenges relating to transport and post-operative management, as well as financial. May result in distress (diagnosing causes of cough and weight loss) and outcome may not incorporate removal of the oral mass (e.g. if systemic disease identified elsewhere) *Do nothing:* owner remains concerned about the oral mass, which might become bigger or more prone to bleeding *Euthanasia:* distressful for client *Modified clinical plan:* a solution that addresses the oral lesion would address immediate needs; in the long term, a solution that addresses the weight loss and cough may prolong the life of the dog
The client's daughter	• (Presumed) concerns about her mother and (to a certain extent) about the dog • (Presumed) responsibilities for transport, which may have impact on wider (unknown) responsibilities	*Do everything:* (presumed) concerns about her mother's financial outlay; impact on daughter for providing transport *Do nothing:* (presumed) concern that her mother's concerns remain unaddressed; she may also be concerned about the dog's cough, weight loss and pain *Euthanasia:* (presumed) may feel this is appropriate and/or may be worried about her mother for this (eventual) scenario *Modified clinical plan:* difficult to identify impact, as this stakeholder's needs are not clear

Table 19.1   (Continued)

	Problem list (needs)	How stakeholder needs are met by each of the possible solutions
The veterinarian	• Need to ensure dog's welfare is met, whatever the decision • May have professional interests surrounding diagnosis of the cough, oral mass and weight loss • Need to maintain positive relationship with the client, at least during the management of this case (and ideally, in the longer term) • To appreciate a sense of satisfaction in one's work and decision-making	*Do everything:* may meet the veterinarian's professional interests in diagnosis and treatment, if these represent his/her professional goals; alternately the veterinarian may feel this is excessive for the dog or may be concerned that it isn't right for the client *Do nothing:* may provide some further time if there are no urgent clinical signs to address; however, the presenting issues remain unresolved and are not likely to improve *Euthanasia:* meets few of the veterinarian's needs in this scenario (although may revisit this at a later date if signs are rapidly progressive) *Modified clinical plan:* if a suitable plan can be identified, this may enable all needs to be met (possibly with the exception of professional interests surrounding definitive diagnosis and treatment)
The practice	• A level of financial income from clinical cases • Positive local reputation amongst pet owners • Support satisfaction of the practice team in their work	*Do everything:* maximum financial income (so long as fees are paid); potential impact on reputation *Do nothing:* minimal financial income; potential impact on staff satisfaction *Euthanasia:* reputational impact may be positive or negative, depending on context and communication *Modified clinical plan:* may enable all needs to be met

In the above analysis, the needs of the veterinarian have been constructed based on a psychology model that frames satisfaction, sense of achievement and self-worth on meeting three personal needs (Ryan and Deci 2000):

1 A need to experience positive human relationships
2 A need to make decisions and take actions that align with one's personal goals and values
3 A need to experience competence in achieving one's goals (or feel that competence is within reach, with appropriate attention on personal learning and development).

As mentioned in the introduction to this chapter, individual veterinarians will construct their professional goals and values in different ways. Some will feel satisfaction and achievement only if they have done everything they can to diagnose and treat the dog's different diseases and underlying conditions. Others will feel a sense of satisfaction if they have explored different solutions and identified a clinical plan that meets the client's needs and addresses the immediate welfare needs of the patient, even if the specific diagnosis remains unresolved. Most veterinarians will want to avoid an inflammatory or argumentative interaction with the client (or colleagues), and therefore high-quality communication (particularly in a context of conflicting needs) is vital and will be discussed next.

Refining the problem: ongoing communication and collaboration

The analysis in Table 19.1 includes some assumptions that are made about stakeholder needs, indicating a need for ongoing communication to fully understand the needs and values of important stakeholders. During the initial stages of professional reasoning, communication is focused on information-gathering: obtaining the perspective of the client (and other stakeholders) through a combination of open-ended questions, rapport-building and active listening. Although not specifically explored amongst veterinary clients, evidence from other healthcare areas demonstrates patients' concerns with being perceived as foolish or difficult, and as a consequence, being reluctant to share their concerns with their healthcare provider (Frosch et al. 2012).

Although challenging in an emergency context, time spent building trust and focusing not only on obtaining pertinent clinical information but also understanding clients' wishes for an acceptable outcome, as well as their concerns and fears about their limitations (financial or logistical), will help the veterinarian to make an informed, empathic decision about appropriate clinical care. Effective communication strategies include building a positive relationship with the client and expressing empathy, as well as addressing non-verbal elements, such as negative body language, being rushed or distractions, that might inhibit a client's willingness to talk (Shaw 2006).

Much recent attention has been focused on the concept of shared decision-making, and this is particularly pertinent when the veterinarian is attempting to construct an individualised, modified clinical plan that will meet the needs of patient, veterinarian and client. Shared decision-making lies between a paternalistic approach (in which the veterinarian determines the most appropriate solution and informs the client of this plan) and a client-centred approach (in which the client is afforded the responsibility for the decision, perhaps selecting from a list of provided options, with no guidance from the veterinarian). Shared decision-making is collaborative, and while the onus is not on the veterinarian persuading a client to accept his/her guidance, it also avoids the sense of burnout and fatigue that arises from veterinarians perceiving they have little agency in clinical decisions (Moses, Malowney, and Wesley Boyd 2018).

It is important to note, however, that this collaborative approach is not always appropriate; in some situations, such as in emergencies or in cases of acute refractory pain, a paternalistic approach may be required to ensure animal welfare and a rapid decision. Similarly, where there is genuinely little difference between different clinical options, and the client has valid reasons for his/her preference (perhaps a recent poor experience, such as an anaesthetic death in a previous pet), a more client-oriented approach might be suitable.

With ongoing, high-quality communication, the veterinarian can create a clinical plan that is based on a thorough consideration of all stakeholder needs, which is then discussed with the client. In the case presented at the start of this chapter, there are many clinical plans that might be discussed, some of which include:

- Removing the oral mass but performing thoracic radiography following the anaesthetic pre-medication to eliminate the possibility of advanced metastatic disease (with a plan in place for if this is observed)
- Removing the oral mass and prescribing non-steroidal anti-inflammatory drugs for the orthopaedic pain, with a caution that if the mass recurs it will be important to investigate further (or discuss euthanasia)
- Leaving the oral mass due to concerns that the weight loss and cough are the more significant problem, with a plan to monitor issues arising from the mass becoming ulcerated and a euthanasia discussion when these become significant.

During this conversation, the proposed plan may be agreed by the client, or he/she may express further concerns. Whichever plan is progressed, even a 'do everything' approach will carry some risks and uncertainties, such as surgical complications, incorrect diagnosis or unpredictable treatment responses. The nuances of how this information is presented to the client will vary depending on the context, including the veterinarian's personal approaches to client communication (whether the veterinarian prefer 'tell them straight' or 'soften the blow' communication strategies), and the veterinarian's relationship with and prior knowledge of the client. There is no single correct way to handle this conversation, which tends to represent a balance between informing the client of the risks of the decision and avoiding inciting feelings of guilt if a more comprehensive approach is not feasible.

Solving the problem: identifying, implementing and reviewing the solution

Once a decision is reached, implementation requires an ongoing collaborative approach to case management, which will often incorporate the wider practice team. Complications may arise that are patient related (e.g. deterioration or progression of clinical signs) or client related (regret at the decision, a change in perspective). Ongoing monitoring of both patient and client response is therefore vital, whether this is via recheck appointments or telephone/email updates.

Communication with colleagues is also important, particularly if another veterinarian is likely to see the patient. When decision-making is complicated by the influence of multiple stakeholder needs, the reasons for a particular decision might not be apparent, so documenting not only the decision but also the rationale for the decision (and the client communication) become very important to ensure continuity of care.

It is often the case that, with time (and when the initial emotions associated with the veterinary consultation have subsided) the client reflects on the decision and modifies his/her views. Ongoing communication that reflects this propensity for change (revisiting the gathering of the client's views and wishes for an acceptable outcome) is helpful and might aid the veterinarian, for example, when he/she is trying to persuade the client to consider further diagnostics, treatment or euthanasia. Professional reasoning is therefore typically not completed within a single veterinary visit and may take place over a lengthier process of communication and shared decision-making.

Completing the problem: reflection and analysis

It is important for veterinarians to reflect on cases and their decisions and actions. In many situations, the clinical plan will deviate from the veterinarian's preferred way of managing the case, something that can lead to feelings of dissonance – the feeling that one's actions are not congruent with personal goals and values, which can increase the risk of burnout. Such cases can therefore threaten a veterinarian's resilience to the challenges of veterinary practice, contributing to attrition from the profession. Reflecting on what has been achieved with the case can help veterinarians to identify their strengths in client communication and collaboration (often in very difficult and emotional contexts), as well as the successes they have achieved in managing patient and client welfare and strengthening the client's relationship with the practice, increasing the likelihood clients will return for veterinary advice in the future.

Key points

As a result of reading this chapter we hope that you appreciate that:
- Professional reasoning and decision-making is an important facet of clinical practice if the needs of the patient, client and veterinarian are to be appropriately considered and balanced.
- The professional reasoning framework described will help you to recognise that there is often not a clear 'right or wrong' way to manage a case.
- Identification of the stakeholders involved and the impact of different management options on them is an important step to aid shared decision-making in complex situations.

References

Armitage-Chan, Elizabeth. 2020. Best Practice in Professional Identity Formation: Use of a Professional Reasoning Framework. *Journal of Veterinary Medical Education*.

Armitage-Chan, Elizabeth, and Stephen A May. 2018. Identity, Environment and Mental Wellbeing in the Veterinary Profession. *Veterinary Record*, June, vetrec-2017-104724. https://doi.org/10.1136/VR.104724.

Bell, Melinda A., Martin A. Cake, and Caroline F. Mansfield. 2018. Beyond Competence: Why We Should Talk about Employability in Veterinary Education. *Journal of Veterinary Medical Education* 45 (1): 27–37. https://doi.org/10.3138/jvme.0616-103r1.

Cooke, Suzette, and Jean-Francois Lemay. 2017. Transforming Medical Assessment. *Academic Medicine* 92 (6): 746–751. https://doi.org/10.1097/ACM.0000000000001559.

Crane, MF, JK Phillips, and E Karin. 2015. Trait Perfectionism Strengthens the Negative Effects of Moral Stressors Occurring in Veterinary Practice. *Australian Veterinary Journal* 93 (10): 354–360. https://doi.org/10.1111/avj.12366.

Frosch, Dominick L., Suepattra G. May, Katharine A. S. Rendle, Caroline Tietbohl, and Glyn Elwyn. 2012. Authoritarian Physicians and Patients' Fear of Being Labeled 'Difficult' among Key Obstacles to Shared Decision-Making. *Health Affairs* 31 (5): 1030–1038. https://doi.org/10.1377/hlthaff.2011.0576.

Grimm, Herwig, Alessandra Bergadano, Gabrielle C. Musk, Klaus Otto, Polly M. Taylor, and Juliet Clare Duncan. 2018. Drawing the Line in Clinical Treatment of Companion Animals: Recommendations from an Ethics Working Party. *Veterinary Record* 182 (23): 664. https://doi.org/10.1136/vr.104559.

Ilgen, Jonathan S., Pim W. Teunissen, Anique B.H. de Bruin, Judith L. Bowen, and Glenn Regehr. 2021. Warning Bells: How Clinicians Leverage Their Discomfort to Manage Moments of Uncertainty. *Medical Education* 55 (2): 233–241. https://doi.org/10.1111/medu.14304.

McKenzie, Brennen A. 2014. Veterinary Clinical Decision-Making: Cognitive Biases, External Constraints, and Strategies for Improvement. *Journal of the American Veterinary Medical Association* 244 (3): 271–276. https://doi.org/10.2460/javma.244.3.271.

Moses, Lisa, Monica J. Malowney, and Jon Wesley Boyd. 2018. Ethical Conflict and Moral Distress in Veterinary Practice: A Survey of North American Veterinarians. *Journal of Veterinary Internal Medicine* 32 (6): 2115–2122. https://doi.org/10.1111/jvim.15315.

Mulley, Albert G., Chris Trimble, and Glyn Elwyn. 2012. Stop the Silent Misdiagnosis: Patients' Preferences Matter. *BMJ (Online)*. https://doi.org/10.1136/bmj.e6572.

Ryan, Richard M., and Edward L. Deci. 2000. Self-Determination Theory and the Facilitation of Intrinsic Motivation, Social Development, and Well-Being. *American Psychologist* 55 (1): 68–78. https://doi.org/10.1037/0003-066X.55.1.68.

Shaw, Jane R. 2006. Four Core Communication Skills of Highly Effective Practitioners. *Veterinary Clinics of North America. Small Animal Practice* 36 (2): 385–396, vii. https://doi.org/10.1016/j.cvsm.2005.10.009.

Springer, Svenja, Peter Sandøe, Thomas Bøker Lund, and Herwig Grimm. 2019. Patients Interests First, but . . . – Austrian Veterinarians' Attitudes to Moral Challenges in Modern Small Animal Practice. *Animals* 9 (5): 241. https://doi.org/10.3390/ani9050241.

Index

Note: All index entries refer to small animal practice (dogs, cats) unless otherwise specified (e.g. specific small mammals, or horses). Page numbers in *italics* represent figures; those in **bold** represent tables. *vs.* denotes a comparison, or differential diagnosis.

A

Abdominal enlargement, 89–101
  case example, 100–101
  causes, 89–90
  colic in horses, 357, 364, 366
  define the lesions, 92–94, 95–96, 97, 98
  define the location, 91
  define the problem, 89–91
  diagnostic approach, 90
  fluid, 89, 90
    ascites *see* Ascites
    blood, 96–97
    characterisation/types, 91, 100
    chyle, 98
    distribution, 91
    eosinophilic effusions, 96
    exudates, 95–96
    transudates (pure/modified), 91–94, 101
    urine, 97
  refine the problem, 91–92, 95, 96, 97, 98
Abdominal pain
  in horses, 356, 358, 362–363
    see also Colic, in horses
  jaundice and, case example, 210–211
Abdominocentesis, horses, 365, 367
Abrasions, in horses, colic, 356, 363
Abscess
  pancreatic, 13
  tooth root, 157

Acanthocytes, 190, *190*
Acetylcholine receptor (AChR), 119, 123
ACTH stimulation test, 68, **251**, *295*, 295
  in guinea pigs, 346
Activated clotting time (ACT), 224–225
Activated partial thromboplastin time
  (APTT), 225
Acute haemorrhage, *see* Haemorrhage,
  acute
Acute haemorrhagic diarrhoea syndrome
  (AHDS), **62**, 65
Acute noncompressive nucleus pulposus
  extrusion (ANNPE), 281
Acute renal failure, polyuria in, 252
ADH *see* Antidiuretic hormone (ADH)
Adult respiratory distress syndrome, 176
Alanine aminotransferase (ALT), 206, 207, 211
Albino animals, 307
Albumin, 93, 94
Aleutian disease, 349–350
Alkaline phosphatase (ALP), 206–207, 211
Allergic bronchospasm, 162
Allergic rhinitis, 156, 157, 217
Allergic skin disease, *288*, 289
  of pinna, 298
Alopecia, *288*
  in guinea pigs *see* Guinea pigs
α2 agonists, colic in horses, 363
Alveolar disease, 172
'Alveolar pattern', radiography, 165
Anaemia, 181–197
  assessment, 182, 183
  case example, 195–197
  causes
    anaemia of inflammatory disease, 182, 191
    chronic kidney disease, 191–192
    bone marrow disorders, 192–193
    haemorrhage, 185–186, 383

Clinical Reasoning in Veterinary Practice: Problem Solved!, Second Edition.
Edited by Jill E. Maddison, Holger A. Volk and David B. Church.
© 2022 John Wiley & Sons Ltd. Published 2022 by John Wiley & Sons Ltd.

Anaemia (*cont'd*)
  haemolysis, 186–187, 187–190, 383–384
  iron deficiency, 193
  characteristics, 181
  of chronic disease, in horses, 388
  define the lesion, 187–190, 194, 196
    in horses, 385, **385–386**
    non-regenerative anaemia, 183, 191–193
    regenerative anaemia, 183, 187–190
    see also Regenerative anaemia;
      Non-regenerative anaemia
  define the location, 185–187, 191, 194, 196
    in horses, 383–384
    non-regenerative anaemia, 183, 191
    regenerative anaemia, 183, 185–187,
      383–384
  define the problem, 182, 194, 195, 381–382
  define the system, 183, *184*, 194, 196, 382
  definition, 181, 382
  development rapidity, 182
  diagnostic approach, 182
  false, after sedation, 182
  as haematologic abnormality not
    diagnosis, in horses 380–381
  haemolytic *see* Haemolytic anaemia
  in horses *see* Horses
  measurements, 182
  microangiopathic, 189–190, *190*
  mild to moderate, 181, 182
  non-regenerative *see* Non-regenerative
    anaemia
  normocytic normochromic, 191, 192
  pre-regenerative, 183, 185, 191
  refine the system, 183, 194
  regenerative, *see* Regenerative anaemia
  severity, 181, 182
Anaesthesia, small mammals, 324–325
Anal gland mass, 259
Anchoring bias, **13**
Angiostrongylus vasorum
  bleeding due to, 222, 227, 230
  coughing with dyspnoea due to, 164, 166
  haemoptysis due to, 159
  ocular disease due to, 311
Anisocoria, 307
Anisocytosis, 183, *184*
Anorexia, 20, 75, 78
  prolonged, causes, 78
Anterior chamber
  examination, 317
  opaque eye, causes, **314**
Antibiotics
  diarrhoea due to, **63**, 373
  diarrhoea management, 67, 68, 368
  sensitivity, in eye problems, 319

Anti-diuretic hormone (ADH), 252
  absent, deficient or impaired, 240, 241,
    242, 248
Anti-emetic drugs, 36, 43, 78
Anti-epileptic drugs, 126, 127, 130, 132
Antimicrobials
  diarrhoea induced by, **63**, 373
  diarrhoea in foals, 368
  see also Antibiotics
Anti-RBC antibodies, 187
Appetite
  in chinchillas, 335
  control, factors affecting, 75
  loss/decreased, 75, 77, 78
    weight loss due to *see* Weight loss
    see also Anorexia; Inappetence
  normal/increased, weight loss with *see*
    under Weight loss
Aqueous humour, colour changes, 308
Ascites, 90, 91–94
  define the lesion (causes), 92–94
    hypoproteinaemia, 93–94
    lymphatic obstruction, 94
    portal hypertension, 92–93
  definition, 91
  fluid composition, 91–92, 93
  pure/modified transudates, 91–94
Aspartate aminotransferase (AST), 206
Aspergillosis, 156, 158
  epistaxis due to, 218
  sneezing/nasal discharge due to, 156–157
Aspiration, gastric contents, 37, 41
Aspiration pneumonia, 37
  in horses *see* Horses
Aspirin, 231
Asteroid hyalosis, 308
Asthma, equine, 377, **378**, 380
Ataxia, 104, 106, 265, 309
  observation (hands-off examination), 107
Auscultation, thoracic, 113, 160, 163
  coughing in horses, 376, 377
Autoagglutination, 185, 387
Autoimmune disorders
  haemolytic anaemia *see* Immune-
    mediated haemolytic anaemia (IMHA)
  immune-mediated thrombocytopenia
    (ITP), 227, 229
  primary, 229
  pruritus due to skin diseases in, 289
  scaling disorders due to, 293–294
  weight loss due to decreased appetite, 77
Automatism, 130, 131
Autonomic dysfunction, 106
Availability bias, **13**
Azotaemia, 246, **247**

B

Babesiosis, 188, 230
Back pain, 278
Bacterial infections
canine otitis due to, *302*
  coughing in horses, **378**, 379, **379**
  coughing with/without dyspnoea, 164
  diarrhoea due to, **61**, **62**, **63**, **64**
  dyspnoea in rats due to, 340, **341**
  enteritis due to, **61**
  in horses (foals), 368
Balance, loss of, 133
Beetroot ingestion (beeturia), 216
Behaviour, hands-off examination of CNS,
    107
Behavioural disorders, 127
  see also Paroxysmal behaviour changes
Bias
  cognitive, 395
  confirmation, **13**, 20, 324
  diagnostic, 13, **13**
Bile acids, serum, 207
Bile peritonitis, 95, 209
Biliary carcinoma, 100–101
Biliary obstruction, 202, 204, 209
Biliary surgery, 209
Biliary tract disease, jaundice due to, 202,
    204, 205, 208
Bilirubin, 199, 200
  conjugated/conjugation, 200, *201*
  excretion, 200, 206
  in horses, 384
  increased *see* Hyperbilirubinaemia
  metabolism, 200, *201*
  unconjugated, 200, 384
  see also Jaundice
Bilirubinaemia, 202, 205
  see also Hyperbilirubinaemia
Bilirubinuria, 200
Biopsy
  bone marrow, in horses, 384, 387–388
  for diarrhoea, 69
  liver, 203, 208
  nasal, 218
  skin, 295–296
Bladder, rupture, 97
Bleeding, 215–235
  case example, 233–235
  causes, 217–221
  of epistaxis, 217–218
  of haematuria, 220–221
    local disorders, 217–221
    of melaena, 219, 235
    systemic disorders, 221–222
  clinical signs, 215–216

define and refine the system, 216, 234
define the lesion, 217–221
define the location, 221
define the problem, 215–216, 233, 234
  red urine, 216
  systemic disorders *see* Bleeding
      disorders, systemic
diagnostic approach, 215–216
  case example, 234
  epistaxis, 218–219
  haematuria, 221
  melaena due to GI ulceration, 219–220
haematuria *see* Haematuria
local disorders, 217–221
melaena *see* Melaena
from nose *see* Epistaxis
systemic disorders, *see* Bleeding
      disorders, systemic
see also Haemorrhage
Bleeding disorders, systemic, 216, 221–227
  clinical signs, 216, 224
  define the lesion, 227–231
    platelet function defects, 230–231
    thrombocytopenia *see*
        Thrombocytopenia
  define the lesion (causes), 227–231
  diagnosis, **223**, 223–227
    activated clotting time (ACT), 224–225
    activated partial thromboplastin time
        (APTT), 225
    buccal mucosal bleeding time, 226
    clot retraction, 226
    platelet count, 224
    platelet function, 226
    prothrombin time (PT), 225
    thrombin time (TT), 225
    thromboelastometry/
        thromboelastography, 225
  epistaxis with, 218
  physiology, 221–222, *222*
Bleeding time, buccal mucosal, 226
Blindness, 306, 309, 310
Blood
  effusions (intra-abdominal), 96–97
  in faeces *see* Melaena
  loss *see* Bleeding; Haemorrhage
  in urine *see* Haematuria
  vomiting *see* Haematemesis
Blood samples, obtaining, small mammals,
    324
Blood smears, *184*, 387
Blood tests, 10, 14–15
  limitations and over-reliance on, 14
BOAS complex, 160, 168
Body system, 23–27

Body system (*cont'd*)
 defining *see under* Problem-based
   inductive clinical reasoning
 primary (structural), 24
 secondary (functional), 24
Bone marrow biopsy/aspirate, 382, 387–388
Bone marrow disorders
bleeding due to, 228
 non-regenerative anaemia due to,
   192–193
 primary, thrombocytopenia due to, 228
Bone marrow failure, thrombocytopenia in, 228
Borborygmi, in horses, 364
 absent, 364, 366
 hypermotile, 357, 364
Bowel necrosis, horses, 358
Brachycephalic obstructive airway syndrome
   (BOAS complex), 160, 168
Brain
 gait abnormalities and, 266–267
 in paroxysmal episodic disorders, 132
 seizure origin, 130–131
 see also Central nervous system (CNS)
Brainstem, 37, 266–267
Breathing
 in rats, 338
 through mouth, 155
Bronchial disease, 160–161, 171, 172
 coughing with minimal dyspnoea due to,
   160, 161, 162, 171
 dyspnoea with minimal coughing due to,
   171, 172
 inflammation (constrictive), 160, 161, 171,
   172
Bronchial sounds, 163
Bronchial washings, 166
Bronchitis, chronic, 179, 180
Bronchoalveolar disorders, 163
 causes, 164–165
 coughing with dyspnoea, 159, 162–163
 diagnostic procedures, 165–166
Bronchoalveolar lavage (BAL), 166, 380
Bronchoconstriction, 160, 161, 163, 171, 172
Bronchoconstrictive disorders
 diagnostic approach, 172
 coughing with/without dyspnoea due to,
   164–165
 dyspnoea with minimal coughing due to,
   171–172
 dyspnoea without coughing due to, 164
Bronchopulmonary disease, diagnosis,
   165–166
Bronchospasm, allergic, 162
Brush border enzyme deficiency, 81
Brush border protein transport, defect, 80

Buccal mucosal bleeding time, **223**, 226
Buphthalmos, **316**

C
Caecotrophs, 326, 329
Caloric requirements, 73–74
Capillary refill time (CRT), 11, 182, 195, 233
 in horses with colic, 362
Cardiac arrhythmia, 25
Cardiac disease
 acquired, pulmonary oedema in, 175–176
 coughing with dyspnoea due to, 164
 dyspnoea with minimal coughing due to,
   173, 175
 pulmonary oedema due to, 175–176
 weakness due to, 105, 112, **115**, **116**
Cardiac failure *see* Heart failure
Cardiomyopathy, 164
Case examples
 abdominal enlargement, 100–101
 anaemia, 195–197
 bleeding, 233–235
 coughing with dyspnoea, 178–180
 diarrhoea, 71–72
   large bowel diarrhoea, 71–72
 dyspnoea, 178–180
 epileptic seizure, 149–151
 immune-mediated haemolytic anaemia
   (IMHA), 195–197
 jaundice, 210–213
 malutilisation of nutrients, 100, 101
 neurological examination, 122
 polyuria/polydipsia (PU/PD), 257–259
 vomiting, 53–54
 weakness, 121–123
 weight loss, 86–87, 100
Cataplexy, 126, 131
 characteristics, **128–129**
Cataract, true, 308
Central nervous system (CNS), 104
 dysfunction, 104
   gait abnormalities due to, 264,
     265–267, 283
   skeletal disorders concurrent with,
     105–106, 107
   weakness due to, 105, 106, 111
 examination *see* Neurological examination
 neuroanatomical localisation, 107–111
 paroxysmal episodic disorders, 132
 primary (structural) disorders, 104, 105, 111
 secondary (functional) disorders, 105, 111
 see also Brain
Cerebrospinal fluid (CSF) examination
 in gait abnormalities, 278, 283
 in inflammatory CNS disease, 283

in seizures, 148, **148**, 151
in vestibular attacks, 145
Chemoreceptor trigger zone (CRTZ), 36–38,
    42, 42, 44
Cheyletiella, 289, 290
Chinchillas
  body condition, assessment, 334
  dental disease, 335, 336, 337, 338
  diet and diet history, 334–335
  'gut stasis', 334
  weight loss, 334–338
    can't eat, 335
    decreased/absent appetite, 335, 336
    define and refine the problems,
        334–336
    define the lesion, 337–338
    define the location, 337
    define the system, 336–337
    investigations, 337
    normal/increased appetite, 336–337
    won't eat, 335–336
Cholangiohepatitis, 203, 208
Cholangitis, 203, 204
Choledochitis, 204
Cholestasis, 64, 205, 206, 207, 211, 212, **250**
Cholesterol, 206, 207
Chondromalacia, 161
Chromodacryorrhea, 338
Chronic kidney disease (CKD)
  anaemia in, 191–192
  azotaemia, impaired urine concentration, **247**
  polyuria/polydipsia due to, 241, **245**
  mechanisms, **247**
Chronic respiratory disease (CRD), in rats,
    341–342
Chyle, causes and characteristics, 98
Chylous effusions, pleural, 170
Client issues
  analysis of the problem, **398**
  communication with veterinarian, 400–402
  compliance, 32, 300
  financial *see* Financial issues
  frustrating/complex cases and, 9, 10, 393,
      400
  needs/wishes, 395, *396*, **398**
    clinical plan and, 401–402
    modification of views with time, 403
  professional reasoning and *see*
      Professional reasoning
  shared decision-making, 401
Clinical cases
  complex, frustrating, 9–10
  professional reasoning skills *see*
      Professional reasoning
  solving, 10–11, 393–395

see also Clinical reasoning; Pattern
    recognition
Clinical decision-making *see*
    Decision-making
Clinical education, 8
Clinical plan, shared decision making
    401–402Clinical problem-solving,
    logical *see* Logical clinical problem-
    solving (LCPS)
Clinical reasoning, 1–6, 8–9, 16, 395
  learning buddy, benefits, 5, *5*
  repetition and consistency, 3
  robust method needed, 8–9
  steps, *16*, *34*
    see also Problem-based inductive
        clinical reasoning
Clinical signs, 1, 8, 17
  chronology of, 19
  define the system involved, 23–24
  in defining the problem, 16–17, 22–23
    prioritising, 17, 20
    specificity, 17–21
    see also Problem-based inductive
        clinical reasoning
  'hard findings' *vs.* 'soft findings', 17
  multiple, 10, 12, 15, 30
    pattern recognition use, 10, 11–12
    flawed, in multiple clinical signs, 12
    problem-based approach, *see* Problem-
        based inductive clinical reasoning
  related to more than one problem, 19
  see also individual clinical signs
Clopidogrel, 231
Clostridiosis, diagnosis, 374
Clostridium, **61**, **64**
Clostridium botulinum, 358
Clostridium perfringens, **64**
Clot formation, 222, *222*
Clot retraction, 226
Clotting factor deficiencies, 222, 224
Clotting times, prolongation, 224
Coagulation system, 222, *222*
  disorders, **223**, 227
  intravascular activation, DIC, 229
  tests, in bleeding disorders, **223**, 224–227
Cobalamin, 68, 80
Cognitive bias, 395
Colic, in horses, 355–367
  borborygmi in, 357, 364, 366
  causes, 357–359, **360–361**
    *see also pathophysiological mechanisms
        (below)*
  define and refine the system, 357–359
  define the lesion, 359, **360–361**
  define the location, 359

Colic, in horses (*cont'd*)
  define the problem, 356
  diagnostic approach, 361–367
    abdominocentesis, 365, 367
    basic examination, 361, 362
    cardiovascular status, emergency, 362,
      364
    history taking, 363
    'immediate needs' assessment,
      362–363
    investigations, 365
    physical examination, 363–364
    rectal examination, 364, 367
    ultrasonography, 365
  emergency, assessment, 362
  'false', 357, 359, **360**, **361**
  in foals, 356, **361**, 364
  frequency and response to therapy, 355
  gas (flatulent), 357, **360**, 366
  gastric reflux in, 365, 367
  management, 357, 365–366
  mild/moderate, 358, 363
  pain, 356, 358, 362–363
    referral indication, 366
    severity assessment, 362–363
  pathophysiological mechanisms, 357–359
    fluid distension, 357–358, 365
    impaction, 357, **360**, 364, 365
    inflammation of bowel, 358, **360**, **361**
    intestinal displacement, 357, **360**, 364
    intra-luminal obstruction, 357, **360**, **361**
    non-GIT, 357, 359, **360**, **361**
    non-strangulating infarctions, 358, **360**
    simple distention, 357, 359, **360**, 364,
      365, 366
    simple obstruction, 357–358, **360**, **361**
    strangulating obstructions, 357, 358,
      360, **361**
    toxic causes, 358–359, **360**
  referral/surgery, 355–356, 361
    indications, 365–367
  severe, 357, 358, 363, 366–367
  spasmodic, 357, **360**
  systemic deterioration, 367
Colitis, acute, in horses, 370
  see also Horses, diarrhoea
Collaboration, shared decision-making, 401
Collapsing episodes, 103, 126
  see also Paroxysmal episodic disorders;
    Seizures
'Collapsing trachea', 168
Collecting tubules, in primary polyuria, 240–241
Communication
  with clients, 400–402
  with colleagues, 403

Competence
  conscious, *8*, 9
  unconscious, 8, *8*, 9
Compliance (owner/client), 32, 300
Computed tomography (CT)
  constrictive bronchial inflammation, 172
  epistaxis, 219
  eye problems, 320
  gait abnormality assessment, 283
  sneezing and nasal discharge, 158
Confirmation bias, **13**, 20, 324
Congestive heart failure, 82
Consciousness
  impairment, 130
  loss, in seizures, 127
Constipation, 57
Constrictive bronchial inflammation,
    171–172
  dyspnoea with minimal coughing due to, 171
  diagnostic approach, 172
Coombs test, 187, 196, 387
Cornea
  blind eye causes, **315**
  colour categories, 308
  colour change, opaque eye,
    307–308, **313**
  cytology, 319
  oedema, 320
  perforation, 309
  ulcer, 319
Corneocytes, orthokeratotic/parakeratotic, 292
Cornification, 291
Cortisol/creatinine ratio, 295
Coughing, 158–162
  aspiration of gastric contents and, 41, 51
  case example, 178–180
  define the problem, 158–159
  definition, 158, 375
  with dyspnoea, 159, 162–166
    bronchoalveolar disease, 164–165
    bronchoconstrictive disease, 164,
      171–172
    case example, 178–180
    define the lesion/causes, 164–165
    define the location, 162–163
    define the system, 164
    diagnostic procedures, 165–166
    in horses, 377
  in example clinical scenario, 392, 393
  gagging after, or confused with, 39, 40, 158
  harsh, differential diagnoses, 179
  in horses *see* Horses
  minimal, dyspnoea with *see under*
    Dyspnoea
  with minimal dyspnoea, 159–162

define the lesion (causes), 160–161
define the location, 159–160
degenerative disorders, 161
diagnostic approach, 161–162
inflammatory disease, 160–161
malformations, 161
neoplasia, 161
in rats, 339
refine the problem, 159
retching after, 158, 159
vomiting *vs.* 39–40
without dyspnoea, 178, 179
Cough receptors, 158, 161, 171, 375, 376
Cough reflex, 158–159, 375–376
Crackles (lung sounds), 163
coughing in horses and, 377
Cranial drawer, 269–270
Cranial nerve, examination, 108, **110**, 122, 300
C-reactive protein, 166
Creatinine, 97
Cricopharyngeal achalasia, 76
Cruciate ligament, integrity, assessment, 270
Crusting, of pinnae, 298
Cryptococcosis, 157, 158
Culture
in eye problems, 319
faecal, 66
in jaundice, 208
in vestibular attacks, 145
Cushing's syndrome, 173, 253
see also Hyperadrenocorticism
Cyanosis, 167
Cyathostomiasis, larval, **371**, **372**, 373, 374
Cyst(s)
granular iridica, 321
ovarian, guinea pigs, 345
uveal, 308
Cystic ovarian disease, guinea pigs, 345
Cytokines
anaemia of inflammatory disease, 191
bronchoconstriction stimulated, 171, 172
inflammatory, 171, 191, 204
pruritic, 286
Cytology
abdominal enlargement case, 100, 101
canine otitis, 299
coughing with minimal dyspnoea, 161
eye problem diagnosis, 319
hepatic *vs.* post-hepatic jaundice, 208, 212
vestibular attack diagnosis, 145

D
DAMNIT-V scheme, 27, 328
equine practice, 370, 378, 385

musculoskeletal disorders, 275, **276–277**
neurological disorders affecting gait, 275
Decision-making, 9, 391–404
challenges/complex situations, 392, 393
factors to consider, 392, 394
influences on, 395–396, *396*
shared, 401
see also Professional reasoning
Defecation, pattern and frequency, 57
Dehydration, 182
azotaemia and, 246, **247**
diabetes insipidus and, 252
impaired urine concentration and, **247**, 248
Demodicosis, 289, 293, 294
Dental disease, 218
chinchillas, 335, 336, 337, 338
Dermatitis, *see* Otitis/dermatitis
Dermatological disease *see* Skin disorders
Dermatophytosis lesions, guinea pigs, 343, 345
Detrusor function, 254
Developing an illness script, 10
see also Pattern recognition
Developmental disorders, coughing in
horses, **378**
Diabetes insipidus
partial central/nephrogenic, 252
polyuria/polydipsia due to, 242, **244**, 249, **249**, 252
Diabetes mellitus, 31
malutilisation due to, 82
polyuria/polydipsia due to, 242, **245**
Diagnosis, 'balance of probabilities', 32
Diagnostic bias, 13, **13**,
'Diagnostic hooks', 17–19, 73
small mammals, 326
Diagnostic tests, 28–29
blood tests *see* Blood tests
primary (structural) *vs.* secondary
(functional) systems, 24–25
see also under specific clinical signs
Diarrhoea, 55–72
acute, 55, 56, 65, 67
fulminating, 65
in horses, 367–368, **371**, 373
small bowel diarrhoea, 65
antibiotic-responsive, 68–69
assessment, 57
case example, 71–72
causes, 60, **60–65**, 370, **371–372**
chronic, 55, 56, 60, 65
in horses, 368, **371**, 373–374
investigations, indications for, 65–69
therapeutic trials, 56
classification, 56–57
define and refine the system, 59–60, 72, 369

Diarrhoea (*cont'd*)
  define the lesion, 60, **60–65**, 370,
    371–372
  define the location (before system),
    57–58, 71, 370
    characteristics (large *vs.* small bowel),
      58, **58–59**
  define the problem, 57, 71, 369
  definition, 57, 369
  diagnostic approach, 56, 65–69
  in exocrine pancreatic insufficiency, 81
  history-taking, 58, 66
  in horses *see* Foals; Horses
  intermittent but repetitive, 55, 66
  large bowel diarrhoea *see* Large bowel
    diarrhoea
  malabsorption with, 80, 84
  maldigestion with, 81, 84
  malutilisation with, 80
  pathophysiology, 56
  profuse watery, polydipsia, 237–238
  in rabbits, 326
  small bowel diarrhoea *see* Small bowel
    diarrhoea
  vomiting association, 44
Diet
  in chinchillas, 334–335
  diarrhoea due to, **60, 62, 64**
  diarrhoea management approach, 66, 67
  in ferrets, 348
  in foals, 368, 370
  history, small mammals, 326
  intolerances in foals, 368
  in rabbits, 329–330
Differential diagnoses, 12–13
  defining the list (define the lesion), 16, 21,
    27, 27–28
Digestion, 79, 82
  in rabbits, 329, 330
Dim light test, 307
Direct Coombs test, 187, 196, 387
Dirofilaria immitis (dirofilariasis), 164, 166, 173
Disseminated idiopathic myofasciitis,
    ferrets, 350
Disseminated intravascular coagulation
    (DIC), 191, 222, 229
  bleeding due to, 222, 229
  thrombocytopenia due to, 229
  pre-hepatic jaundice due to, 205
Drinking, excessive *see* Polydipsia; Polyuria/
    polydipsia (PU/PD)
Drug(s)
  bone marrow disorders due to, 193
  dyscrasias, weight loss and, 77
  haemolytic anaemia due to, 188–189

  hepatic jaundice due to, 203
  platelet dysfunction due to, 227
  primary polydipsia due to, 241
  thrombocytopenia due to, 228
  vomiting due to, 38, 46
  see also specific drug groups
'Dynamic airway disease', 162
Dyscoria, 307
Dysfibrinogenaemia, 225
Dysphagia, 75
  causes, 76
Dyspnoea, 162–177
  case example, 178–180
  with coughing *see* Coughing, with
    dyspnoea
  define the problem, 162
  expiratory, 162, 168, 377
  in horses, 377
  inspiratory, 162, 168, 377
  with minimal coughing, 166–177
    adult respiratory distress syndrome, 176
    bronchial disease causing, 171–172
    cardiac disorders, 173
    constrictive bronchial inflammation,
      171–172
    define the lesion, 168–177
    define the location, 167–168
    define the system, 166
    hypoproteinaemia, 176
    laryngeal disorders *see* Laryngeal
      dysfunction
    neurogenic pulmonary oedema, 176
    normal delivery of abnormal
      haemoglobin, 173, 177
    primary alveolar disease, 172
    pulmonary oedema, 174–176
    pulmonary thromboembolism, 173–174
    reduced delivery of normal
      haemoglobin, 173–176
    secondary disorders, 173–177
    space-occupying disorders, pleural
      cavity, 169–171
  nasal cavity obstruction in cats, 155
  in rabbits, 327, 328
  in rats *see* Rats, dyspnoea
  respiratory sounds in, 167, 169, 171, 174
  without coughing, 168
Dysrhythmias, physiological, in horses, 354
Dysuria, 16, 17, 220, 221, 253

E
Ear, examination, 300–301
Ear canal
  black mucoid material from, 298
  sampling, 301

Ear disease, 297
  see also Otitis/dermatitis
Ecchymosis, 224
Ectoparasites
  in guinea pigs with alopecia and pruritus,
    344, 345
  otitis due to, 298
  pruritus due to, 287, *288*, 289, 290, 294
  scaling disorder due to, 293
Effusions
  abdominal, 90, 91
  see also Abdominal enlargement, fluid
    eosinophilic, 96
    haemorrhagic, 97
  neoplastic, 95
  pleural, *see* Pleural effusion
  pseudochylous, 98
Electroretinogram (ERG), 320
Emergency cases, 18, 20
  communication issues, 401
  horses, 362, 364, 368
  shared decision-making inappropriate,
    401
Emesis *see* Vomiting
'Emetic complex', 37
Emetic reflex, 36, 37, *42*
Emphysema, 165
Endocrine disorders
polydipsia due to, 240
see also specific endocrine disorders
Endocrine function tests, 119
Endocrinopathy
  keratinisation disorder due to, 291, 293
  otitis due to, 298
  weakness due to, 113
Endoscopy, 27, 69
Endothelium, abnormal, microangiopathic
  anaemia, 189
Endotoxemia, polyuria/polydipsia due to,
    242
Endotoxic shock, in horses, 362, 365–366
Endotoxin, 358, 368
Enophthalmos, **316**
Enterocyte defects, 80
Eosinophilic effusions, 96
Epilepsy
  breeds predisposed to, 143, 148
  genetic, 143
  idiopathic, primary, 140, 142, 143
  progressive myoclonic, 148
  structural, 140
Epileptic seizures, 130–132
  atonic, 131
  case example, 149–151
  characteristics, **128–129**, 131–132, 150

define the lesion, 140–143, 151
  extra-cranial causes, 140, *142*, 143–144
  flow-chart, *143*
  intra-cranial causes, 140–143, *141*
define the location, 132–133, 134–135, 151
define the problem, 131–132, 150
define the system, 132, 150
diagnostic approaches, 147–148, **148**, 151
extra-cranial causes, 135, 140, *142*, 143–144
  clinical signs, 144
  diagnostic approach, 147, **148**
focal-onset asymmetrical, 135
generalised onset (symmetrical), 141–142
intra-cranial causes, 135, 140–143, *141*
  asymmetric neurological deficits, 141
  diagnostic approach, 148, **148**
  functional diseases, 140
  structural diseases, 140–141
  symmetrical deficits, 141
origin, focus, 130–131, 150
paroxysmal dyskinesma *vs.*, 127
post-ictal dysfunction, 131–132, 135
stages, 131
stereotypical, 131
symptomatogenic zone, 130–131
tonic–clonic, 131
see also Seizures
Epiphora (tearing), 306, 308–309
  causes, **314**
  nasolacrimal duct flush, **315**
Episodic disorders *see* Paroxysmal episodic
    disorders
Episodic falling, 139
Epistaxis, 25, 155, 156, 215
  define the lesion (causes)
    fungal and neoplastic, 217, 218, 219
    local disorders, 217–218
    systemic disorders, 218
  diagnostic approach, 217–219
  site of bleeding, 217
Equine practice, 353–389
  colic (abdominal pain) *see* Colic, in horses
  coughing *see under* Horses
  define and refine the problem, 354
  define the location, 355
  diagnostic tests/procedures, 355
  diarrhoea *see under* Horses
  emergencies
    acute diarrhoea, 368
    colic, assessment, 362
  monetary value of horses, 354
  pallor and anaemia *see under* Horses
  problem-based clinical reasoning, 353–389
  significance of problems by purpose of
    horse, 354

Erythema, macular-papular, on pinna, 298
Erythrophagocytosis, 97
Escherichia coli, 13, **61**, **64**, 242, **245**
Euthanasia, *396*, 397
Exercise, increased levels, polydipsia, 238
Exercise-induced weakness *see* Weakness
Exocrine pancreatic insufficiency (EPI), 59
  diarrhoea due to, 59, 60, 67, 81
  maldigestion due to, 81
Exophthalmos, 309, **316**
Exotic animals, problem-based clinical
        reasoning, 325
Extra-hepatic bile duct obstruction
        (EHBDO), 204
Exudates, 95–96
  in abdominal enlargement, 95–96
  in bronchopulmonary disease, 161, 163,
        165
  causes, 95–96
  characteristics, 95
  in constrictive bronchial inflammation, 171,
        172
  non-septic, 95–96, 101
    pleural fluid, 170
  septic, 95, 96
Eye problems, 305–322
  abnormal-sized eye, 309
    causes, **316**
  abnormal-sized pupil, 307
    causes, **312–313**
  blind eye, 309, 320
    causes, **315–316**
    testing, 320–321
  causes (systemic), 310–311
  classification, 305–306
  define and refine the problem, 305–309
  define and refine the system, 310–311
  define the lesion, 311–321
  diagnostic approach, 316–321
    ancillary tests, 317
    culture and sensitivity, 319
    cytology, 319
    electroretinogram (ERG), 320
    fluorescein staining, 318–319
    gonioscopy, 320
    imaging, 320
    nasolacrimal duct flush, 319–320
    ophthalmic examination, 317
    Schirmer tear test, 317–318
    tonometry, 318
    visual testing, 320–321
  differential diagnosis, 310–311
  opaque eye, 307–308
    causes, **313–314**
    examination, 317

  pain, 305
  red eye, 305–307
    causes, **311–312**
  'runny' eye, 306
  'sore' eye, 305, 306
  wet eye, 308–309
    causes, **314–315**

F

Facial sensation, reduction, 135
Factor VII deficiency, 222
Factor XII deficiency, 222
Faecal culture, 66
Faecal output
  chinchillas, 335
  horses, 369
  rabbits, 329
  reduced, 329, 330, **332–333**
Faecal water syndrome, 369
Faeces
  blood in *see* Melaena
  horses, diarrhoea, 369
Fatigability, 104
Feline immunodeficiency virus (FIV), **61**,
        228, 229
Feline infectious peritonitis (FIP)
  exudates, abdominal enlargement due to,
        91, 95, 101
  jaundice due to, 203
  large bowel diarrhoea due to, **64**
  myelopathy due to, **280**
  vestibular disease and, **138**
  weight loss due to, 78, 82
Feline leukaemia virus (FeLV), **61**, 78, 192,
        228, 229, 293
Ferrets
  clinical examination, 347
  hindlimb weakness, 346–350
    Aleutian disease, 349–350
    causes, 347, 348–350, **350**
    define and refine the problems, 347
    define the lesion, 348–350
    define the location, 348
    define the system, 347–348
    disseminated idiopathic myofasciitis, 350
    insulinoma, 349
    investigations, 348, 349
    musculoskeletal causes, 347, **350**
    neurological causes, 347, **350**
    pain response, 347
Fibrinolysis, 222
Fibrocartilaginous embolism (FCE), 281
Financial issues, 14
    consideration in decision-making, 392, 394
    costs of non-discriminatory blood tests, 14

Fine needle aspiration (FNA), liver, 203, 208, 212
'Fishing expeditions' (diagnostic), 13, 14
Fistula, hepatic arteriovenous, 93
Fits *see* Epileptic seizures; Seizures
Five-finger rule, 111, *112*, 136, *136*, 137, 275, 278
Fluid, intra-abdominal *see under* Abdominal enlargement
Fluorescein staining, eye, 318–319
Fluoroscopy, 39
Foals
    abdominal distension, 364
    acute/chronic blood loss, **385**
    colic, 356, **361**, 364
    coughing, causes, **379**, 380
    diarrhoea, 368–370
        causes, **372**, 373
        diagnostic approach, 373
        faecal consistency, 369
    decreased red cell production, **386**
    diet, 368, 370
    dietary intolerances, 368
    haemolysis causes, **386**
    heat diarrhoea, 368, 373
    neonatal
        cough, 376, **379**
        diarrhoea, 368, 369, **372**, 373
Follicular pustules, 289
Food
allergy/hypersensitivity, **62**
    aversion, 36
    intolerance, **62**
    weight and caloric value, 74
    Food-responsive enteropathy (FRE), **62**, **64**
Forebrain dysfunction, 134, 135, 150
    see also Epileptic seizures
Foreign body
gastric, 48
    inhaled, 164
    intestinal, 24, 28, 44, 46, 47, 204, 235
    in rabbits, 329, **332**
    jaundice due to, 204
    nasal, 156, 217
    otitis due to, 298
    tracheal, coughing in horses, **378**, 380
Framing bias, **13**
Fungal disease
effusions due to, 96
    epistaxis due to, 217, 218, 219
    eye disease due to, 311
    in guinea pigs, 344, **344**
    in horses, **371**, **372**, **378**, **379**, **385**, **386**
    skin disease due to, 286, *288*, 289, 292, *302*

sneezing and nasal discharge due to, 156–157
vestibular disease due to, **138–139**, *141*
Fusi coli, 330

G
Gagging, 39, 40–41
    coughing and, vomiting *vs.*, 39, 40, 158
Gait abnormalities, 261–284
    assessment
        cranial drawer, 269–270
        diagnostic tools/investigations, 282–283
        diagnostic work-up, *271*
        distant examination, 267
        gait analysis, 268
        general observation, 262, 267
        hands-off examination, 107–108, **110**, 273
        history taking, 262, 267
        neurological examination, 270, *272*, 273
        orthopaedic examination, 267–269
        palpation/manipulation, 268–269
        tibial thrust, 269–270
    causes, 264–265, 275–281
    musculoskeletal disorders, 264, 275, **276–277**
    myelopathic spinal diseases, 278, **279–280**, 281
    neurological disorders, 264, 275
    painful non-myelopathic spinal diseases, 278
    clinical signs, 265, *266*
    define and refine the system, 264–266
        musculoskeletal *vs.* neurological, 264, *266*
        primary structural problem, 264–265, **276–277**
        secondary functional problem, 264, **277**
    define the lesion (pathology), 275–281, **276–277**, **279–280**
    define the location, **110**, 266–273
        in neurological system, 266–267, 272, *272*, **274**
        in neuromuscular system, 267
        in orthopaedic system, 266–267, *271*
        spinal lesions, 267, 273
    define the problem, 262–263, *263*
    diagnostic tools, 282–283
    in seizures (post-ictal), 132
    stilted gait, 265
    in vestibular attack, 127
    weakness and, 264, 265
    see also Weakness
Gastric reflux, 35, 39–41
    horses with colic, 365, 367
    'silent', 39
    vomiting *vs. see under* Vomiting

Gastric ulceration, 46, 48
  melaena due to *see* Melaena
Gastritis, 46, 238
Gastrointestinal (GI) disorders, primary, 24,
    42, *42*, 43
  in chinchillas with weight loss, 336, 337
  colic in horses due to, 357
  diarrhoea due to, 57, 59, 369
  'gut stasis' in rabbits due to, 331, 332, **332**
  malabsorption due to, 81–82
  melaena due to, 219, 233–235
  secondary disorders *vs.*, 42–43, 51
    clues to differentiate, 44–45
    importance of differentiating, 43–44
  vomiting due to, 43–45
    causes, 46–47, 50
    clinical pathology, 50–51
    clues to suspect, 44
    define the lesion, 46–48
    define the location, 45–46
    diagnostic approach, 43, 45, 49, 50
    management, 43
Gastrointestinal (GI) disorders, secondary,
    24, 42, 43
  in chinchillas with weight loss, 336
  diarrhoea due to, 58–59
    acute diarrhoea, **62**
    chronic diarrhoea, **64**
    diagnostic approach, 67–68
  'false' colic in horses, 357
  malabsorption due to, 82
  melaena due to, 219
  primary disorders *vs. see* Gastrointestinal
      (GI) disorders, primary
  vomiting due to, 43–46, 53
    causes, 42, 43, 47, **47**
    clinical pathology, 50–51
    clues to suspect, 45, 53
    define the lesion, 47
    define the location, 45, 46, 54
    diagnostic approach, 43, 45–46, 49, 50
    pancreatitis in dogs, 44, 45
Gastrointestinal haemorrhage, chronic, 186
Gastrointestinal (GI) motility, control in
    rabbits, 329
Gastrointestinal (GI) obstruction
  in horses, 357–358
  in rabbits, 331
  vomiting due to, 47, 51
Genetic testing, 119, 139, 147
Ghost cells, *184*
Giardia, 67
Glaucoma, 310, **316**, 318
Glioma, 148
Glomerular disease, **247**
Glomerular filtrate, altered osmolarity of, 241

Glomerular filtration rate (GFR), decreased,
    azotaemia, 246
Glomerular perfusion, decreased, 246
Glomerular renal disease, malutilisation due
    to, 83
Glomeruli, decreased numbers, 246
Glomerulopathies, 173
Glucose, blood, 144, 349
Glucosuria, 31, 242, **251**
  'Going fishing', 13, 14
  'Gold standard' care, 393–394
  wider professional priorities, 394–395
Gonioscopy, 320
Granular iridica cyst, 321
Granulomatous colitis, **64**
Grass sickness, 358–359
Guinea pigs
  alopecia, 342–346
    causes, **344**
    define and refine the problems,
      342–343
    define the lesion, 344
    define the location, 343
    define the system, 343
    diagnostic approach, 344–346
    normal/abnormal location, 342
    pruritus with, 343, **344**, 345
    primary dermatologic disorders, 343, **344**,
      344–345
  PU/PD in, 346
  secondary dermatologic disorders, 343,
      344, 345–346
  seizure-like behaviour, 343
  weight loss and inappetence, 326
Gut motility *see* Intestinal motility
Gut sounds, rabbits, 330
'Gut stasis'
  in chinchillas, 334
  in rabbits *see* Rabbits

H
Haemangiosarcoma, 186, 252
Haematemesis, 41, 48
  causes (primary/secondary), 46, 48
Haematocrit (HCT), 181, 182
Haematological disorders, weakness due
    to, 113
Haematology (diagnostic)
  coughing with dyspnoea, 166
  diarrhoea in horses, 374
Haematuria, 17, 27, 187, 216
  define the lesion (causes)
    local disorders, 220–221
    systemic disorders, 221
  define the location, 221
  diagnostic approach, 221

Haemoabdomen, 97
Haemoglobin
  abnormal, disorders with normal delivery,
    173, 177
  breakdown, 200
  normal, disorders with reduced delivery,
    173–176
  unoxygenated, 162, 173
Haemoglobinaemia, horses, 384
Haemoglobinuria, 187, 216
  horses, 384
Haemogram, 181, 183, 192, 194, 228
Haemolysis, 186–187
  anaemia due to, 185, 186–187, 187–190
    horses, 382, 383–384, **386**, 387
  cholestasis and jaundice due to, 201,
    205–206
  extravascular, 186–187, 384
  haemorrhage *vs.* anaemia due to, 185
  intravascular, 187, 384
  pre-hepatic jaundice due to, 201–202
Haemolytic anaemia, 187–190, 202
  causes, 187–188, 202
    drugs/toxins, 188–189
    infections, 188
  hereditary, 189
  hyperbilirubinaemia in, 197
  immune-mediated (IMHA) *see* Immune-
    mediated haemolytic anaemia (IMHA)
  microangiopathic anaemia, 189–190, *190*
Haemoplasmosis, 188
Haemopoietic neoplasia, 193
Haemopoietic system, 183
Haemoptysis, 159
Haemorrhage, 185–186
  acute, 185–186, 228
    in horses, 383, **385**
  anaemia due to, 185–186
    in horses, 382, 383, **385**
  body cavity, 224
  chronic, in horses, 383, **385**
  chronic external, 186, 193
  haemolysis *vs.*, anaemia due to, 185
  intestinal, with jaundice, 205
  intra-abdominal, 97, 186
  intra-thoracic, 186
  jaundice due to, 202, 205
  local *vs.* systemic disease, 185–186
  PU/PD due to, 252
  renal/ureteral, 221
  retroperitoneal, 186
  thrombocytopenia causing, 225, 228, 229
  thrombocytopenia due to, 228
  see also Bleeding
Haemorrhagic effusions, 96–97
Hair plucks, guinea pigs, 344

Hands-on/off examination, *see* Neurological
    examination
Hansen type-I disc disease, 281
Hansen type-II disc disease, 281
Head, ventral flexion, in cats, 113
Head nod, 268
Head tilt, 127, 133
Head tremor, idiopathic, 127, **128–129**
Heart disease *see* Cardiac disease
Heart failure, 170
  congestive, malutilisation due to, 82
  pulmonary oedema due to, 175
Heart murmurs, 175
  horses, 354, 382
Heinz bodies, 189, 387
Hepatic arteriovenous fistula, 93
Hepatic disease *see* Liver disease
Hepatic encephalopathy, 241
Hepatic failure, fulminant, 203
Hepatitis, 93, 203
Hepatocellular disease, jaundice in, 202,
    205, 206
Hepatocutaneous syndrome, 294
Hepatomegaly, 90, 93
Hindlimb weakness, in ferrets *see* Ferrets
Horses
  abdominal distension, 357, 364
  abdominal pain, 356, 358, 362–363
  anaemia, 380–388
    acute, 381–382, 383
    blood loss causing, 382, 383, **385**, 387
    causes, 382, 385, **385**, **386**
    chronic, 381
    decreased red cell production, 382, 384,
      386, 387–388
    define and refine the system, 382
    define the lesion, 385, **385**, **386**
    define the location, 383–384
    define the problem, 381–382
    diagnostic approach, 382, 386–388
    haemolysis causing, 382–384, **386**, 387
    pallor due to, 380, 381
    pathophysiological mechanisms, 382
  aspiration pneumonia, **378, 379**
  blood loss, 382, 383
    acute, or chronic, 383, **385**
  colic *see* Colic, in horses
  coughing, 375–380
    acute, 379–380
    causes, 375–376, 377, **378, 379**, 379–380
    chronic, 379, 380
    define and refine the system, 375–376
    define the lesion, 378, **378, 379**
    define the location, 376–377
    define the problem, 375
    diagnostic approach, 379–380

Horses (*cont'd*)
  dyspnoea with, 377
  diarrhoea, 367–374
    acute, 367–368, 369, **371**, 373
    age-specific diseases, 373
    causes, 358, **371**, 372, 373
    chronic, 368, 369, **371**, 373–374
    define and refine the system, 369
    define the lesion, 370, **371–372**
    define the location, 370
    define the problem, 369
    diagnostic approach, 372–374
    infectious, **371**, 372, **372**
    investigations, 374
    osmotic, 369
    pathophysiological mechanisms, 369
    risk factors, 373
    therapeutic approach, 372
  endotoxic shock, 362, 365–366
  faecal water syndrome, 369
  heart murmurs, 354, 382
  hypovolaemic shock, 382
  hypoxia, 381
  pallor, 380–388
    causes, 381
    define and refine the system, 382
    define the problem, 381–382
  pharyngeal/laryngeal paralysis, cough, 376
  tachycardia, in colic, 362
  see also Equine practice; Foals
Howell-Jolly bodies, *184*
Husbandry, small mammals, 326
Hydrocephalus, 148
Hyperadrenocorticism, 30, 31
  abdominal enlargement due to, 90
  guinea pigs with alopecia, 346
  polyuria/polydipsia due to, 241, 242, **243**, **249**
  scaling disorder in, 293
  weakness due to, **116**
  see also Cushing's syndrome
Hyperbilirubinaemia, 197, 199, 204, 211
  horses, 384
  see also Jaundice
Hypercalcaemia, 13
  azotaemia, impaired urine concentration, **247**
  polyuria/polydipsia due to, 242, **244**, **247**, 258
  weakness due to, **116**
Hypercholesterolaemia, 211
Hyperfibrinolysis, 222, 227, 230
Hyperkalaemia
  seizures due to, 144
  weakness due to, **115**, **116**
Hyperparathyroidism, secondary, in ferrets, 348
Hyperpigmentation, 298
Hypersalivation, 40
Hypersthenuria, 239
Hypertension, systemic, 176

eye problems due to, 311
Hyperthyroidism, 12, 87
  guinea pigs with alopecia, 346
  malabsorption and weight loss due to, 80, 82
  malutilisation due to, 80, 82
  mild hyperbilirubinaemia due to, 202, 204
  primary polydipsia due to, 241, **243**
  vomiting due to, 45, **47**
Hyphaemia, 308
Hypoadrenocorticism, 59, 60, 68
  polyuria/polydipsia due to, 242, **245**
Hypoalbuminaemia, 94
  in horses, 374
Hypocalcaemia, weakness due to, **116**
Hypochromasia, 193
Hypocretin, 147
Hypofibrinogenaemia, 225
Hypoglycaemia
  seizures due to, 144
  weakness due to, **116**
Hypokalaemia, 31
  polyuria/polydipsia due to, 242, **244**, **251**
  vomiting due to, **47**
  weakness due to, **116**
Hyponatraemia
  azotaemia, impaired urine concentration, **247**, 248
  polyuria/polydipsia due to, 242, **251**
Hypoproteinaemia, 65, 69, 83, 91, 176
  ascites due to, 93–94
  in bleeding case example, 234, 235
  in horses, blood loss with, 383, 386–387
Hypopyon, 308
Hyporexia, causes, 78
Hyposthenuria *see under* Urine, impaired concentration
Hypothermia, 327
Hypovolaemic shock, horses, 382
Hypoxia, 174
  horses, 381

I
Ichthyosis, 292–293
Icterus *see* Jaundice
Idiopathic head tremor, 127, **128–129**
Immune-mediated haemolytic anaemia (IMHA), *184*, 187–188
  associative/non-associative, 187, 188
  case example, 195–197
  detection, 187
  in horses, **386**, 387
  jaundice in, 205
  secondary, 187
Immune-mediated thrombocytopenia (ITP), 227, 229, 231, 310, **312**
  in horses, **385**

Immunosuppressive-responsive enteropathy
    (IRE), **63**
Impaired urine concentration, *see* Urine
Inappetence, 19, 44, 78–79
Incontinence *see* Urinary
    incontinence (UI)
Infections
  in bone marrow disorders, 193
  coughing in horses due to, **378**, **379**
  dyspnoea in rats due to, 340
  eye problems due to, 311
  myelopathic spinal disease, **280**, 283
  otitis due to, 299, 301
  pruritus due to, *288*, 289, 290, 294
  scaling disorders due to, 293, 294
  see also specific infections,
      microorganisms
Infectious enteritis, 47
Infectious haemolytic anaemia, 188
Infectious thrombocytopenia, 228, 230
Inflammation/inflammatory disease
  airways, in cats, 160, 161
  anaemia of, 182, 191
  bowel, in horses, 358
  brain, epileptic seizure due to, 152
  bronchial/tracheal, 160–161, 171, 172
    radiography, 165
  bronchoalveolar, 164
  cutaneous, pruritic mediators in, 286
  of ear, 299, 301
  eye problems due to, 310
  hepatic jaundice in, 203
  lower urinary tract disease, 220
  mastication, prehension or dysphagia due
    to, 76, 77
  myelopathic spinal disease, **280**, 283
  sneezing and nasal discharge due to, 156,
    157
Inflammatory arthropathies, 265
Inflammatory bowel disease, 47, **63**, **65**
Inflammatory cytokines, 171, 191, 204
Insulinoma, 264
  ferrets with hindlimb weakness, 349
Interleukin 31 (IL-31), 286
Intervertebral disc
  extrusion, 281, 283
  protrusion, 281
Intestinal disease
large bowel, colic in horses, 361, 366
small bowel, *see* small bowel disease
  vomiting caused by, 47
  see also Gastrointestinal (GI) disorders
Intestinal motility, in rabbits, 329–330, 331
Intestinal obstruction, 47, 51
Intra-abdominal haemorrhage, 186
Intra-hepatic pre-sinusoidal portal
    hypertension, 93

Intra-ocular pressure, 318
  high, glaucoma, 318, 320
  low, uveitis, 318
Intra-thoracic disease, dyspnoea with
    minimal coughing, 167–168
Intravascular haemolysis, 187
in horses, 384
Intuition, 9
Investigations
  chronic diarrhoea, 65–69
  colic, in horses, 365
  diarrhoea in horses, 374
  dyspnoea in rats, 340, 342
  gait abnormalities, 282–283
  'gut stasis' in rabbits, 333–334
  hindlimb weakness, ferrets, 348, 349
  primary *vs.* secondary systems, 24–25, 43
  regurgitation, 40, 43
  vomiting, 26, 27, 42
  weight loss, chinchillas, 337
Iridocorneal angle, 320
Iris, abnormal-sized pupil, **312**
Iron deficiency, 186, 193
Isosthenuria, 239, 252
Itch threshold, 286

J
Jaundice, 18, 199–213
  abdominal pain with, case example, 210–211
  in anaemia, 186
  anaesthesia and surgery cautions, 208, 209
  case example, 210–213
  causes, 201–202, 202–204
    hepatic, 203
    non-hepatic, 204
    pancreatitis, case example, 211–213
    post-hepatic, 204
    pre-hepatic, 202
  define the lesion, 202–204
  define the problem, 199–200, *201*
  define the system and location, 25, 201–202
  definition, 199
  differentiating causes/types, 205–209
    clinical pathology, 206–207
    clinical signs and examination, 206
    cytology, culture, histopathology, 208
    diagnostic imaging, 207–208
    hepatic *vs.* post-hepatic, 201, 202,
      205–209
    pre-hepatic *vs.* hepatic/post-hepatic,
      205, 211
    reasons for, 209
    signalment and history, 206
  haemolysis and, 186
  hepatic, 202, 203, 205–206
    vs. post-hepatic, 201, 202, 205–209
  in horses, 384

Jaundice (*cont'd*)
  intestinal haemorrhage with, 205
  physiology, 200, *201*
  post-hepatic, 202, 204–206
  pre-hepatic, 201–202, 205
  specificity of problem, 18, 19
  treatment, 209
  vomiting and, 18, 206, 211
Jerk nystagmus, 133
Joint pathology, in gait abnormality, 282
Jones test, 309, 319
Junctionopathy, weakness due to, **110**, **115**,
  117, 122

K
Kennel cough, 161
Keratinisation, 291
Keratinisation disorders, 291, 292, 294
  clinical presentation, 291
  define and refine the system, 291–292
  primary, or secondary, 291, 292
Keratoconjunctivitis sicca (KCS), 318

L
L2-hydroxyglutaric aciduria, 148
Lafora body storage disease, 148
Lameness, 261, 265, 268, 275
Laminitis, acute, 359
Laparotomy, 69
Large bowel diarrhoea, 56–59
  case example, 71–72
  causes, 59, **64–65**
    systemic diseases, 59–60
  in horses, 370
  small bowel diarrhoea *vs.*, 57–58, **58–59**
Large bowel disease, colic in horses due to,
  359, 364
Laryngeal disease/dysfunction, 167, 168–169
  causes, 168
  cyanosis and respiratory distress in, 167
  diagnostic procedures, 168–169
  dyspnoea and coughing due to,
    162–163, 168
  dyspnoea with minimal coughing due to,
    167, 168
Laryngoscopy, 168–169
Learning
  effective, 1–2
  sequence, 2–3, *3*
  theory, relevance to current book, 4–5, *5*
  what and how, 2–3
Learning buddy, benefits, 5, *5*
Left atrial hypertension, 164, 170, 175
Lens
  abnormal-sized pupil, **312**
  blind eye causes, **315**

  opacity, 308, **314**
Leptospirosis, 230
Leukaemia, 192
Leukogram, peripheral, 166
Leukopenia, 374
Lichenification, 292
Limb(s)
  gait abnormalities, neuroanatomy, **274**
  malalignment, 267
  musculoskeletal disorders, **276–277**
  reflexes and postural reactions, **274**
Liver biopsy, 203, 208
Liver disease, 93
  bleeding due to, 225, 227, 231
  decreased appetite in, 83
  diarrhoea due to, 59, **64**
  hypoproteinaemia due to, 94
  increased appetite in, 84, 85
  malabsorption and weight loss due to, 82
  malutilisation due to, 83
  polyuria/polydipsia due to, 242, **243**, **250**
  vomiting due to, 47, 48, **48**, 54
Liver enzymes, 13
  cholestatic patterns, 206
  hepatic *vs.* post-hepatic jaundice,
    206–207
Logical clinical problem-solving (LCPS), 4–5,
  7–34
  see also Problem-based inductive clinical
    reasoning
Lower motor neuron disorders, urinary
  incontinence, 254
Lower respiratory tract disease, 154
  coughing in horses, 376, 377
  in rats, 339
  see also Bronchoalveolar disorders
Lung consolidation, rats, 340
Lung sounds *see* Respiratory sounds
Lymphangiectasia, **63**, 80
Lymphatic obstruction, 80, 94
Lymphoma, hepatic, 13
Lymphopenia, 192

M
Macrocytosis, 183
Magnetic resonance imaging (MRI), 283, 320
Malabsorption, 79
  in chinchillas, 336
  define the lesion (causes), 81
    primary GI diseases, 81–82
    secondary GI diseases, 82
  in horses, 374
  weight loss due to, 80, 81–82
Malassimilation of nutrients, 80
  in chinchillas, 336
  see also Malabsorption; Maldigestion

Maldigestion, 79
  in chinchillas, 336
  in hepatic disease, 82
  weight loss due to, 80, 81
Malutilisation of nutrients, 80
  case example, 86, 87, 100, 101
  in chinchillas, 337
  define the lesion (causes), 82–84, 86–87
  weight loss due to, 80, 82–84
Mammary carcinoma, 87
Mast cell neoplasia, 219
  case example, 233–235
Mastication difficulties, 75, 76
Maze testing, 320, 321
Mean corpuscular haemoglobin
        concentration (MCHC), 384
Mean corpuscular volume (MCV), 182, 384
Meconium impaction, in foals 364, 356
Medulla oblongata, 36, 37
Megaoesophagus, 40, 43, 45, **49**
Melaena, 26, 48, 216
  case example, 233–235
  define the lesion (causes)
    bleeding disorders, 219
    GI ulceration, 219–220
    primary GI diseases, 219
    secondary GI diseases, 219, 235
  diagnostic approach, 219–220
Memorisation
  sequence of actions to improve, 2–3, *3*
  'staircase' of, 2, *3*
  structure of current book to improve, 4–5, *5*
  through subvocalization, 5, *5*
Menace response, 108, 131, 135
Meningoencephalomyelitis, 148
Meningo(encephalo)myelitis of unknown
        origin (MUA), 281
Mentation
  changes in epileptic seizures, 135
  hands-off examination of CNS, 107, **110**
M:E (myeloid:erythroid) ratio, horses, 384,
        387–388
Metabolic disorders
  scaling disorders due to, 294
  seizures due to, 143, 144
  weakness due to, 105, **115, 116**
Methaemoglobinaemia, 189
Methimazole, 228
Microangiopathic anaemia, 189–190, *190*
Microcytosis, 193
Microphthalmos, **316**
Micturition *see* Urination (micturition)
Middle ear disease, in cats, 300
Minimum database, 10, 14
Miosis, 132, 307, **312–313**
Mononuclear cells, 95

Motilin, 330
Mouth disorders, 76
Movement disorder, breed-specific, 127, 130
Mucous membranes
  colour, assessment in horses, 362, 381
  pale/pallor, 17, 182, 195, 233, 234
    in horses, 381
    in rabbits, 334
Muscle
  atrophy, 74, 267
  rhythmic alternating contractions in
        seizures, 131
  tone
    assessment, 106, 109, **110**
    in epileptic seizures, 131
  wasting, 74
Musculoskeletal system disorders, 264
  gait abnormalities due to, 261, 264
    define the lesion, 275, **276–277**
    define the location, 267
    diagnostic tools, 282–283
    diagnostic work-up, *271*
    examination, 267–270
    neurological gait abnormalities *vs.*, 261,
        264, *266*
    primary structural disorders causing,
        276–277
    secondary functional disorders causing,
        277
  hindlimb weakness in ferrets, 347, 349,
        350
  see also Weakness
Myasthenia gravis
  case example, 122–123
  regurgitation due to, 45, **49**
  weakness due to, 114, 115, **117**
Mycoplasma haemofelis, 188
Mycoplasma pulmonis, 341
Mycoplasmosis, 188
  in dyspnoeic rats, 340–342, **341**
Mydriasis, 106, 307, **312–313**
Myelodysplasia, 192, 193
Myelofibrosis, 193
Myelography, 283
Myeloid:erythroid (M:E) ratio, horses, 384,
        387–388
Myelopathic spinal diseases, 273, 278, 281
  differential diagnoses, **279–280**
Myelophthisis, 228
Myofasciitis, disseminated idiopathic, in
        ferrets, 350
Myoglobinuria, 216
Myopathy, 265
  weakness due to, **110, 115, 118**
Myotonia, 265
Myringotomy, 146

Myxomatosis, in rabbits, 351
Myxomatous degenerative mitral valve
  disease (MMVD), 175–176

N

Narcolepsy, 126, 134
  cause, 134
  clinical characteristics, **128–129**
  diagnostic approach, gene test, 147
  familial, 147
  triggering, 126, 139
Nasal biopsy/washings, 218
Nasal discharge *see* Sneezing and nasal
  discharge
Nasal disease/disorders, 155
  clinical signs, 155
  epistaxis due to, diagnostic approach,
    218–219
Nasal examination, epistaxis, 217–218
Nasogastric tube, passing, in horses, 365, 376
Nasolacrimal duct, blockage, 308–309
Nasolacrimal duct flush, 319
Nasopharyngeal polyps, 157
Nasopharynx, coughing in horses and, 376
Nausea, 36, 41
Neck, ventral flexion, in cats, 113
Neoplasia
  bone marrow disorders in, 193
  coughing with dyspnoea due to, 161, 165
  coughing with minimal dyspnoea due to, 161
  epistaxis due to, 217, 218, 219
  haematuria due to, 220
  haemopoietic, 193
  large bowel diarrhoea due to, **65**
  mast cell, 219, 233–235
  melaena due to, 219, 235
  myelopathies due to, **279**
  nasal discharge and sneezing due to, 157
  pulmonary, 165
  renal, PU/PD due to, 242
  scaling disorders due to, 294
  weight loss due to, 77
Nephrocalcinosis, polyuria/polydipsia due to,
  242
Nephrons
  impaired function, primary polyuria, 240, 242
  reduced number, primary polyuria, 240,
    241–242, 248
Nerve growth factor (NGF), 286
Neurogenic lesions, urinary incontinence in,
  253, 254, 255
Neurogenic pulmonary oedema, 176
Neurological disorders
  eye problems due to, 310
    abnormal-sized pupil, **313**
  gait abnormalities due to, 261, 264, 265
    define the lesion, 275

define the location, 266–267, *272*, **274**
diagnostic tools, 283
musculoskeletal causes *vs.*, *263*, 264, 265
neurological examination, 270, *272*, 273
hindlimb weakness in ferrets due to,
  347, 348, 349, **350**
primary (structural) *vs.* secondary
  (functional), 24, 104
Neurological examination, 106, 107, 122
  case example, 122
  in epileptic seizure, 133, 134–135, 140
  in ferrets with hindlimb weakness, 347
  in gait abnormalities, 270, *272*, 273
  hands-off examination (observation),
    107–108, 270, 273
    mentation and behaviour, 107, 108, **110**,
      122
    posture and gait, 107–108, **110**, 122
  hands-on examination, 107, 108–111, 273
    cranial nerve examination, 108, 122
    palpation (muscle tone), 109, **110**
    postural reactions, 108, 122
    sensory evaluation, 109, 111
    spinal reflexes, 109, 122
  in neuromuscular disease, 107–111, **110**
  in paroxysmal episodic disorders,
    132–133, 134
Neurological system, 24, 104
  see also Central nervous system (CNS)
Neuromuscular lesions/disorders, 24, 104
  affecting mastication, 76
  clinical pathology, 119
  concurrent with skeletal disorders, 105–106
  dysphagia due to, 76
  gait abnormalities due to, 267, 275
    see also Gait abnormalities
  neurological examination, 106–108
    see also Neurological examination
  pain deficits, symmetry, in weakness, **115**
  primary (structural), 24, 104, 111
    weakness due to, 104, 105, 111, 113,
      114, **115**, **116–117**
  secondary (functional), 24, 104
    weakness due to, 104, 105, 111,
      113–114, **115**, **116–117**
  spinal reflexes in, 109
  weakness due to, 104, 105, 111
    define and refine the system, 104–105,
      106
    define the lesion, 111–114
    define the location, 106–111
    episodic/exercise-induced weakness,
      113–114, **115**, **128–129**
    neuroanatomical localisation, 107–111,
      110
    neurological examination findings,
      106–107

persistent weakness, 114, **116–118**, 120
  see also Weakness
Neuromuscular system, 24, 104
Neuronal ceroid lipofuscinosis, 148
Neuropathy, **115**, **117**, 168
assessment, 106
peripheral, **110**, 114
polyradiculoneuropathy, **110**
weakness due to, 114, **115**, **117**
Neutropenia, 77, 192
Neutrophils, 95, 98
Nitric oxide, 204
Nociceptive deficits, 109, **110**
Non-hepatic jaundice, 204
Non-regenerative anaemia, 183, 191, 382
  define the lesion (causes), 191–193
    anaemia of inflammatory disease, 182, 191
    bone marrow disorders, 192–193
    chronic kidney disease, 191–192
    iron deficiency, 193
  define the location, 191
  diagnostic approach, in horses, 384, 388
  in horses, 382, 384, 388
  microangiopathic anaemia as, 190
Non-responsive chronic enteropathy (NRE), **63**
Non-specific problems, 20, 73
Non-steroidal anti-inflammatory drugs
    (NSAIDs), toxicity, 46, 48, 219, 231
Nuclear sclerosis, 308
Nutrients, assimilation, 79
  pathophysiology, 79–80
Nutritional abnormalities, scaling disorders
    due to, 294
Nystagmus, 127

O
Ocular discharge, 306, 308–309
  causes, **314–315**
  in chinchillas, 336
Oesophageal disorders, regurgitation due to, **49**
Oesophagitis, secondary, 41
Oestrogen, toxicity, 228
Oncotic pressure, 94, 176
Ophthalmic examination, 317
Ophthalmoscopy, 317
Oral disease, chinchillas, 335, 336
Oral tumours, 77
Orthopaedic disorders, 261, 265
  see also Musculoskeletal system
Orthopaedic examination, 268–269
  in ferrets with hindlimb weakness, 347
Osmolarity, of glomerular filtrate, 241, 242, 249
Osmotic diuresis, 242
Osmotic injury, 189
Otitis/dermatitis, 296–302
  canine, 298–300, *302*
  causes, 298–300

primary factors, 298
  secondary factors, 299
clinical signs, 296–297
define the lesion, 298–300
define the location, 297
define the problem, 296–297
define the system, 297
definition, 296
diagnostic approach, 300–302
  flowchart, *302*
feline, 300
perpetuating factors, 299–300
predisposing factors, 299
Otitis externa, 297–299, 300
  proliferative necrotising, 300
  recurrent, 300
Otitis media, 145, 297, 299, 300
  in cats, 300
Otoscopy, 301
Ovarian cysts, guinea pigs, 345
Oxygen exchange, impaired, 162, 167, 173

P
'Pacemaker' of gut, 330
Packed cell volume (PCV), 181, 182, 195
  acute haemorrhage, 185
  bone marrow disease, 192
  in horses with anaemia, 383, 386
Pain
  abdominal *see* Abdominal pain
  assessment, neuromuscular disease
    causing weakness, **110**
  episodic, behavioural response, 126
  eye, 305
  in ferrets with hindlimb weakness, 347
  in horses with colic, 356, 362
  non-myelopathic spinal disease, 278
  spinal diseases causing gait
    abnormalities, 273
Pale mucous membranes/pallor, 17, 182,
    233, 234
  case example, 195
  in horses, *see* Horses
  in rabbits, 334
Palpation
  abdominal, 11, 210, 332, 345
  in gait abnormalities, *263*, 267, 268–269
  in neuromuscular disorders, 109
  in otitis, 301
Pancreatic abscess, 13
Pancreatic enzymes, 79, 81
Pancreatitis, 44, 45
  acute, case example, 211–213
  in cats, 45, 79, 204
  diarrhoea due to, 59, **62**, **64**
  in dogs, 42, 44, 45, 204, 212–213
  effusion due to, 96

Pancreatitis (*cont'd*)
  haematemesis due to, 48
  jaundice due to, 204, 211–213
  platelet dysfunction in, 231
  testing, 47, 211
  vomiting due to, 44, 45
Panosteitis, 275
Papules, 289
Parasites
  bronchoalveolar disease due to, 164, 166
  coughing in horses due to, **378, 379**, 380
  diarrhoea due to, **60, 63, 64, 66**, 67, 68, 73
  melaena due to GI ulceration from, 219
  pruritus due to, 289
Paresis, 106, **110**, 261, 265
  definition, 106, 108, 261, 265
  flaccid, 108, **110**
  lameness *vs.*, 265
  laryngeal disorder due to, dyspnoea in, 168
  observation (hands-off examination), 108
  spastic, 108
Paroxysmal behaviour changes, 126–127, 134
  characteristics, **128–129**
  diagnostic approaches, 147
  seizure differential diagnosis, 139
Paroxysmal dyskinesias, 127, **128–129**
Paroxysmal episodic disorders, 125
  characteristics, **128–129**
  define and refine the problem, 126–127, 130
  define and refine the system, 132
  define the lesion, 136–144
  define the location, 132–135
  diagnostic approach, 145–148
  onset and clinical course, 137, *137*
  see also Epileptic seizures; Narcolepsy;
    Syncope; Vestibular attacks
Paroxysmal movement disorders, 127,
    128–129, 130, 134, 139
  diagnostic approaches, 147
Pathology, types, 27
Pattern-based tunnel vision, 13, 16, 20
Pattern recognition, 9–14, 29–30, 32,
    323–324
  after defining the problem, 30
  combined with diagnostic tests, 14–15
  criteria for success/benefits, 13, 30, 323
  disadvantages, 14, 20, 323–324
  flawed and unsatisfactory, 12, 25, 30,
    323–324
  small mammals, 323–325, 351, 324
  use and indications for, 11–12, 29–30
PCR (polymerase chain reaction) testing, 342
Perennial itch, 290
Peripheral neuropathy, weakness due to, **110**
Peripheral perfusion, poor, 182
Peritoneal fluid analysis, horses with colic,
    358, 365, 367

Peritonitis, 13
  bile, non-septic exudates due to, 95
  septic exudates due to, 96
Petechiation, 224
Pharynx, disorders, 76
Phenobarbitone, 77, 228, 241
Phosphofructokinase deficiency, 189
Plasma protein, concentration, 185, 186
Platelet(s)
  count, 224, 228
  dysfunction, 227, 230–231
  excessive consumption, 229
  excessive destruction, 229
  function, *222*, 231
    acquired disorders, **223**, 231
    assessment, 226
    defects, 227, 230–231
    inherited disorders, **223**, 230–231
  inadequate production, 228
  reduced, 192, 224, 226, 227, 228
    see also Thrombocytopenia
Plegia, 108, **110**, 261
Pleural cavity, space-occupying disorders,
    169–171
  diagnostic approach, 170–171
Pleural effusion, 90, 91, 169–171
  ascites with, post-hepatic obstruction, 93
  causes, 170
  chylous, 170
  diagnostic approach, 170–171
  transudates, 170
Pleural fluid
  characterisation, 170, 171
  volume, and removal, 171
Pleural friction rubs, 377
Pneumonia, aspiration, 37
Poikilocytosis, 193
Pollakiuria, 220, 221, 238
Polychromasia, 183, *184*
Polydipsia, 10, 11, 12
  appropriate physiological response,
    237–238
  compensatory, 239, 240
  confirmation, measurement, 238
  definition, 238
  primary, 25, 240, 247
    causes, 240, 241, **243**
  psychogenic, 240, **243, 249**
    see also Polyuria/polydipsia (PU/PD)
Polyphagia, 10, 12, 30, 84, 239
Polyradiculoneuropathy, weakness due to, **110**
Polyuria, 237, 238, 239
  in acute renal failure, 252
  incontinence and, 238, 253
  pollakiuria *vs.*, 238
  primary, 25, 240–241, 241–242, 247
    causes, 240, 241–242, **244–245**, 247–248

Polyuria/polydipsia (PU/PD), 11, 237–249
    azotaemia and, 246, **247**
    case example, 257–259
    causes/pathophysiology, 239–242,
        243–245, 249–251, 252
        ADH impairment/deficiency causing,
            240–241, 248, 252
        altered glomerular filtrate osmolarity,
            241, 248
        chronic kidney disease (CKD), 241,
            247, 251
        diabetes insipidus, 242, **244, 249**, 252
        diabetes mellitus, 242, **245, 251**
        hepatic disease, **243, 250, 251**
        hyperadrenocorticism, 241, 242, **243,
            249, 251**
        hypercalcaemia, 242, **244, 247, 249, 251**
        hyperthyroidism, 241, **243**, 252
        hypoadrenocorticism, 242, **245, 251**
        hypokalaemia, 242, **244, 251**
        impaired nephron function, 240, 242
        primary polydipsia, 240, 241, **243**
        primary polyuria, 240–241, 241–242, **244**
        psychogenic polydipsia, **243**
        pyelonephritis, 241, 242, **245**, 248, **250,
            251**
        pyometra, 242, **244, 245, 250, 251**
        reduced nephron number, 240,
            241–242, 248
        renal tubule damage, 240, 241–242
    define and refine the system, 247–249, 258
        functional (extra-renal) abnormality, 248,
            258
        structural renal abnormality, 248
    define the lesion, **249–251**, 252, 259
    define the problem, 237–239, 258
        as specific problem, 20
    diagnostic approach, 247–249, 259
    differential diagnosis, 20, 248–249, **249–251**
    in guinea pigs, 346
    incontinence and, 238, 252
    internal haemorrhage with, 252
    mechanisms, classification, 239–240
        primary polydipsia, 240
        primary polyuria, 240–241
    polyphagia with, 30
    urine SG determination, 238–239, 248, 258
    see also Polydipsia; Polyuria
Porphyrin pigments, 338
Portal hypertension
    ascites due to, 92–93
    intra-hepatic pre-sinusoidal, 93
    malabsorption due to, 80
    post-hepatic, 93
    pre-hepatic, 92
Portal vein obstruction, 92
Post-hepatic jaundice, 202, 204–206

Post-hepatic obstruction, 93
Post-hepatic portal hypertension, 93
Postural reactions, 108, **110**, 122
    deficits, in epileptic seizures, 135
    gait abnormalities, **274**
Posture, hands-off examination, 107–108,
        110, 122
Prehension difficulties, 75, 76
    in chinchillas, 335
Pre-hepatic jaundice, 201–202, 205
Pre-hepatic portal hypertension, 92
Premature closure (of case), **13**
Primary GI disease see Gastrointestinal (GI)
        disorders, primary
Primary polydipsia, see Polydipsia
Primary polyuria, see Polyuria
Problem-based inductive clinical reasoning,
        4, 10, 15–34, *16*, *34*
    approach variations, 21
    benefits of structured approach, 32–33
    clinical sign combinations, 30
    define and refine the problem, *16*, 16–21,
        22–23, 395
        clinical sign confusion, 21, 22, 326
        diagnostic methods for, 28
        equine practice, 354
        failure, implications, 23
        importance, 16–17, 23
        list construction and benefits, 16–18, 327
        non-specific problems to refine, 20
        prioritizing problems, 17, 18, 20, 21,
            326, 327
        refining the problem, 20, 22
        small mammals, 326–327
        specificity of problem see below
    define and refine the system, *16*, 22, 23,
        23–26
        diagnostic methods for, 28–29
        failure, implications, 25
        importance, 24–26
        local *vs.* systemic problems, 25–26
        primary (structural), 23, 24
        primary *vs.* secondary system, 25, 26, 327
        refining the system, 23, 24, 25
        secondary (functional), 24
        small mammals, 329
    define the lesion, *16*, 21, *27*, 27–28
    define the location, *16*, 21, *26*, 26–27
        small mammals, 329
    definition and description, 15–16
    diagnosis, likelihood, 21
    diagnostic methods, 28–29
        small mammals, 333, 335
    equine practice, 353–389
    example clinical scenario, 391–393
    exotic animals, 325
    frustrating cases 9–10

Problem-based inductive clinical reasoning
  (cont'd)
  making sense of, 31
  pathophysiological thinking, 31
  skill acquisition, 8, *8*, 32, 33
  small mammals, 325, 351
    see also Small mammals
  solving clinical cases, 10–11
  specificity of problems, 17–19
    deciding on specificity, 19–21
  steps and components, *4*, 15, *16*, 16–21,
    22, 28–29
    making sense, 31
    order, and changing, 29
  tedious but important, 32
  as time waster *vs.* time saver?, 33
  wider professional priorities *see*
    Professional reasoning
Professional reasoning
communication and collaboration, 400–402, 403
  completing the problem (reflection/
    analysis), 403–404
  define the problem, 395–396, *396*
    analysis by each stakeholder, 396–400,
      397–399
    doing everything, *396*, 396, **397**, **398**,
      399, 402
    doing nothing, *396*, 396–397, **397**, **398**,
      399
    euthanasia, *396*, 397, **397**, **398**, **399**
    modified clinical plans, *396*, 397, **397**,
      398, **399**, 401–402
    stakeholders, *396*
  example clinical scenario, 391–393, 397,
    400–402
  holistic client/patient needs, 394–395
    monitoring, reviewing the solution, 403
  multi-stakeholder, 395–396, **397–399**, 403
  optimal solution not always 'gold
    standard', 393–394
  principles, 391–404
  refining the problem, 400–402
  skills, importance, 393–395
  solving the problem (identifying/
    implementing), 402–403
  wider professional priorities, 394, **399**
Progressive retinal atrophy (PRA), 321
Proptosis, 309, **315**
Prostatitis, 221
Protein-losing enteropathy, 63, 94, 374
Prothrombin time (PT), 225
Protozoa
  coughing in horses due to, **378**, **379**
  diarrhoea due to, **60**, **63**, **64**
  see also Parasites
Pruriceptors, 286
Pruritic mediators, 286

Pruritus, 285–290
  aural, 298
  behavioural signs, 287
  causes, 289, 290
    allergic skin disease, *288*, 289
    ectoparasites, 287, *288*, 289, 290, 294
    infection, *288*, 289, 291, 294
    psychogenic, 290
  chronic, control difficulty, 286
  define and refine the system, 287
  define the lesion, 289–290
  define the location, 287, 289
  define the problem, 287
  definition, 285
  diagnostic approach, *288*
  in guinea pigs with alopecia, 343, **344**, 345
  pathophysiology, 285–287
  perennial, 290
  primary skin lesions, 289
  rate of onset, 290
  scaling disorder and, 294
  seasonality, 290
  secondary skin lesions, 289–290
  self-trauma, 290
  in small mammals, 342, **344**, 345
  stress and, 287
Pseudochylous effusion, 98
Pseudohaematuria, 216
Pseudohyperreflexia, 109
Pulmonary granular cell tumours, 380
Pulmonary neoplasia, 165
Pulmonary oedema, 174–176
  causes, 174, 175, 176
  adult respiratory distress syndrome, 176
  cardiac disease, 175–176
  reduced oncotic pressure, 176
  clinical signs, 174
  coughing secondary to, 375
  coughing with dyspnoea due to, 164–165
  dyspnoea with minimal coughing due to,
    174–176
  high-output, 175
  in horses, 375
  neurogenic, 176
Pulmonary parenchymal disease,
  inflammatory, 165
Pulmonary thromboembolism, 173–174
Pulmonary tumours, 165
Pulmonary venous hypertension, 164, 174, 175
Pulmonary venous pressure, 176
Pupil(s)
  abnormal-shaped, 307
  abnormal-sized, 307, **312–313**
Pustules, on medial pinna, 298
Pyelonephritis, PU/PD due to, 241, **245**,
  248, **250**
Pyloric disorders, 46

Pyoderma, 289, 290, 293
Pyometra, polyuria/polydipsia due to, 242,
    244, **245**, **250**
Pyruvate kinase deficiency, 189

R
Rabbits
  diarrhoea, 326
  dyspnoea, 327, 328
  'gut stasis', 329–334, **332–333**
    causes, **332–333**
    define and refine the problem, 326,
      330–331
    define the lesion, 332, **332–333**
    define the location, 332
    define the system, 331–332
    investigations and indications for,
      333–334
    physiology, role of diet, 329
    primary GI disease, 331, 332, **332**
    secondary GI disease, 331
  hypothermia and enlarged stomach, 327
  moult, 331, 333
  sneezing, 326, 327
  upper respiratory tract disease, 327, 328
Radiography
  epistaxis, 219
  gait abnormality assessment, 282–283
  spinal, 283
  stressed, in gait abnormality assessment,
    282
  thoracic, 161, 165, 172
Rats
  chronic respiratory disease (CRD),
    341–342
  dyspnoea, 338–342
    causes, 340, **341**
    define and refine the problems,
      338–339
    define the lesion, 340–342
    define the location, 339–340
    define the system, 339
    investigations, 340, 342
  nasal discharges, 338
  respiratory noises, 339
Rectal examination, horses, 359, 364, 367
Recurrent airway obstruction (RAO), 380
Red blood cells (RBCs), 181, 183
  agglutination, 387
  anaemia due to, 186, 187, 189, 190, 191, 196
  microangiopathic anaemia, 189, 190
  antibodies to, 187
  in bone marrow disease, 192
  break down, 186, 196, 202
  decreased/ineffective production, 191,
    196
    horses, 382, 384, **386**, 387–388

haemolysis, 186, 187, 201–202
    see also Haemolysis
  jaundice due to haemolysis of, 202
  metabolism, congenital defects, 189
  nucleated, 183, *184*
  staining and size variations, 183
Red eye *see under* Eye problems
Red urine, 216
Reference ranges, lacking, small mammals, 324
Reflex dyssynergia, 255
Reflexes, assessment, 109
  gait abnormalities, **274**
Reflux *see* Gastric reflux
  Regenerative anaemia, 183, 185–190,
    196, 202, 382
    haemolysis, 185, 186–187, 382–384
    haemorrhage, 185–186, 382, 383
    in horses, 382, 383, 384, 387–388
    pre-hepatic jaundice, 202, 205
    testing/diagnosis, 183, 384, 387–388
    see also Haemolysis; Haemolytic
      anaemia; Haemorrhage
Regurgitation, 36, 40–41
  aspiration pneumonia after, 37, 41
  causes, 40, 47, **49**
    oesophageal disorders, 43, **49**
    secondary GI disease, 43–44
  define and refine the system, 42
  define the location before system, 46
  investigations, 40, 43
  treatment, 44
  vomiting *vs. see under* Vomiting
  vomiting with, 41
Renal disease, malutilisation due to, 83
Renal glucosuria, 31, 242, **251**
Renal neoplasia, polyuria/polydipsia due to,
  242
Renal tubule damage, primary polyuria due
  to, 240–242
Repetition, to improve memorisation, 3
Respiratory distress, 167
Respiratory rate, colic in horses, 364
Respiratory sounds, 160, 163, 167
  abnormal lung sounds, 163
  increased, constrictive bronchial-
    inflammation, 171
  'muffled', 169
  normal lung sounds, 163
  in rats, 339
Respiratory system/tract, 154
  disease/disorders, 153–154
    degenerative, 172
    lower tract *see* Lower respiratory tract
      disease
    primary, 153–154, 167, 179
    primary, in rats, 339–340
    secondary, 154, 173–177

Respiratory system/tract (*cont'd*)
  upper tract *see* Upper respiratory tract
    disease
  weakness due to, 112, 113, **115**
  subdivisions/areas, 154, 167
  see also Sneezing and nasal discharge
Retching, 36
  after coughing, 158, 159
Reticulocytes, 183, *184*
Reticuloendothelial system (RES), 200
Retina
  blind eye causes, **316**
  opaque eye, causes, **314**
Retinal detachment, 310
Retroperitoneal haemorrhage, 186
Retroviral infections, 228
Rhodococcus equi, 373, 380
Right atrial hypertension, 170
Ronidazole, 72
Rotavirus, 372, 374

S
Salmonella, **61**
Salmonellosis, 372, 374
Sarcoma, soft-tissue, in middle ear, 145
Scabies, 287, 289
Scale production, 292
Scaling disorders, 291–296
  classification, 292
  clinical presentation, 291
  define and refine the system, 291–292
    important clues, 292
  define the lesion (causes), 292–294
  define the problem, 291
  diagnostic approach, 294–296, *295*
    flow diagram, *295*
    skin biopsy, 295–296
  keratinisation disorders *see* Keratinisation
    disorders
  of pinnae, 298
  primary disorders, 292–293
    focal, 293
    generalized, 292–293
  pruritus in, 294
  secondary disorders, 292, 293–294
Schirmer tear test, 308–309, 317–318
Schistocytes, 190, *190*
Sclerae, examination, jaundice, 199
Scratching, 285, 287
  see also Pruritus
Seborrhoea, 291, 298
Secondary GI disease *see* Gastrointestinal
  (GI) disorders
Sedation
  small mammals, 324–325
  splenic relaxation after, false anaemia, 182

Seidel test, 319
Seizures, 22, 26, 104, 125–152
  breeds predisposed to, 143, 148
  causes and forms, 130
  define and refine the problem, 130–132
  define and refine the system, 132
  define the lesion, 140–144, *141, 142,*
    143
  extra-cranial (reactive) causes, 135, 140,
    142, 143–144
  intra-cranial causes, 140–143, *141*
  define the location, 132–133, 134–135
  diagnostic approaches, 147–148, **148**
  focal, 126, 127, 135
  nystagmus and gait abnormalities with, 127
  semiology, 130–131
  see also Epileptic seizures
Self-mutilation, 106, **110**
Sensory dysfunction, 106
Sensory evaluation, in weakness, 109, 106,
  110
Sepsis, 60, 229
Serology
  in coughing with dyspnoea, 166
  in sneezing and nasal discharge, 158
  in weakness, 119
Shock
  endotoxic, in horses, 362, 365–366
  haemorrhagic, in horses, 383
  hypovolaemic, in horses, 382
Signalment, 15, 206, 326
Skeletal disorders, 105–106, 107
  see also Musculoskeletal system,
    disorders
Skill acquisition pathway, 8, *8*
Skin biopsy, 295–296
Skin disorders, 285
  guinea pigs, 342, 343
    primary in, 343, **344**, 344–345
    secondary in, 343, **344**, 345–346
  see also Pruritus; Scaling disorders
Skin scrapes, guinea pigs, 344
Skull radiography, 145
Small bowel diarrhoea, 56, 58–59
  causes
    acute diarrhoea, **60–62,** 65
    chronic diarrhoea, **62–64,** 81
  characteristics, 58, **58–59**
  diagnostic approach, 65–69
    acute *vs.* chronic, 65
  in foals, 370
  large bowel diarrhoea *vs.* 57–58, **58–59**
Small bowel disease, in horses, 370
  colic, 359, 364, 367
  diarrhoea, *see* Small bowel diarrhoea
  enteritis, 358

Small mammals, 323–352
  anaesthesia/sedation risk/benefits, 324–325
  clinical scenarios
    chinchilla with weight loss, 334–338
    dyspnoeic rats, 338–342
    ferret with hindlimb weakness, 346–350
    guinea pig with alopecia, 342–346
    'gut stasis' in rabbits, 329–334, **332–333**
    see also Chinchillas; Ferrets; Guinea pigs; Rabbits; Rats
  define and refine the problem, 326–327, 351
  define the lesion, 328
  define the location, 328
  define the system, 327
  delay in diagnosis, advanced conditions, 325
  diagnostic methods, 327, 328, 337
  diagnostic testing, challenges, 324
  hiding disease by animals, 325, 326
  pattern recognition flawed approach, 324, 351
  problem-based inductive clinicalreasoning, 325
    application to all cases?, 351
  treatment trials, 325
  'wait and see' inappropriate, 336
Smell, loss of sense of, 75
Sneezing and nasal discharge, 155–158
  acute, 156
  chronic, 156–157
  clinical signs, 155
  define and refine the system, 156
  define the lesion (causes), 156–157, 217
  define the location, 155
  define the problem, 155
  diagnostic approach, 157–158
  discharge type/character, 155, 156, 157, 217
  discharge with/without sneezing, 156
  epistaxis with, 217, 218
  haemorrhagic or mucopurulent, 217, 218
  in rabbits, 326, 327
  in rats, 338, 339
Sodium retention, 94
Space-occupying disorders, pleural, see Pleural cavity
Specific gravity (SG), urine, 238–239, 248, **251**, 258
Specificity of problems, 17–21
Spherocytes, spherocytosis, *184*, 187
Spinal diseases, 267, 273
  diagnostic workup, 283
  myelopathic, 278, **279–280**, 281
  painful non-myelopathic, 278
Spinal reflexes, assessment, 109, **110**, 122
Splenic haemangiosarcoma, 252
Splenomegaly, 90

'Staircase' for memorisation, 2, *3*
Stakeholders in veterinary care, *396*
  define the problem, 395–396, *396*
    analysis by each stakeholder, 396–400, **397–399**
  influences on professional reasoning, 395–396, *396*
  see also Client issues; Veterinarians
Stercobilinogen, 200
Steroid-responsive meningitis arteritis (SRMA), 278
Stomach, diseases, vomiting caused by, 46
Strange episodes see Paroxysmal episodic disorders
Strangles, horse, 380
Streptococcus equi subsp. *equi*, 380
Stress-induced colitis, **65**
Stridor, 167
Subalbinotic patients, 307
Subvocalisation, 5, *5*
Swallowing, difficulty see Dysphagia
Synchysis scintillans, 308
Syncope, 104, 126
  characteristics, **128–129**
  diagnostic approach, 147
  differential diagnosis, **140**
Synechia, 310
Synovial arthrocentesis, 283
Syringomyelia, 278
Systemic bleeding disorders see Bleeding disorders, systemic

T
Tachycardia, 11, 12, 175
  case example, 233, 234
Tapetal reflection, assessment, 317
Tear(s)
  abnormal drainage, **315**
  over-production, 308–309, **315**
  Schirmer tear test, 317–318
Tearing (epiphora), 306, 308–309
  causes, **314**
Tendon reflexes, assessment, 109
Tensilon test, 122
Tetraparesis, 106
Thermal injury, 190
Thoracic radiography, 161, 165, 172
Thoracocentesis, 171
Thrombi, formation, 173
Thrombin time (TT), 225
Thrombocytopathia, 227, 230–231
Thrombocytopenia, 192, 224, 226
  causes, 228–231
    excessive consumption of platelets, 229
    excessive destruction of platelets, 229
    inadequate production of platelets, 228

Thrombocytopenia (*cont'd*)
  infectious, 230
  miscellaneous, 230
  immune-mediated (ITP, IMT), 227, 229
Thrombocytosis, 193
Thromboelastometry/thromboelastography,
  225
Thromboemboli, 173
Thromboembolism, pulmonary, 173–174
Thromboxane, 231
Tibial thrust, 269–270
Tick-borne disease, thrombocytopenia due
  to, 230
Tongue disorders, 76
Tonometry, 318
Tonopen (applanation tonometer), 318
Tonovet (rebound tonometer), 318
Tooth root abscess, 157
Toxins
  acute small bowel diarrhoea due to, **61**
  bone marrow disorders due to, 193
  colic in horses due to, 358–359
  extra-cranial cause of seizures, *142*,
    143–144
  haemolytic anaemia due to, 188–189
  hepatic jaundice due to, 203
  vomiting due to, 35, 37, 38, 42, 44, *47*
  weakness due to, 105, 122
Tracheal disease, 159, 160
  collapsing, 162, 168, 179
  inflammatory, 160–161
Tracheal hypoplasia, 159–160
Tracheal squeeze test, 376
Tracheobronchial disease, 167
Tracheobronchitis, infectious, 161
Transtracheal washings, 165–166
Transudates, 91–92, 93
  case example, 100, 101
  pleural fluid, 170
Trauma
  gait abnormalities, 267, **276**, 282, 283
  self-, pruritus due to, 290
Trichobezoar, 331
Tritrichomonas, 68, 72
Trixacarus caviae, 343
Tubular renal disease, weight loss, 83
Tympanic bullae, 145

U

Ulcer, corneal, 319
Ultrasound
  abdominal, 68, 101, 259
    horses with colic, 365
  in eye problems, 320
  hepatic *vs.* post-hepatic jaundice, 207,
    208, 212

pleural cavity, space-occupying disorders,
  170
Uncertainty, 395
Unconjugated bilirubin, 200
  in horses 384
Unconscious competence, 8, *8*, 9
Undergraduate education, veterinary, 8
Upper airway obstruction, prolonged, 169
Upper motor neuron disorders, urinary
    incontinence, 254
Upper respiratory tract disease, 154
  coughing in horses, 376
  small mammals
    rabbits, 327, 328
    rats, 339
  see also Sneezing and nasal discharge
Uraemia, 60
Urea, 97
  decreased, PU/PD due to, 242
Urethral sphincter, incompetence, 252–253
Urethral tone, 254
Urinary incontinence (UI), 252–255
  causes, 252, 253, 254, 255
  neurological, 253, 255
  urinary tract, 253, 255
  constant, 253, 254
  define and refine the location, 253–254
  define and refine the problem, 252–253
  define and refine the system, 253–254
    urogenital *vs.* neurological, 253–254
  define the lesion, 255
  inappropriate urination *vs.*, 253
  intermittent, 253, 254, 255
  in polyuria, 238, 253
  urination not initiated, 253, 255
  urination not successful, 253, 254, 255
Urinary tract obstruction, 254
Urination (micturition), 253, 254
  bleeding during, 221
  incontinence and, 254
  not initiated, 253, 255
  unsuccessful, 253, 254, 255
Urine
  in abdomen, 97–98
  concentration, 239, 240, **251**
  impaired concentration (dilute urine,
    hyposthenuria), 20, **247**, 248–249
    azotaemia and, 246, **247**
    case example, 257–259
    causes, **243–245**, **249–251**, 252
    definition (SG level), 239
    dehydration and, 246, **247**, 248
    diagnostic approach, 247–249
    differential diagnosis, 248, **249–251**, 252
    functional (extra-renal) abnormality, 248
    mechanisms, 240–241, 246, **247**

pathophysiology, 240–241
  structural renal disease, 248
inappropriate concentration
  (hypersthenuria), 239, **251**
isosthenuria, 239, 252
output failure, post-renal azotaemia, 246
red, 216
  small volumes passed, 254
  specific gravity (SG), 238–239, 248,
    251, 258
Urine dipsticks, 216
Urobilin, 200
Urobilinogen, 200
Uvea, blind eye causes, **315**
Uveal cysts, 308
Uveitis, 310, 318

V
Vascular damage, clot formation, 221–222, *222*
Vasculitis, 80
Vesicular sounds, 163
Vestibular apparatus, vomiting and, 38, 42
Vestibular attacks, 127, 132
  characteristics, 127, **128–129**
  define the lesion, 137, **138–139**, 145–147
  define the location, 133–134
  define the problem, 127
  define the system, 132
  diagnostic approach, 145–147
    algorithm, *146*
  diagnostic work-up, 137, **138–139**, *146*
  transient ischaemic, 146
Vestibular nuclei, 133
Vestibular syndrome, 'central', 133
Vestibular system, 133
  disease, 133
    central, 134, *134*, **138**
    clinical signs, 133–134, *134*
    diagnostic approach, 145–147
    differential diagnosis, **138**, **139**
    groups, 137, **138–139**
    peripheral, 134, *134*, **138–139**
  paradoxical signs, *134*
  peripheral and central parts, 133, 134,
    134
  unilateral nature, 133
Veterinarians
  burnout and fatigue 401, 403
  collaborative approach (with clients),
    400–402
  communication, 400–402
    with clients, 400–402
    with colleagues, 403
    presenting risks and uncertainties, 402
  frustrating cases, reasons, 9–10
  'gold standard' care preference, 393–394

learning *see* Clinical cases; Learning
  needs of, other stakeholder needs and,
    393, 394, **398**
  personal needs, **399**, 400
  'problem list', 395, *396*, **397**
  solutions, **399**
  professional goals/values, 394, 400
  reflection/analysis after the problem
    completed, 403–404
  shared decision-making (with client), 401
  see also Professional reasoning
Viral infections
  coughing in horses due to, **378**, 379, **379**
  diarrhoea due to, **61**, **63**, **64**
  dyspnoea in rats due to, 340, **341**
  enteritis, **61**
  laryngeal disorders causing dyspnoea, 168
  thrombocytopenia due to, 228
  weight loss due to, 76, 78
Vision deficits, 135
Visual disturbances, 306, 309, 320
Visual testing, 320
Vitamin K, deficiency disorders, **223**, 227
Vitreal opacities, 308
Vitreous, opaque eye, causes, **314**
Vomiting, 35–54
  assessment, 38–41
  of bile, 11
  of blood *see* Haematemesis
  case example, 53–54
  coughing *vs.*, 39
    importance of differentiation, 39–40
  define and refine the system, 24, 27,
    42–46, 50, 53
    clues for primary *vs* secondary, 44–45
    exceptions to 'rules', 45
    primary *vs* secondary disorders, 42–45
    see also Gastrointestinal (GI) disorders
  define the lesion (causes), 46–49
    primary diseases, 46–47
    secondary diseases, 47, 48
    see also Gastrointestinal (GI) disorders
  define the location, 26–27, 45–46
  define the problem, 38–41, 53
    specificity, 18, 19
  definition, 35–36
  diagnostic approach, 49–51
    clinical pathology, 50–51
    fuller work-up *vs.* symptomatic therapy, 51
  diarrhoea associated, 44
  gagging *vs.*, 39–41
  gastric reflux *vs.*, 39
    differentiating clues, 40–41
    importance of differentiation, 39–40
  hypersalivation, 40
  initiation and process, 36, 37–38, *42*

Vomiting (*cont'd*)
  central stimulation, 37–38, *42*
  CRTZ, 36, 37, 38, *42*, 42, 44
  peripheral receptors, 36, 38, 42
  vestibular apparatus, 38, 42
  vomiting centre, 36, 37, 38, *42*
  jaundice and, 18, 206, 211
  nausea, 36, 41
  neurological components, 36–38
  pathophysiology, 35–38, *42*
  as priority problem, 17
  regurgitation *vs.*, 36, 38
    differentiating clues, 40–41
    importance of differentiation, 39–40
  regurgitation with, 41
  stages, 36
Vomiting centre, 36, 37, 38, *42*
Vomitus, 41, 45
Von Willebrand disease (vWD), **223**,
  230–231
Von Willebrand factor (vWF), 230

W
Wasting, of muscle, 74
Water intake
  excessive *see* Polydipsia
  normal, 238
Weakness, 24, 103–123
  case example, 121–123
  in cats, 113
  causes, 104–106, 107, 111–113, **115**,
    116–118
  define and refine the problem, 103–104, 121
    other presenting complaints, 104
  define and refine the system, 104–106,
    107, 121
    primary (structural) *vs.* secondary
      (functional), 104, 105
    skeletal disorders, 105–106, 107
  define the lesion, 111–114, 122
    primary CNS/neuromuscular disorders,
      111, **115**, **117–118**, 121
    secondary disorders, 111–113, **115**,
      116–117, 121
  define the location, 106–111, 122
    see also Neurological examination
  diagnostic approach to, 114, 119
  episodic, 103, 104, 113–114
    causes, 113–114, **115**, 121
    characteristics, **128–129**
  exercise-induced, 104, 108, 109, 113,
    110, 121
    potential diagnoses, **115**, 121

gait abnormalities, 264, 265
hindlimb, 27, 120
  in ferrets *see* Ferrets
persistent, 104
  aggravated by exercise, 113
  causes, 114, **116–118**
spastic or flaccid, 104, 108
Weight
distribution, gait abnormalities and, 267
failure to gain, 73
Weight loss, 73–87
  can't eat, 75–77
    in chinchillas, 335
    define the lesion, 76–77
    define/refine the problem, 75
    dysphagia, 75, 76
    inflammation assessment, 76–77
    prehension and mastication, 75, 76
    systemic pathology, 76–77
  case example, 86–87, 100
  in chinchillas *see* Chinchillas
  decreased appetite, 75–79, 84
    can't eat, *see can't eat (above)*
    in chinchillas, 335, 336
    define and refine the problem, 75, 77
    define the lesion, 76–77, 78–79
    won't eat, *see won't eat (below)*
  define and refine the problem, 73–74, 75,
    77, 86
  define the lesion, 76–77, 78
    can't eat, 76–77
    malabsorption, 81–82
    maldigestion, 81
    malutilisation, 82–84
    won't eat, 78–79
  diet and caloric intake, 73–74
  normal/increased appetite, 79–84, 85, 100
    define the system, 79–80, 86
    see also Malabsorption; Maldigestion;
      Malutilisation of nutrients
  polydipsia/polyuria with, 239
  won't eat, 75, 77–79
    in chinchillas, 335, 336
    define the lesion, 78–79
    define/refine the problem, 75, 77
Wheezes/wheezing, 163, 179
  coughing in horses and, 377
  in rats, 340
White blood cell (WBC) count, 192
Withdrawal (flexor) reflexes, 109

Z
Zinc, metabolism alterations, 293